NEW ACTIONS OF PARATHYROID HORMONE

NEW ACTIONS OF PARATHYROID HORMONE

Edited by

Shaul G. Massry

University of Southern California
Los Angeles, California

and

Takuo Fujita

Kobe University School of Medicine
Kobe, Japan

PLENUM PRESS • NEW YORK AND LONDON

Library of Congress Cataloging-in-Publication Data

International Conference on New Actions of Parathyroid Hormone (1st :
  1987 : Kobe-shi, Japan)
    New actions of parathyroid hormone / edited by Shaul G. Massry and
  Takuo Fujita.
        p.   cm.
    "Proceedings of the First International Conference on New Actions
  of Parathyroid Hormone, held October 26-31, 1987, in Kobe, Japan"-
  -T. p. verso.
    Includes bibliographical references.
    ISBN 0-306-43418-0
    1. Parathyroid hormone--Physiological effect--Congresses.
  I. Massry, Shaul G. II. Fujita, Takuo. III. Title.
    [DNLM: 1. Parathyroid Hormones--physiology--congresses.   WK 300
  I615n 1987]
  QP572.P3I56   1987
  612.4'4--dc20
  DNLM/DLC
  for Library of Congress   89-71051
                                                                  CIP

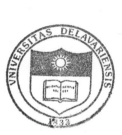

Proceedings of the First International Conference on
New Actions of Parathyroid Hormone,
held October 26–31, 1987, in Kobe, Japan

© 1989 Plenum Press, New York
A Division of Plenum Publishing Corporation
233 Spring Street, New York, N.Y. 10013

Printed in the United States of America

TO OUR PATIENTS
WHO STIMULATED OUR INTEREST IN PARATHYROID HORMONE

CONTENTS

IV. METABOLIC EFFECTS OF PARATHYROID HORMONE

V. PARATHYROID HORMONE AND THE NERVOUS SYSTEM

VI. AGING AND PARATHYROID HORMONE

VII. CLINICAL TOPICS

VIII. MISCELLANEOUS

INTRODUCTION

Shaul G. Massry

Division of Nephrology, The University of
Southern California, School of Medicine
Los Angeles, California

In the last two decades evidence has accumulated indicating that parathyroid hormone may exert a multitude of effects on many cells and a variety of organs beyond its classical targets: the kidney and the bone. These efforts have been spearheaded by nephrologists. The interest of this group of clinicians-scientists stems from the fact that patients with renal failure have secondary hyperparathyroidism and markedly elevated blood levels of PTH (1,2). If this hormone does act on various organs, it becomes plausible that excess blood levels of PTH may be harmful in these patients.

Indeed, in an Editorial published in 1977, Massry suggested that the elevated blood levels of PTH in patients with renal failure may exert deleterious effects on many systems and as such may participate in the genesis of many of the manifestations of the uremic syndrome (3). Thus, the essence of the Massry hypothesis is the notion that PTH may act as a major uremic toxin.

The search for uremic toxins did not yield successful results. In the last three decades many compounds have been implicated as uremic toxins. However, a cause and effect relationship between these compounds and the manifestations of the uremic syndrome has not been established in most cases.

Several reasons may be responsible for the failure to identify a uremic toxin that could clearly be considered the culprit in the genesis of the clinical manifestations of the uremic syndrome. First, the tendency to extrapolate an adverse effect of uremic sera in an in vitro system to the clinical level has resulted in erroneous conclusions. Second, rigorous criteria were not used before considering a substance to be a toxin. A compound should satisfy at least five criteria before being considered responsible for the genesis of one or more of the uremic signs and symptoms (4). These criteria include that: a) the nature and structure of the compound should be known, b) its blood level should be elevated, c) a relation between it and the uremic manifestations must be demonstrated, d) an improvement in the signs and symptoms of uremia should follow a reduction in its blood levels, and e) its administration to experimental animals with normal renal function should produce derangements similar to those seen in uremic patients. Third, the emphasis was placed on products of protein breakdown as the possible uremic toxins while the role of the hormonal disturbances in the genesis of the uremic syndrome is not fully explored.

It is evident, therefore, that the exploration of uremic toxicity must employ a more critical approach which must encompass an integrated research endeavor utilizing at least three levels of investigations. First, one must examine the effect of a potentially toxic compound on in vitro system to understand the mechanisms of its action on various organs and to explore whether such effects have relevance to any of the uremic manifestations. Second, one must investigate the effect of excess amount of the compound in question on the genesis of the various components of the uremic syndrome in experimental animals with chronic renal failure, and examine, whenever feasible, its effect on the function of various organs in animals with normal renal function. Third, one must evaluate in patients with renal failure the consequences of the reduction in the blood levels of the toxic compound.

In the last decade and a half, efforts have been directed to explore the potential toxicity of PTH in the genesis of uremic syndrome. These studies have utilized a more critical approach and attempted to satisfy the rigorous criteria for a toxin mentioned above. PTH, indeed, satisfies the first two criteria since its nature and structure are known and its blood levels are elevated in patients with renal failure. At present a large body of evidence exists indicating that PTH satisfies the other criteria of a uremic toxin and demonstrating the toxic effects of PTH on the nervous system, the myocardium, the skeletal muscle, the pancreatic islets, B cell function and antibody production, erythropoietic system, leucocyte function and sexual function (5).

These new actions of PTH may have important clinical implications beyond the patients with renal failure. Both the blood levels of PTH and its biological actions increase in the elderly subjects (6). This is not surprising, since loss of renal function occurs with aging and one can consider many of the elderly subjects as having valuable degrees of renal insufficiency; the latter is associated with secondary hyperparathyroidism (1,2). It is possible, therefore, that this state of secondary hyperparathyroidism in elderly subjects exerts harmful effects on many body organs and as such participates in the pathogenesis of aging and is, at least, partly responsible for many of the clinical manifestations associated with old age. The potential role of excess PTH in the process of aging have been suggested by others as well (10,11).

Theoretically, the adverse effects of excess PTH may be mediated through a variety of pathways. These may include: a) increasing intracellular calcium concentrations, b) altering the intracellular: extracellular calcium ratio, c) affecting phospholipid turnover, d) internalization into cells and acting on subcellular structures, e) affecting cellular membrane permeability and/or integrity, f) exaggerated stimulation of cyclic AMP, g) causing soft tissue calcification, and h) augmenting protein catabolism. Evidence supporting these potential actions has been reviewed elsewhere (12).

REFERENCES

1. Berson SA, Yalow RS: Parathyroid hormone in plasma in adenomatous hyperparathyroidism, uremia and bronchogenic carcinoma. Science, 154:907-909, 1966.
2. Massry SG, Coburn JW, Peacock M, Kleeman CR: Turnover of endogenous parathyroid hormone in uremic patients and those undergoing hemodialysis. Trans. Am. Soc. Artif. Intern. Organs. 8:410-412, 1972.
3. Massry SG: Is parathyroid hormone a uremic toxin? Nephron 19:125-130, 1977.
4. Massry SG: Parathyroid hormone and the uremic manifestations. Contrib. Nephrol. 20:84-91, 1980.
5. Massry SG: Parathyroid hormone as a uremic toxin. In Textbook of Nephrology. Eds. Massry SG and Glassock RJ. Williams and Wilkins, Baltimore, MD, 2nd Edition pp 1126-1144, 1988.
6. Roof BS, Piel CF, Hanson J, Fadenberg HM: Serum parathyroid hormone levels and serum calcium levels from birth to senescence. Mech. Ageing Dev. 5:289-294, 1976.
7. Wiske PS, Epstein S, Bell N, Queener SF, Edmonson J, Johnston CC, Jr.: Increases in immunoreactive parathyroid hormone with age. N. Engl. J. Med. 300:1419-1421, 1979.
8. Gallagher JC, Riggs BL, Jerpbak CM, Arnaud C: Effect of age on serum immunoreactive parathyroid hormone in normal and osteoporotic women. J. Lab. Clin. Med. 95:373-385, 1980.
9. Inogna KI, Lewis AM, Lipinski BA, Bryant C, Baran D: Effects of age on serum immunoreactive parathyroid hormone and its biological effects. J. Clin. Endocrinol. Metab. 53:1072-1080, 1981.
10. Avioli LV: Calcium, cell function and cell death. Adv. Exptl. Med. Biol. 208:9-15, 1986.
11. Fujita T: Aging and calcium. Miner. Elect. Metab. 12:149-156, 1986.
12. Massry SG: The toxic effects of parathyroid hormone in uremia. Semin. Nephrol. 3:306-328, 1983.

KEYNOTE ADDRESS:

FIRST INTERNATIONAL CONFERENCE ON NEW ACTIONS OF PARATHYROID HORMONE

John T. Potts, Jr.

General Medical Services
Massachusetts General Hospital
Boston, Massachusetts 02114

The convening of this international meeting to review the non-mineral ion actions of parathyroid hormone reflects a growing realization of the potential significance of the actions of parathyroid hormone on such diverse tissues as vascular endothelium, cardiac muscle, hematopoetic cells and nerve and muscle tissue, as well as lipid metabolism. There are obvious questions regarding the mechanism whereby PTH causes these diverse actions, the biological significance and/or the therapeutic potential. With peptide hormones the initial event that results in the physiological actions characteristic of the peptide are now universally understood to involve interaction with specific receptors on target cells. Hormone/receptor interaction generates an intracellular signal or signals which transduce hormone binding into a series of specific cellular biochemical changes and, ultimately, the physiological actions at the tissue and organ level.

The traditional actions of parathyroid hormone, increased renal phosphate clearance, increased urinary cyclic AMP excretion, reduced renal calcium clearance, increased renal 1,25-dihydroxyvitamin D production, and increased calcium and phosphate release from bone involve a series of interactions with discrete target cells in the two tissues.(1) The receptors for the renal action of the hormone are localized to small regions of the renal tubule, different regions and therefore different target cells being responsible for each of the three principal renal actions: phosphate transport, calcium transport, and vitamin D synthesis.(1) The actions of the hormone on bone involve complex interactions among several cell types (osteoblasts, osteoclasts) and a series of still poorly understood cellular biochemical events. The osteoclast, one of the principal mediators of the bone resorptive action of parathyroid hormone, is now believed to be stimulated only indirectly through products that result from interaction of parathyroid hormone with specific receptors on osteoblasts. Thus the osteoclast, although physiologically a target cell for parathyroid hormone, lacks specific receptors.

New Actions of Parathyroid Hormone
Edited by S. G. Massry and T. Fujita
Plenum Press, New York

It is useful to consider this background when analyzing the physiological significance and/or biological importance of the actions of parathyroid hormone on its non-traditional target tissues and biological responses; even the traditional responses involve heterogeneity of target cells and perhaps receptors. As outlined in the many papers collected in this symposium, the dose of parathyroid hormone required to elicit non-mineral ion responses in vivo and in vitro usually exceeds, sometimes considerably, the doses required to detect hormonal responses on the traditional targets in bone and kidney. Certain of the actions, such as the vascular actions, occur at doses much closer to the hormonal doses required to elicit changes in calcium and phosphate ion flux.(2,3)

It is difficult to compare the dose response curves needed to elicit various non-mineral ion actions of parathyroid hormone because of confusing differences in the types of hormone preparations available to be used, the lack of standardized assay design and potency estimates, and the great variation in units in which the concentration of hormone is described. Clearly, as can be seen from a survey of reported results and summaries presented in this meeting, some of the non-mineral ion effects other than the vascular action, actions which include effects on cardiac and hematopoeitic cells, (3,4,5,6,7) require doses of at least an order of magnitude greater than those required for traditional actions.

What is the meaning of the non-mineral ion effects of PTH in light of the above considerations? One possibility is that the actions, particularly those requiring higher doses, are of a non-specific type. By this is meant that some of the actions of the peptide are not the result of a specific hormone/receptor interaction, but are an indirect consequence of multiple actions of high doses of peptide. Such effects would presumably not be of physiological or potential pharmacologic interest. The extensive characterization of the vasodilating actions of parathyroid hormone points toward a direct, receptor-mediated action that involves blockade of calcium entry (8) as does the likelihood of direct actions with other non-traditional actions, evident through responses in vitro with purified hormone preparations. (6,7) There are two variations of specific actions to be considered, that is, the interaction of parathyroid hormone with a specific receptor or receptors. One possibility is that parathyroid hormone activates not only the traditional receptors coupled to mineral ion transport changes, but also receptors of a structurally and functionally distinctive type in vascular, hematopoietic, nerve and muscle cells. In this postulate, these receptors are normally activated by a different agonist than PTH, an agonist that is the usual effector of the observed, non-mineral ion response. In this view parathyroid hormone is acting as a surrogate for the normally active agonist; it should be appreciated that the PTH effect need not involve the same active site or conformation that is involved in the mineral actions of the hormone. For example, a different region of the primary sequence of parathyroid hormone than that vital for stimulation of bone and renal parathyroid hormone receptors might be involved, as has been suggested by some of the studies of Pang and collaborators. In addition, the peptide's conformation rather than primary sequence may satisfy receptor activation requirements.

An alternate possibility is that the receptor activated by PTH in the non-traditional actions is structurally and functionally related to

the parathyroid hormone receptor but is present at lower concentration
or works through alternate second messenger pathways.

It seems likely that current research directions in the parathyroid
field will soon provide explanations for these non-mineral ion effects
of PTH and help to distinguish among the several possibilites. Analysis
of the comparative endocrinology of parathyroid hormone structure and
function is continuing through efforts in our laboratory and others.
Parathyroid hormone is known to be present as early in evolution as
amphibians and much recent data, although indirect, supports the
possibility that a polypeptide structurally similar to parathyroid
hormone may be found in fish.(9) It is clear that the biological role
assigned to peptide hormones varies throughout evolution. An
outstanding example is prolactin, which has principal effects on salt
and water excretion in amphibians and certain fish, whereas its
principal role in mammals is on mammary gland function and milk
production.(10) Primitive prolactin molecules do reveal mammotrophic
activity when tested in appropriate mammaliam assays and some effect on
receptors involved in salt and water metabolism in amphibians can be
demonstrated with mammalian prolactin molecules.(10) The role of
parathyroid hormone may also have changed in emphasis throughout
evolution. Current work in our group has led to the identification of
the sequence of chicken parathyroid hormone; these findings will be
followed by the synthesis of the molecule and its extensive biological
testing. Subsequently, the power of recombinant DNA techniques should
lead to cloning, structural analysis, and, eventually, chemical
synthesis and biological testing of amphibian parathyroid hormone.

A survey of the spectrum of biological actions, not only on
traditional targets for mineral ion metabolism, but on the multiple
effects ascribed to mammalian parathyroid hormone in vascular, muscle,
nerve and hematopoietic cells with these bird and amphibian forms of PTH
may be quite revealing. Perhaps the "non-traditional" actions of the
hormone will be displayed by these evolutionarily distinct forms of PTH
with much greater potency relative to potency on mineral ion
metabolism. In this speculation therefore, effects seen with mammalian
parathyroid hormone may be explained by an earlier evolutionary
role represented more weakly in parathyroid hormone in humans and cows
than in birds and amphibians. There may have been parallel evolutionary
changes in the hormone and its receptor. Studies of relevant cells and
tissues from birds and amphibians as well as parathyroid hormone from
these species may ultimately clarify the role of non-mineral ion actions
of the hormone across evolutionary time, analogous to our present
knowledge of changing biological emphasis in the role of prolactin.

The alternate possiblity is that the receptors involved in vascular
and other tissues differ significantly from those involved in calcium
and phosphate metabolism in response to parathyroid action. Recently,
recombinant DNA technology in concert with peptide sequencing and
immunologic approaches has been used to define the primary peptide
structure of many receptors. Several general patterns of receptor
structure have emerged. Growth factor and insulin receptors share
common features (11); and their properties differ markedly from those of
receptors coupled to G proteins, the latter sharing among themselves
many common characteristics.(12,13,14,15,16,17) Although no primary
sequence of any G protein-coupled peptide hormone receptors has been
determined (only G-protein coupled receptors with non-protein ligands),
it seems likely that all G-protein receptors will share some common

structural and functional properties. A survey of the similiarities and differences in the G-protein receptors that have already been isolated, such as the muscarinic acetylcholine receptor, the rhodopsin receptor, and the beta adrenergic receptor, reveal interesting features that are pertinent to this discussion of the actions of parathyroid hormone.(12,13,14,15,16) Since parathyroid hormone action is associated with increased cyclic AMP production, it seems likely that the parathyroid hormone receptor will prove to be more closely related to the guanyl nucleotide binding group of receptors as typified by the beta-adrenergic receptor. These receptors have a similar overall chemical topography and display a complex series of structural domains.(12,13,14,15,16,) The proteins are some eighty to ninety thousand in molecular weight, are glycoproteins, and are believed to have an extracellular domain, 7 intra-membranous domains, and an intracellular domain of varying length.(13,14,15,16) It has not been as easy with the guanyl nucleotide-related receptors as it was with the somewhat structurally simpler growth factor receptors to identify regions associated with ligand binding and signal transduction. Much has been learned, by analysis of the structures of closely related receptor families such as in the muscarinic acetylcholine group (13) or the beta adrenergic receptor.(15,16) The theme observed is one of overall topographical similarity with numerous amino acid sequence changes that, in ways not yet understood, account for the discriminate function among the various receptors. Of particular interest has been the discovery that each of the receptor types identified on careful cloning and structural analysis is revealed to be a family of closely related receptors. This has been shown recently, for example, with the muscarinic acetylcholine receptor(13); in this case results suggest that slightly different ligand affinity properties and biological responses will be demonstrable with these receptor subtypes. A clear example of this concept of closely related families of receptors is evident with the rhodopsin group. Cloning and structural analysis has revealed the particular structural features whereby color vision is transmitted through differential receptivity of similar but distinctive rhodopsins associated with each primary color transmission.(18)

Further complexity is evident in the second messengers used by receptors for signal transduction. Several distinctive but interconnected pathways have been described including increased cyclic AMP production through stimulation of adenylate cyclase resulting activation of cyclic AMP-dependent protein kinase or protein kinase-A; stimulation of the polyphosphoinositol pathway with generation of diacylglycerol and inositoltriphosphate and with activation of protein kinase-C; and direct, channel-mediated enhanced calcium uptake.(19) It remains at this point unclear whether these second messenger pathways identified in target cells for various hormones are activated exclusively by different receptors. This is highly possible, however, since a number of structurally and functionally distinctive subsets of guanyl nucleotide-binding proteins that presumably link receptor occupancy with biological response have been identified.

As the primary work aimed at identifying the receptor for parathyroid hormone develops and the receptor is cloned and structurally analyzed much information pertinent to understanding the extra mineral ion actions of the hormone will be clarified, presumably rapidly. It will be pertinent to determine how many types of parathyroid hormone receptors can be distinguished in the traditional target cells of bone and kidney, and how their actions are accomplished via second messenger pathways. It will then be important to identify the number and content of parathyroid-like receptors on vascular, muscular, and hematopoietic cells, for example. Receptor content can be related to the dose response curve evident for the activating ligand. It may be revealed that receptors identical to parathyroid hormone receptors are found on vascular or hematopoietic cells, but that they are present at much lower concentration than on traditional target cells in kidney and bone. This would explain the rightward shift in dose response curve noted when parathyroid hormone effectiveness is analyzed in in vitro or in vivo assays. This could be consistent, for example, with a change in the relative importance of the parathyroid-mediated biological response in evolutionary history. A given response might be found to be mediated more readily and to be associated with higher parathyroid hormone receptor content in tissues in cells from amphibians, reptiles, or birds, for example, than in mammals, thus, explaining the significance of the biological effect, but placing it in an evolutionary context.

If the application of recombinant DNA techniques with cloned DNA representing the parathyroid hormone receptor(s) fails to reveal any evidence of detectable PTH-like receptors in vascular, hematopoietic, or other potential parathyroid target cells then it may yet develop that the hormone is indeed acting as a surrogate for another type of ligand, unrelated in primary sequence or physiological role to parathyroid hormone. Such a view might also be supported independently by further studies with parathyroid hormone-related peptides. If indeed different regions of the PTH sequence are responsible for the vascular versus hypercalcemic actions of mammalian PTH, it may become apparent that PTH is merely sharing actions with another system of ligand/receptor actions. Suggestions derived from recent findings that there are immunoreactive substances in fish pituitary and even mammalian brain that react with some antisera to PTH would then need to be explored in efforts to identify the presumed true agonist for these vascular and other non-mineral actions.

The two apparently dissimilar concepts, 1) PTH actions on non-traditional targets are a reflection of an earlier evolutionary role versus 2) the view that PTH actions reflect merely an accidental surrogate role for another ligand, need not be viewed as totally divergent. Recent studies with insulin and IGF-1 and their respective receptors reveal that both ligands and receptors share strong structural homology even though the biological role of the two systems is now clearly different in mammals. (11) Such true evolutionary linkage yet divergence could prove true with parathyroid hormone's multiple actions.

It is difficult to make predictions regarding the resolution among these possibilities and the ultimate significance, both physiological and therapeutic, of the 'multiple' biological responses ascribed to parathyroid hormone. It seems highly likely, however, that at the time of convening another international conference of this type we will understand much more about the chemical basis of the multiple biological responses now ascribed to the hormone. It seems highly possible that exciting new leads in comparative endocrinology may emerge from further exploration of these non-traditional biological actions of parathyroid hormone. It is conceivable that analogs of the hormone may find useful physiological and even therapeutic roles that, at the present time, are only hinted at.

References

1. Habener JF, Rosenblatt MR, Potts JT Jr. Parathyroid hormone: Biochemical aspects of biosynthesis, secretion, action, and metabolism. Physiol Rev 64:985-1053, 1984.

2. Pang PKT, Janssen HF, Ye JA. Effects of synthetic parathyroid hormone on vascular beds of dogs. Pharmacology 21:213-222, 1980.

3. Pang PKT, Yang MCM, Khosla MC, Bumpus FM. Vascular action of parathyroid hormone fragments and analogs. Proceeding Seventh International Conference on Calcium Regulating Hormones. Elsevier Publishers, 1980.

4. Baczynsky R, Massry SG, Cohan R, Magott M, Saglikes Y, Brautbiar N. Effect of parathyroid hormone on myocardial energy metabolism in the rat. Kidney Int 27:718-725, 1985.

5. Akmal M, Telfer N, Ansari AN, Massry SH. Erythrocyte survival in chronic renal failure. J Clin Invest 76:1695-1698, 1985.

6. Levi J, Besler H, Hirsh I, Djaldetti MD. Increased RNA and synthesis in mouse erythroid precursors by parathyroid hormone. ACTA Hemat 67:125-129, 1979.

7. Remuzzi G, Dodesini P, Livio M, Mecca G, Benigni A, Schieppati A, Poletti E, Degaetono G. Parathyroid hormone inhibits human platelet function. Lancet 1321-1323, 1981.

8. Pang PKT, Yen L, Yang MCM. Parathyroid hormone: A specific potent vasodilator. Karger: Contr Nephrol Vol 41, #26, 1984.

9. Harvey S, Zeng Y-Y, Pang PKT. Parathyroid hormone-like immunoreactivity in fish plasma and tissues. Gen & Comp Endcrinol, in press.

10. Niall HD. Peptide hormone homologies and evolution in peptide hormones. Parsons JA ed, MacMillan Press, London, 9-32, 1976.

11. Ulrich, Gray, Tam, Yang-Feng, Stsubokawa, Collins, Henzel, LeBon, Kathuria, Chen-Jacobs, Francke, Ramachandran, Fujita-Yamaguchi. Insulin-like growth factor 1 receptor primary structure: Comparison with insulin receptor suggests structural determinants that define functional specificity. EMBO J 5:2503-2512, 1986.

12. Kubo T, Fukuda K, Mikami A, Maeda A, Takashi H, Mishina M, Haga T, Haga K, Ishiyama A, Kangawa K, Kojima M, Matsuo H, Hirose T, Numa S. Cloning, sequencing and expression of complementary DNA encoding the muscarinic acetylcholine receptor. Nature 323:411-416, 1986.

13. Bonner TI, Buckley NJ, Young AC, Brann MR. Identification of a family of muscarinic acetylcholine receptor genes. Science 237:527-532, 1987.

14. Benovic JL, Mayor F, Somers RL, Caron MG, Lefkowitz RJ. Light dependent phosphorylation of rhodopsin by beta-adrenergic receptor kinase. Nature 321:869-872, 1986.

15. Dixon RAF, Sigal IS, Rands E, Register RB, Candelore MR, Blake AD, Strader CD. Ligand binding to beta-adrenergic receptor involves its rhodopsin-like core. Nature 326-73-77, 1987.

16. Strader CD, Sigal IS, Register RB, Candelore MR, Rands E, Dixon RAF. Identification of residues required for ligand binding to the beta-adrenergic receptors. Proc Natl Acad Sci USA 84:4384-4388, 1987.

17. Stryer L, Bourne HR. G proteins: A family of signal transducers. Ann Rev Cell Biol 2:391-419, 1986.

18. Nathans J, Thomas D, Hogness DS. Molecular genetics of human color vision: The genes encoding blue, green, and red pigments. Science 232:193-202, 1986.

19. Yoshimasa T, Sibley DR, Bouvier M, Lefkowitz RJ, Caron MC. Cross talk between cellular signalling pathways suggested by phorbol ester induced adenylate cyclase phosphorylation. Nature 327:67-70, 1987.

PARATHYROID HORMONE SECRETION, METABOLISM AND MODE OF ACTION

CHEMISTRY, MOLECULAR BIOLOGY AND MODE OF ACTION OF

PARATHYROID HORMONE

J.T. Potts Jr., S. Nussbaum, K. Wiren, M. Freeman,
T. Igarashi, T. Okasaki, J. Zajak, A.B. Abou-Samra,
R. Bringhurst, G. Segre, and H. Kronenberg

Massachusetts General Hospital
Boston, Massachusetts 02114

The impact of molecular and cell biology on endocrinology, as on many other fields of biomedical science, has been immense over the last decade. Genes for most of the peptide hormones have been cloned and analyzed over the last three years; more recently, the difficult task of cloning hormone receptors has been accomplished at least for several hormonal systems. Development of bacterial or mammalian cell systems to express the cDNA and genes for hormones and receptors, coupled with oligonucleotide directed mutagenesis, is permitting wide exploration of structure/activity relations for peptide hormones in endocrine signaling. The techniques of peptide chemistry can now be combined with those of molecular biology to investigate in detail the contribution of primary structure to endocrine function.

Work by our group, as well as that of others, in the chemistry, molecular biology, metabolism, and mode of action of parathyroid hormone have led to several important advances that, in turn, permit more central and fundamental questions in parathyroid physiology to be asked. Cloning, structural characterization, and expression of genomic and cDNA for human, bovine, rat and, in preliminary phases, chicken parathyroid hormone have been accomplished. These advances, coupled with the expression of mutant parathyroid hormone genes, have led to definition of critical features in the regulation of transcription, translation, posttranslational processing, transport, and secretion of parathyroid hormone. Systematic studies of parathyroid hormone structure/activity relations through synthesis of analogs of the native peptide have led to definition of pure antagonists of parathyroid hormone, analogs that bind to parathyroid hormone receptors in both bone and kidney yet do not activate them and hence block PTH action at receptors in these tissues. Receptors for parathyroid hormone have been selectively radiolabeled, purified, and chemically characterized. We and others are intensively involved in efforts to clone the parathyroid hormone receptor. Recently we have been successful in transfecting parathyroid hormone target cells with mutant forms of the regulatory subunit of the cyclic AMP-dependent protein kinase. This work provides exciting new opportunities to block specific second-messenger pathways associated with parathyroid hormone action, thereby making possible analysis of alternate pathways of hormone action within cells.

The present effort in our group is focused on four main areas: structure, function and evolution of the parathyroid hormone gene; structural basis of the biological action of parathyroid hormone; initial events in the cellular response to parathyroid hormone: receptor structure, function, and regulation; and intracellular responses of target cells to parathyroid hormone: alternate pathways, second messengers, and protein kinases. In work just recently completed, other efforts in our group were focused on the metabolism of parathyroid hormone. The effort was to determine whether biologically active fragments of parathyroid hormone arose from peripheral degradation of the hormone once it entered the circulation. We have now established, to our satisfaction, that the high capacity, peripheral metabolic pathways that dispose of parathyroid hormone are largely catabolic; no active amino-terminal fragment of hormone reenters the circulation.(1) This advance helps in turn with efforts to improve the radioimmunoassay of parathyroid hormone; the use of double antibody methods to measure only the intact hormone, approaches which have several practical advantages, are made more feasible when it becomes clearer that there are no active fragments in the circulation. (2)

Our group has spent considerable effort in developing a variety of systems that are suitable to express the parathyroid hormone gene in vitro. The systems can be used in several significant applications. They are useful for the efficient production of full length parathyroid hormone for various biochemical and chemical applications and will be helpful in analysis of transcriptional defects in naturally occurring, mutant, parathyroid hormone genes isolated from patients with parathyroid disease. A major use of the systems, however, has been to study the role of the signal sequence and the prohormone portion of the peptide in post-translational processing of the precursor molecule to the secreted form of the hormone.(3,4,5,6) The inserted parathyroid hormone cDNA is deliberately altered by oligonucleotide directed mutagenesis; effects of experimentally produced mutations in the hormone precursor can then be analyzed. The normal parathyroid hormone cDNA produced under vital vector control in mammalian cell system was faithfully transcribed and translated and the parathyroid hormone precursor was accurately processed, resulting in parathyroid hormone, indistinguishable from the natural product, extracted from glands, entering the secretory pathway and being secreted from cells.(6)

Use of the mutants in these cell culture systems has advanced knowledge of the rules that govern the intracellular processing not only of parathyroid hormone but of the biosynthetic precursors of all proteins destined for secretion from cells. For example, the consequences of amino-terminal deletions of the preproparathyroid hormone signal sequence have been analyzed by a series of 5' terminal truncations of the corresponding region of the parathyroid hormone cDNA.(5) These studies have established the critical nature of the hydrophobic core of the leader sequence in the orderly processing of parathyroid hormone through the secretory pathway.(5) More complex mutations which affect the nucleotide sequence encoding the site of cleavage by the signal peptidase, that is, the region between the leader sequence and the proparathyroid hormone portion of the molecule, have helped greatly to clarify the rules that govern recognition of precursor proteins by signal peptidases.(3,4) The expression of several of these mutant forms of parathyroid hormone interfered with the efficiency of transport of the precursor across the endoplasmic reticulum and/or cleavage of the precursor molecule by signal peptidase. In addition,

some of these mutant forms of preproparathyroid hormone are secreted
with either amino-terminal extensions or, in the majority of cases, with
amino-terminal truncation of the processed product, the secreted
protein; products PTH 2-84 and PTH 4-84 are secreted (3,4). These
analogs, incidentally, are of considerable interest as potential
antagonists of parathyroid hormone since studies by chemical peptide
synthesis established that such amino-terminally truncated peptides are
competitive inhibitors of parathyroid hormone action in vitro.

Drs. Igarashi, Okazaki, and Zajac, working with Dr. Kronenberg,
have made exciting breakthroughs recently in definition of genetic
control elements that determine the activity of the parathyroid hormone
gene. Their findings include detection of a specific upstream promotor
element that interacts with 1-25 dihydroxy D_3 and is a site of negative
transcriptional regulation.(7) Several thousand nucleotides upstream
from the vitamin D binding site, two silencer elements and sequences
responsive to the level of extra-cellular calcium have been identified;
it is not clear whether the silencer sequences and the site of calcium
regulation are identical.(8,9) In these studies, the control elements
of the parathyroid gene have been linked to a "reporter element" a
bacterial enzyme, chloramphenicol acetyl-transferase, that permits
effects on transcription to be studied free of the influence of
complicating factors such as the turnover of PTH messenger RNA or the
rate of secretion of the hormone itself.(8,9)

In our continuing studies of the structural basis of the biological
action of parathyroid hormone, we face a formidable task in a molecule
the size of parathyroid hormone, since so many potential sequences could
be studied in the search for optimum binding analogs. Substitution of
tyrosine for the C terminal phenylalanine and amidation of the alpha
carboxyl function of the PTH fragment 1-34 brought about significant
enhancement of potency. Deletion of two or more amino-terminal amino
acids was associated with the loss of the usual post-receptor activation
of adenylate cyclase, i.e., resulted in the formation of a competitive
inhibitor of parathyroid hormone action. This compound, however,
although devoid of agonist activity in vitro, was an agonist in
vivo.(10) It was then necessary to delete more of the amino-terminal
sequence of the molecule in order to remove residual agonist activity.
Several bioassay systems were designed to test the action of the
compound, 7-34-PTH-1-34 tyrosine amide in inhibition of parathyroid
hormone action on phosphate transport in the kidney and bone calcium
release.(11,12) The compound was found to be an effective and complete
antagonist of PTH stimulation of both urinary cyclic AMP production and
phosphaturia in rats.(11) Although the compound was effective, a 30-100
to 1 ratio of inhibitor to peptide was necessary to demonstrate full
antagonism.(11) In an assay which detects calcium mobilization from
bone within one to two hours of parathyroidectomy, it could be shown
that somewhat higher doses of the inhibitor also blocked the skeletal as
well as renal actions of the hormone.(12) We have concluded that the
antagonist was at the limit of receptor binding affinity necessary to
produce blockade of hormone action. Thus, the studies, although
encouraging, have merely provided impetus to the effort to design more
potent agonists with a better affinity for the receptor and a longer
metabolic half life in the circulation. More potent agonists would
allow design of more effective antagonists through use of amino-terminal
truncations of the more potent agonist.

Given the complexity of analog design, it has proven useful, to the
search for structural variants of parathyroid hormone that bind much

more tightly to the receptor and therefore serve as either better
agonists, or, in amino-terminally truncated form, better antagonists.
The recent determination of a portion of the sequence of chicken
parathyroid hormone (cPTH) (13) plus the finding that the peptide
responsible, at least in part, for the hypercalcemia of malignancy, the
humoral hypercalcemia of malignancy factor (HHM)(14), also shares
striking homologies with the parathyroid hormone in the first 13 amino-
terminal residues of both molecules, has provided several clues to
potency enhancing amino acid substitutions. These are now being
evaluated by undertaking a series of syntheses based upon these
structural features. Of particular interest is the finding that
residues 25-27, ARG-LYS-LYS, a highly basic region, is substituted for
by non-conservative amino acid changes that eliminate the positive
charge at each of these sites in PTH if the structural changes in cPTH
and HHM are combined.(13,14) Since the vascular actions of parathyroid
hormone have been correlated with this 25-27 sequence region, it may be
very helpful in efforts to understand the biological significance of
non-mineral ion effects of PTH, as discussed elsewhere throughout this
symposium, to synthesize and test new analogs that lack basic charge in
this critical region of the molecule.(15)

As the work proceeds, it becomes increasingly clear that the
receptors for parathyroid hormone may differ somewhat in both structure
and function in different tissues. Furthermore, more than one second
messenger may be involved in mediating the action of the hormone. As
new parathyroid hormone analogs are designed by the strategies outlined
above, drawing clues from forms of parathyroid hormone found earlier in
evolution or parathyroid-like peptides, we may uncover molecules with an
altered spectrum of action differentially stimulating one target cell
vs. another in renal or bone tissue. It will be quite intriguing as we
build upon our interests in the evolution of parathyroid hormone to
develop more potent agonists, antagonists and analogs of altered
spectrum of action on traditional target cells, to provide certain of
these peptides to our colleagues who study the less traditional actions
of the parathyroid hormone. These studies may help in understanding the
ultimate physiological significance and pharmacologic potential of
actions of the hormone on tissues other than kidney and bone.

Efforts to clone the receptors for peptide hormones have greatly
advanced in the last several years. Several different types of
receptors have been cloned and structurally
characterized.(16,17,18,19,20) Receptors for insulin and other growth
factors act through autophosphorylation of tyrosine kinase.(16) A
second large and functionally diverse group of receptors including the
rhodopsin family, the muscarinic acetylcholine receptor group, and the
beta adrenergic receptor group, use guanyl nucleotide proteins of
several subtypes with discrete functional capacities to link surface
signaling from a receptor to specific, cellular biochemical response to
the hormone. (21) The muscarinic acetylcholine receptor, B adrenergic
receptor, and rhodopsin all have a rather complicated structure with
seven intramembranous domains as well as intracellular and extracellular
domains.(17,18,19,20) Surprising heterogenity in structure within these
closely related families has been uncovered as recombinant DNA
techniques are applied to examine potential receptor variations. These
structural variations imply greater functional heterogeneity than was
suspected.(17,19)

These receptors must undergo complex conformational changes during their interaction with the binding ligand and the guanyl nucleotide protein effector (17,18,19,20,21). It seems plausible that parathyroid hormone belongs to this category of receptors. Efforts, as yet not successful, are being undertaken through a number of parallel approaches to clone the receptor and initiate the functional characterization of the various domains associated with receptor activation and function. Once a parathryoid receptor molecule is cloned, it should be possible, in analogy with the muscarinic acetylcholine and β-adrenergic receptor, to quickly establish the identity or differences in parathyroid hormone receptors found in various cells in bone and kidney, that is, whether the identical parathyroid hormone receptor mediates the actions of the peptide in all tissues or whether different actions are associated with functionally distinctive receptors. Receptor clones would be of great assistance in looking for the presence of parathyroid hormone receptors in the other tissues that seem to be targets for parathyroid hormone.(22,23,24,25)

Closely related to the efforts to characterize the receptor are efforts to analyze second messengers for the hormone. Stimulated by the recent discovery that, like several other hormones, parathyroid hormone activates multiple intracellular signals in addition to cyclic AMP, including phosphoinositol hydrolysis and increase in intracellular calcium, protein kinase C activity and arachidonate metabolism (26,27,28), Drs. Bringhurst and Abou-Samra have initiated an intensive effort to develop and characterize novel PTH target cell systems with which to examine the roles of different intracellular signals in the specific cellular actions of the hormone. They have established a series of mutant sub-clones from PTH responsive osteoblastic and renal cell lines in which the cyclic AMP dependent protein kinase can be suppressed in a controlled manner by regulated transcription of transfected genes stably incorporated in the genome whose products prevent activation of the kinase. (29) It has also been demonstrated by these workers that in PTH target cells derived from rat osteosarcoma cells (ROS cells), PTH causes translocation of protein kinase C activity from the cytosol to the membranes (30). Also, parathyroid hormone modulates the phosphorylation of endogenous protein kinase C substrates. These findings, together with the reports of others that PTH increases phosphoinositol breakdown (26,27,28), suggest an important role of the phosphoinositol/protein kinase C pathway in the action of PTH. Thus the relative importance of cyclic AMP dependent and independent pathways in PTH action should be largely clarified in the next few years ahead through the combination of studies involving receptor cloning and application of unique cell lines which amplify or diminish the effectiveness of specific second messengers. Parathyroid hormone analogs may be developed that exploit these different pathways, if they can be shown to exist, to bring about differential PTH biological actions in vivo such as osteoblastic stimulation without corresponding osteoclastic stimulation.

These studies outlined above, should contribute greatly to our understanding of the physiological role and therapeutic potential of parathyroid hormone. At the same time, much of the current uncertainty that has been generated by discovery of the multiple non-traditional actions of parathyroid hormone on target tissues other than bone and kidney may also be clarified by the advances in parathyroid chemistry that provide new parathyroid hormone agonists and antagonists, cloned receptors, and test cell systems that utilize selective second messenger pathways.

References

1. Bringhurst FR, Stern AM, Yotts M, Mizrahi N, Potts, JT Jr. Peripheral metabolism of parathyroid hormone: fate of the biologically active amino-terminus *in vivo*. Am J Physiol. (submitted).

2. Nussbaum SR, Zahradnik RJ, Lavigne JR, Brennan GL, Nozawa-Ung K, Kim LV, Keutman HT, Wang CA, Potts JT Jr., Segre GV A Highly Sensitive Two-Site Immunoradiometric Assay of Parathyroid Hormone and its Clinical Utility in Evaluating Patients with Hypercalcemia. Clin Chem 33,1364-1367, 1987.

3. Wiren KM, Ivashkiv L, Ma P, Freeman MW, Hellerman J, Potts JT Jr, Kronenberg HM. Mutations in Signal Sequence Cleavage Domain of Preproparathyroid Hormone Induce Stop-Transfer Function and Alter Protein Translocation and Signal Sequence Clevage. Mol Cell Biol. (submitted)

4. Wiren KM, Potts JT Jr, Kronenberg HM. Functional consequences of precise deletion of the pro sequence from preproparathyroid hormone. J Cell Biol. (submitted).

5. Freeman MW, Wiren KM, Rapoport A, Lazar M, Potts JT Jr, Kronenberg HM. Consequences of amino-terminal deletions of preproparathyroid hormone signal sequence. Molec Endocrinol. (in press).

6. Hellerman JG, Cone RC, Segre GV, Potts JT Jr, Rich A, Mulligan RC, Kronenberg HM. Secretion of human parathyroid hormone from rat pituitary cells infected with a recombinant retrovirus encodling preproparathyroid hormone . Proc Natl Acad Sci USA. 1984; 81:5340-5344.

7. Igarashi T, Muramatsu OA, Ogata E, Okazaki T, Kronenberg HM. Functional analysis of the promoter region of the humanparathyroid hormone gene: sequences responsible for basal expression and for responsiveness to $25(OH)_2$ vitamin D. Nature. (submitted).

8. Okasazi T, Kronenberg HM. Unpublished results.

9. Zajac J, Kronenberg HM. Unpublished results.

9A. Maniatis T, Goodbourn S, Fischer JA. Regulation of inducible and tissue-specific gene expression. Science 236:1237-1245, 1987.

10. Segre GV, Rosenblatt M, Rully GL III, Laugharn J, Reit B, Potts JT Jr. Evaluation of an *in vitro* parathyroid hormone antagonist *in vivo* in dogs. Endocrinology. 1985, 116:1024-1029.

11. Horiuchi N, Holick MF, Potts JT Jr, Rosenblatt M. A parathyroid hormone inhibitor *in vivo*: design and biological evaluation of a hormone analog. Science. 1983; 220:1053-1055.

12. Doppelt SH, Neer RM, Nussbaum SR, Federico P, Potts JT Jr, Rosenblatt M. Inhibition of the *in vivo* parathyroid hormone-mediated calcemic response in rats by a synthetic hormone antagonist. Proc Natl Acad Sci USA. 1986; 83:7557-7560.

13. Khosla S, Kronenberg HM. Unpublished results.

14. Suva LF, Winslow GA, Wettenhall REH, Hammonds RG, Moseley JM, Diefenbach-Jagger H, Rodda CP, Kemp BE, Rodriguez H, Chen EY, Hudson PJ, Martin TJ, Wood WI. A parathyroid hormone-related protein implicated in malignant hypercalcemia: cloning and expression. Science, August, 1987 237:893-896.

15. Pang PKT, Yang MCM, Keutmann HT, Kenny AD. Structure activity relationship of parathyroid hormones: separation of the hypotensive and hypercalcemic properties. Endocrinology. 1983; 112:284-289.

16. Ulrich, Gray, Tam, Yang-Feng, Stsubokawa, Collins, Henzel, LeBon, Kathuria, Chen-Jacobs, Francke, Ramachandran, Fujita-Yamaguchi. Insulin-like growth factor 1 receptor primary structure: Comparison with insulin receptor suggests structural determinants that define functional specificity. EMBO J 5: 2503-2512, 1986.

17. Bonner TI, Buckley NJ, Young, AC Brann MR. Identification of a family of muscarinic acetyl choline receptor genes. Science 237:527-532, 1987

18. Benovic JL, Mayor F, Somers RL, Caron MG, Lefkowitz RJ. Light dependent phosphorylation of rhodopsin by beta-adrenergic receptor kinase. Nature 321:869-872, 1987.

19. Dixon RAF, Signal IS, Rands E, Register RB, Candelore MR, Blake AD, Strader CD. Ligand binding to beta-adrenergic receptor involves its rhodopsin-like core. Nature 326:73-77, 1987

20. Strader CD, Signal IS, Register RB, Candelore MR, Rands E, Dixon RAF. Identification of residues required for ligand binding to the beta-adrenergic receptors. Proc Natl Acad Sci USA 84:4384-4388, 1987

21. Styer L, Bourne HR. G proteins: a family of signal transducers. Ann Rev Cell Biol 2:391-419, 1986.

22. Pang PKT, Yang M, Oguro C, Phillips JG Ye JA. Hypotensive actions of parathyroid hormone preparations in vertebrates. J GenComp Endocrinol 1980.

23. Baczynsky R, Massry SG, Cohan R, Magott M, Saglikes Y, Brautbiar N. Effect of parathyroid hormone on myocardial energy metabolism in the rat. Kidney Int 27:718-725, 1987

24. Meytes D, Bogin E, Ma A, Dukes PP, Massry SG. Effect of parathyroid hormone on erythropoesis. J Clin invest 67:1263-1269, 1981.

25. Remuzzi G, Dodesini P, Livo M, Mecca G, Benigni A, Schieppati A, Poletti E, Degaetono G. Parathyroid hormone inhibits human platelet function. Lancet 1321-1323, 1981.

26. Yoshimasa T, Sibley DR, Bouvier M, Lefkowitz RJ, Caron MC, Cross-talk between cellular signalling pathways suggested by phorbol ester induced adenylate cyclase phosphorylation. Nature 327:67-70, 1987.

27. Hruska KA, Moskowitz D, Esbrit P, Civitelli R, Westbrook S, and Huskay M. J Clin Invest 79:230-239, 1987.

28. Civitelli R, Reid Ir, Dobre V, Shen V, Halstead L, Avioli LV, and Hruska K. J Bone Min Res 2 (Suppl 1): Abstr. 233, 1987.

29. Bringhurst FR, Zajac JD, Daggett As, Clegg C, McNight GS, Kronenberg HM Osteoblastic cell lines genetically engineered to express nonresponsive cAMP-dependent protein kinase. (American Society for Bone and Mineral Research, Annual scientific Meeting, 9th Indianapolis, Indiana,June 6-9, 1987. J Bone Min Res. 1987; 2 (Supp. 1), Abst. 235.

30. Abou-Samra AB, Jueppner H, Westerberg D, Potts, JT Jr, Segre GV. Parathyroid hormone modulates protein kinase-C activity in rat osteosarcoma cells. J Biol Chem. (submitted).

SYNTHETIC SIGNAL PEPTIDES OF PARATHYROID HORMONE: PROBES FOR

COMPONENTS OF THE SECRETORY APPARATUS

Michael P. Caulfield, Le T. Duong, and Michael Rosenblatt

Parathyroid Hormone Laboratory
Department of Biological Research and Molecular Biology
Merck Sharp and Dohme Research Laboratories
West Point, Pennsylvania, USA

INTRODUCTION

Parathyroid hormone (PTH), like the vast majority of secreted proteins and peptide hormones, is initially biosynthesized as a larger precursor, preproPTH (1,2). These precursor proteins have a cleavable N-terminal extension termed the signal sequence or leader sequence (3,4). This sequence is only transiently associated with the secreted protein and is rapidly removed by an enzyme, signal peptidase (located on the lumenal face of the endoplasmic reticular membrane (ER)), once the initiation of secretion has been effected (3). It is generally assumed that secreted proteins all use the same secretory machinery to achieve passage through the ER, although their subsequent passage through the cellular secretory pathway may be different.

Parathyroid hormone is no exception to this secretory pathway. It is initially synthesized on membrane-bound ribosomes and preproPTH is synthesized and sequestered within the lumen of the RER. The signal sequence is cleaved during this sequestration. The pro peptide is removed subsequently during the passage from the RER to the golgi stack and from there to the secretory vesicles, where it is stored prior to release. The function of the pro peptide has recently been investigated by Kronenberg and his co-workers. They have found that the PTH molecule is secreted even in the absence of the pro region, however, it is more slowly secreted and has erroneous processing (5). This suggests that the function of the pro region in this protein, and in others (6), may be to act as a spacer between the signal peptide and the mature protein, allowing for proper processing of the signal sequence.

The currently accepted hypothesis of the initial stages of protein secretion, targeting to the endoplasmic reticulum, interaction with the secretory apparatus, and translocation across the ER membrane, is outlined in the signal hypothesis (3,7). Briefly, an 11S ribonucleoprotein particle, termed signal recognition particle (SRP), composed of a 7S RNA species and six proteins, interacts with the ribosome in the cytoplasm (8). Upon the emergence of the signal sequence of a secretory protein from the ribosome, the signal sequence interacts with SRP, resulting in a 6,000-fold increase in affinity of SRP for the ribosome and causing an arrest of further protein translation by that ribosome (7). The

New Actions of Parathyroid Hormone
Edited by S. G. Massry and T. Fujita
Plenum Press, New York

SRP-arrest of translation is released by a SRP-receptor (9), or docking protein (10), present in the membrane of the rough endoplasmic reticulum (RER) (11). The signal sequence is presumed at this stage to interact with the membrane either directly with the lipid environment or via an interaction with a protein(s). Recent work has indicated an additional component in the membrane that interacts with the signal sequence (12). This component could function as a second receptor for the signal peptide (after SRP) and could be involved in the insertion of the protein into the membrane (13). The nature of this last step and the mechanism of the subsequent passage of the secretory protein through the membrane remain to be elucidated. At present, there is some evidence suggesting the involvement of a protein channel in this process (14).

The cleavage of the signal sequence from the mature protein occurs on the lumenal face of the RER and is mediated by the enzyme signal peptidase (15). This enzyme has recently been purified from rough microsomes isolated from the canine pancreas (16) and hen oviduct (17). In both cases, the peptidase was initially purified as a complex of six proteins. The signal peptidase activity has been purified further (18) from this complex resulting in a preparation containing three of the initial six proteins, two of which are glycosylated and may actually be the same protein with different glycosylation states. However, it is not yet known which of these three subunits is responsible for the peptidase activity.

From the lumen of the RER, the secretory protein then passes to the golgi apparatus. During this passage further processing, such as glycosylation, acylation, proteolytic cleavage, etc., of the secretory protein, can occur. After passage through the golgi stack, the secretory protein is transferred to a secretory vesicle which transports the protein to the plasma membrane, where it is released by exocytosis. Secretory proteins, including PTH, may also be stored in secretory granules until a suitable stimulus for release is received by the cell, in the case of PTH, for example, this would be low serum calcium.

It is worth mentioning that although the cell has an elaborate process to ensure correct processing and secretion, the irreversible commitment to secretion by the cell occurs at a very early stage in the biosynthesis and secretory pathway: once the protein has been vectorially transferred across the RER membrane, it is in essence secreted since all subsequent events that occur in the secretory pathway are within a membraneous compartment and are totally distinct from the cytoplasm.

In this paper, only the initial stages of protein secretion are to be considered, i.e. interaction of the signal sequence with components in the cytoplasm and cleavage of the signal sequence by signal peptidase.

We have used the synthetic signal and pro region of bovine pre-pro-parathyroid hormone, [D-Tyr^{+1}]preproPTH-(-29-+1)amide (native sequence), and its sulfur-free analog, [Nle-(-25,-21,-18),Ala-(-14),-D-Tyr-(+1)]preproPTH-(-29-+1)NH2, as probes to study the initial steps involved in protein secretion. In particular, we have used this peptide to inhibit translocation in a mammalian cell-free translation system, the rabbit reticulocyte lysate containing canine pancreatic rough microsomes, and to inhibit protein translation in a plant system, the wheat germ lysate, in a SRP-dependent manner. These studies with the synthetic peptide have shown that there is a major difference in the secretory systems present in the mammalian and plant lysates, the two systems generally employed in eucaryotic in vitro secretory studies. The iodinated synthetic sulfur-free analog of the native sequence peptide was found to be a substrate for the eucaryotic signal peptidase isolated from hen oviduct rough microsomes. Analogs of the sulfur-free peptide with altered hydrophobic cores do not appear to be substrates for this enzyme but appear to interact with the enzyme as they can inhibit cleavage of the iodinated sulfur-free peptide.

The effect of the synthetic signal peptides on in vitro translation and translocation. The in vitro assays used here have been previously described (19). Briefly, both the rabbit reticulocyte lysate and the wheat germ lysates are membrane-free cell extracts that contain all the necessary components for protein synthesis. Specific mRNA (total cellular RNA was used from specific tissues) encoding a particular protein, such as human placental prelactogen is added to the lysate. Protein synthesis is monitored, on SDS-polyacrylamide gel electrophoresis, by the incorporation of [35S]methionine into the specific protein. For translocation assays, canine pancreatic rough microsomes (20) (RM) are also added. For assays involving SRP, purified canine SRP (21) is added prior to the mRNA and signal peptides. Synthetic signal peptides were added in a solution of 35% glycerol at final concentrations ranging from 3-10 μM. For release of SRP-arrest, salt-washed RM are added to the lysate at various times after initiation of protein synthesis. In the wheat germ lysate cytoplasmic protein synthesis is also monitored by the inclusion of globin mRNA in the incubation mixture. Translations were carried out at 37°C for 60 min or 25°C for 120 min in the rabbit reticulocyte lysate or wheat germ lysate, respectively.

The native sequence preproPTH peptide was the first synthetic signal peptide to be synthesized (22,23) and was shown to display a bioactivity in vitro in the rabbit reticulocyte lysate supplemented with RM. In this assay system, the bioactivity of the native sequence peptide was shown by its ability to compete with a component involved in the secretory apparatus resulting in the inhibition of translocation of a number of secretory proteins and inhibits conversion of precursor proteins to their more mature forms. This occurs even with proteins from different species and tissues (24). Thus the native sequence signal peptide of PTH is able to not only inhibit the translocation of preproPTH but is also capable of inhibiting translocation of bovine growth hormone, pre-prolactin, and human placental lactogen. This observation is important for a number of reasons. Firstly, it indicates that a synthetic signal peptide is capable of interacting with a component of the secretory apparatus in a competitive manner. Secondly, it supports the suggestion that the secretory pathway is common to a number of proteins. Thirdly, the signal sequences of many proteins are known to have very little if any primary amino acid sequence homology (4) yet they interact with a common component. The obvious question that these data raise is whether the signal peptides are exerting their effect through an interaction with the membrane or through an interaction with a cytosolic component such as SRP.

The following results discussed below in this section have recently been published (19) and are summarized for convenience in Table 1.

To address the question of a membrane versus a cytoplasmic effect the synthetic signal peptides were assayed in an alternative in vitro system using a wheat germ lysate supplemented with the same membranes used in the rabbit reticulocyte lysate. Presumably if the synthetic signal peptides were exerting their effect through an interaction with the membrane then a similar effect should be observed in the wheat germ lysate. However, when assayed in the plant system, the native sequence peptide and the sulfur-free peptide did not inhibit translocation. This

Table 1. Summary of biological effects of synthetic signal peptides in
the wheat germ and reticulocyte lysate in vitro
translation/translocation systems

	Reticulocyte Lysate			Wheat Germ Lysate		
	Translation Arrest (a)		Inhibition of Translocation	Translation Arrest (c)		Inhibition of Translocation
Peptide	−SRP	+SRP	(b)	−SRP	+SRP	(b)
NS (d)	−	nt	+	−	+	−
SF (e)	−	−	+	−	+	−
AS (f)	−	nt	+	−	−	−

(a) In the reticulocyte lysate translation arrest was determined by the
inhibition of synthesis of human placental prelactogen in the
absence or presence of exogenously added canine SRP.

(b) Inhibition of translocation in both assay systems was determined by
the ability of the synthetic signal peptides to inhibit the processing of the precursor protein to its mature form in the presence
of RM. Processing was followed by mobility of proteins on
SDS−polyacrylamide gel electrophoresis.

(c) Translation arrest in the wheat germ lysate was assayed by the
ability of the synthetic signal peptide to inhibit globin synthesis
in the absence or presence of canine SRP in the absence of
salt−washed RM.

(d) NS = Native sequence; $[D-Tyr-(+1)]$preproPTH$-(-29--+1)NH_2$

(e) SF = Sulfur−free; $[Nle-(-25,-21,-18),Ala-(-14),D-Tyr-(+1)]$prepro-
PTH$-(-29-+1)NH_2$

(f) AS = Asp−substituted; $[Nle-(-25,-21),Asp-(-18),Ala-(-14),D-$
Tyr$-(+1)]$preproPTH$-(-29-+1)NH_2$

nt; not tested

strongly suggests that these peptides are not exerting their effects at
the level of the membrane and in addition, that there is a soluble
factor in the reticulocyte lysate, possibly SRP (10) (L.T. Duong, et al.
unpublished results), that interacts with the signal peptide to cause
the inhibition of translocation.

At present, the only known cytosolic factor involved in protein
secretion is SRP. SRP is known to cause a translational arrest in the
wheat germ lysate via its interaction with the signal sequence as it
emerges from the ribosome (7). If the synthetic signal peptide was able
to mimic the signal peptide emerging from the ribosome, it might be able
to interact with SRP and cause a translational arrest of even a
non−secreted protein.

To address this possibility, the effect of the synthetic signal
peptide in the wheat germ lysate supplemented with purified canine SRP
was examined. In the SRP−supplemented wheat germ lysates, the

sulfur-free peptide caused an SRP-specific inhibition of total translation, as it also inhibited the synthesis of globin. This supports the idea that the synthetic signal peptides are capable of mimicking a native signal peptide. However, unlike a native signal peptide which can only cause the arrest of translation of itself, the synthetic signal peptide could also cause the arrest of translation of a cytoplasmic protein. This observation is most easily explained by presuming that the synthetic signal peptide interacts with the SRP, which in turn interacts with the ribosomes. In this configuration, any protein undergoing biosynthesis, even one not normally secreted, will be subjected to a specific signal peptide-induced arrest of translation. Unlike a normal SRP arrest which can be released by the addition of salt-washed RM, the synthetic signal peptide-induced SRP-arrest was only released at very early times, suggesting that a non-reversible complex forms with time. In addition, in the presence of the synthetic signal peptide-SRP arrest, the addition of salt-washed RM did not result in the synthesis of mature secretory proteins. This strongly suggests that translational arrest was caused by the synthetic peptides directly, rather than the native signal sequence emerging from the ribosome. The arrest caused by synthetic signal peptide and SRP was also dependent on the amount of protein synthesis that had already taken place before the addition of signal peptide. Thus, after synthesis of approximately two thirds of the protein globin (approximately 100 amino acids of a total of 141 amino acids), the synthetic signal peptide could no longer inhibit globin synthesis. Presumably, this length dependence reflects some steric hinderance of SRP interaction with the ribosome due to the presence of the growing peptide chain emerging from the ribosome.

Since SRP has been shown to be present in the reticulocyte lysate (26), the results obtained in the wheat germ lysate were somewhat intriguing. Why does the synthetic signal peptide in the reticulocyte lysate in the absence of membranes not cause a translational arrest? Possibly the concentration of SRP in the lysate is too low for all the ribosomes to become inhibited. This possibility was dismissed by the finding that the synthetic signal peptide did not cause a translational arrest in the reticulocyte lysate in the presence of exogenously added canine SRP. In addition, even in the presence of this excess of SRP the synthetic signal peptide was able to inhibit translocation.

These results taken together indicate a difference between the mammalian (rabbit) and plant (wheat germ) in vitro translation/translocation systems and possibly in the process of protein secretion. As outlined previously, the accepted hypothesis includes an SRP-dependent translation arrest brought about by the interaction of the signal peptide with this particle on the ribosome. In the wheat germ system, this is indeed the case as seen with the synthesis of many secretory proteins (25) and also by the inhibition of globin synthesis in the presence of the synthetic signal peptide. Yet in the reticulocyte lysate in the presence of exogenous canine SRP and synthetic signal peptide, there was no inhibition of protein synthesis. Presumably this result indicates that SRP is not able to inhibit translation in the reticulocyte lysate, yet it is required for protein secretion in this system (L. T. Duong, unpublished observations). Therefore, to account for the ability of the synthetic signal peptides to compete for protein translocation in the reticulocyte lysate, the existence of an additional component that interacts with the signal peptide must be invoked. The presence of this component may account for the lack of a translational arrest by SRP and may mediate the interaction of the ribosome with the membrane. This component is either absent in the wheat germ lysate or does not recognize the canine SRP and, therefore, the SRP arrest phenomenon occurs.

In support of this suggestion, we have found that an analog, [Nle-(-25,-21),Asp-(-18),Ala-(-14),D-Tyr-(+1)]preproPTH-(-29-+1)NH$_2$ (asp-substituted), of the sulfur-free peptide displays differential activities in the plant and mammalian in vitro translation/trans-location systems. Asp-substituted peptide caused an inhibition of translocation in the reticulocyte lysate while in the wheat germ system supplemented with SRP it had no effect on globin synthesis. These results in the wheat germ lysate suggest that SRP does not recognize the asp-substituted analog while in the reticulocyte lysate, the asp-substi-tuted peptide was recognized, presumably by the newly proposed factor. This finding may indicate that the proposed factor has a lower stringency for recognition of a signal sequence than does SRP.

Synthetic preproPTH as a substrate for the eucaryotic signal peptidase. As mentioned previously, secreted proteins have their signal sequences removed at an early stage in biosynthesis by the enzyme, signal peptidase. This enzyme is located on the lumenal face of the RER. A similar type of enzyme is also found in procaryotic organisms on the external face of the plasma membrane. Various signal peptidases have been purified from bacteria (26) and shown to be single poly-peptides. Recently, two signal peptidases have been partially purified from eucaryotic sources, the rough microsomes of hen oviduct (17) and canine pancreas (16). In all likelihood, these two are the same enzyme. Both enzymes, upon initial purification, were found to be a complex of six proteins. It is unlikely that all six proteins are required for enzyme activity. Indeed, in the case of the hen oviduct signal peptidase (HOSP), the complex of six proteins has been purified further to a complex of three proteins in which signal peptidase activity remains intact. Two of the three proteins are glycosylated and may actually be the same protein containing different patterns of glycosylation (18).

The synthetic signal peptide has also been used to study signal peptidase, the enzyme responsible for the cleavage of the signal peptide from the nascent protein. Signal peptidase (HOSP) was purified from the hen oviduct rough microsomes as described (17). The HOSP fraction used in this work was the complex of six proteins. The sulfur-free peptide or its analogs were iodinated using Iodo-Gen and Na[^{125}I]. The iodinated peptide was purified by reverse phase HPLC. The trifluoro-acetic acid eluant was neutralized with triethanolamine, and the solution brought to 1% in bovine serum albumin and frozen in aliquots at -80°C. The iodinated peptide was not concentrated. Acetonitrile (up to 8% final concentration) had no effect on the signal peptidase activity. Enzyme activity was assayed at 25°C for various lengths of time, from 0 to 120 min.

The iodinated sulfur-free peptide was assayed as a potential substrate for the HOSP. Fortuitously, the sulfur-free peptide was insoluble in 5% trichloroacetic acid (TCA) while the pro peptide (residues -6 to +1) was soluble. Therefore, it was easy to monitor cleavage of the sulfur-free peptide by HOSP by following the TCA soluble counts. In this manner, the sulfur-free peptide was found to serve as a substrate for HOSP; up to 70% cleavage of peptide occurs in two hours. The time course of cleavage gave a rectangular hyperbola curve, characteristic of substrate digestion by enzyme.

Three methods were used to demonstrate that the peptide was cleaved accurately at the junction of the "pre" and "pro" regions of the hormone. Firstly, the retention time on HPLC of the cleavage product of the iodinated sulfur-free peptide after treatment with HOSP was compared to a chemically synthesized iodinated pro-peptide, [D-Tyr^{+1}]pro-

PTH-$(-6-+1)$NH$_2$, representing the expected cleavage product. Under the same elution conditions on reverse phase HPLC using a Vydac C-4 HPLC column, both peptides had the identical elution position. Secondly, the iodinated species that remained TCA soluble after treatment with HOSP and TCA was compared to the iodinated pro-peptide on TLC. Both peptides had the same relative mobility and were distinct from the untreated intact iodinated sulfur-free peptide. Thirdly, after cleavage of iodinated sulfur-free peptide with HOSP the cleavage product was isolated from a C-4 HPLC column and submitted for sequential Edman degradation. The cpm eluting at each cycle were determined. The major radioactive peak (iodo-tyrosine) was found at cycle seven, indicating that peptide bond cleavage had occurred in the predicted position, between residues -7 and -6. Thus HOSP is able to faithfully cleave the iodinated sulfur-free peptide. Again this demonstrates the universality of the secretion system: a hen oviduct signal peptidase is able to faithfully cleave an analog of bovine preproPTH. Having a relatively simple assay for signal peptidase should allow rapid screening of potential signal peptidase inhibitors and should also be useful for investigation of the structural requirements for interaction of the signal peptide with signal peptidase.

In this regard, four analogs of the sulfur-free peptide with alterations in the hydrophobic core at residue -18 were assayed for their ability to act as substrates for HOSP. Of these analogs the pro-substituted analog, [Nle-$(-25,-21)$,Pro-(-18),Ala-(-14),D-Tyr-$(+1)$]-prepro-PTH-$(-29-+1)$NH$_2$, was the best substrate but was cleaved very slowly; only 17 % was cleaved in two hrs. The truncated, [N-acetyl Leu-(-17),Ala-(-14),D-Tyr-$(+1)$]preproPTH-$(-17-+1)$NH$_2$, the lys-substituted, [Nle-$(-25,-21)$,Lys-(-18),Ala-(-14),D-Tyr-$(+1)$]-preproPTH-$(-29-+1)$NH$_2$, and asp-substituted peptides were not cleaved. However, when the iodinated sulfur-free peptide was assayed in the presence of an excess of either the sulfur-free peptide or the analogs, cleavage of the iodinated peptide was inhibited. Therefore, the analogs can compete for occupancy of HOSP. The relative order of potencies as determined in one set of assays were asp-substituted (0.15 µM, 42% inhibition) > prosubstituted (0.17 µM, 18% inhibition) > lys-substituted (0.2 µM, 19% inhibition) > truncated peptide (0.38 µM, 14% inhibition). The uniodinated sulfur-free peptide gave 78% inhibition of cleavage at 0.23 µM.

Finally, the iodinated sulfur-free signal peptide and its analogs were examined as substrates for the procaryotic signal peptidase, the Escherichia coli leader peptidase (27). Neither the iodinated sulfur-free signal peptide nor the analogs of this peptide were cleaved by this enzyme. This suggests a difference in the specificities between the procaryotic and eucaryotic enzymes. This observation is in agreement with a recent report that prepro PTH, when expressed in E. Coli and localized to the periplasmic space, is not processed to proPTH (28).

This study demonstrates the usefulness of the synthetic signal peptide of preproPTH in the study of the initial stages of protein secretion. It has given some insight into the differences between the two principal in vitro assays used to study this process and has suggested the presence of an additional component in the reticulocyte lysate that may modulate the interaction of the signal peptide and SRP with the membrane. In addition, this peptide can be used as an affinity label in conjunction with cross-linking techniques to identify this and other components. This work is presently being done in our laboratory. Finally, the last stage of involvement of the signal peptide in secretion is its removal from the growing protein by the signal peptidase.

The iodinated signal peptide of PTH can be used to study this process since it is faithfully cleaved by this enzyme, as if it were part of a nascent precursor protein. In addition, this approach permits a direct examination of the structural requirements for signal sequence recognition by this enzyme. In this respect, the analogs of the sulfur-free peptide which have alterations in the hydrophobic core are not substrates for the HOSP suggesting that the hydrophobic core is involved in the recognition of the signal peptide by the enzyme. Yet, they could inhibit HOSP enzymatic activity. These findings suggest that the hydrophobic core of the signal sequence, a distance of 11 residues from the actual cleavage site, may play a role in the correct recognition of a signal peptide by signal peptidase, and that the "reading frame" of this enzyme is remarkably long and extends (in the N-terminal direction) well beyond the beta-turn present at the junction of the signal sequence with the remainder of the protein.

ACKNOWLEDGEMENTS

We thank Drs. Mark Lively and Keith Baker for providing hen oviduct signal peptidase and Jay Levy for synthesis and cleavage of the sulfur-free analogs.

REFERENCES

1. H. M. Kronenberg, B. E. McDevitt, J. A. Majzoub, J. Nathans, P. A. Sharp, and J. T. Potts, Jr., Cloning and nucleotide sequence of DNA coding for bovine preproparathyroid hormone, Proc. Natl. Acad. Sci. USA. 76:4981 (1979).
2. G. N. Hendy, H. M. Kronenberg, J. T. Potts, Jr., and A. Rich, Nucleotide sequence of cloned cDNAs encoding human preproparathyroid hormone, Proc. Natl. Acad. Sci. 78:7365 (1981).
3. G. Blobel, and B. Dobberstein, Transfer of proteins across membranes. 1. Presence of proteolytically processed and unprocessed nascent immunoglobulin light chains on membrane-bound ribosomes of murine myeloma, J. Cell Biol. 67:835 (1975).
4. M. E. E. Waters, Compilation of published signal sequences, Nucleic Acids Res. 12:5415 (1984).
5. K. Wiren, J. Hellerman, L. Ivashkiv, M. Freeman, E. Amatrude, R. Mulligan, J. T. Potts, Jr., and H. M. Kronenberg, Deletion of signal cleavage site and "pro" sequence results in abnormal cleavage and secretion of preproparathyroid hormone-related peptides, J. Bone Mineral Res. 1:58 (1986).
6. R. J. Foltz, and J. I. Gordon, Deletion of the propeptide from human preproapolipoprotein A-II redirects cotranslational processing by signal peptidase, J. Biol. Chem. 261:14752 (1986).
7. P. Walter, and G. Blobel, Translocation of proteins across the endoplasmic reticulum III. Signal recognition protein (SRP) causes signal sequence-dependent and site-specific arrest of chain elongation that is released by microsomal membranes, J. Cell Biol. 91:557 (1981).
8. P. Walter, and G. Blobel, Signal recognition particle contains a 7S RNA essential for protein translocation across the endoplasmic reticulum, Nature 299:691 (1982).
9. R. Gilmore, P. Walter, and G. Blobel, Protein translocation across the endoplasmic reticulum II. Isolation and characterization of the signal recognition particle receptor, J. Cell Biol. 95:470 (1982).
10. D. I. Meyer, E. Krause, and B. Dobberstein, Secretory protein translocation across membranes -- the role of the docking protein, Nature 297:647 (1982).

11. M. Hortsch, and D. I. Meyer, Immunochemical analysis of rough and smooth microsomes from rat liver. Segregation of docking protein in rough membranes, Eur. J. Biochem. 150:559 (1985).
12. M. Wiedmann, T. V. Kurzchalia, E. Hartmann, and T. A. Rapoport, A signal sequence receptor in the endoplasmic reticulum membrane, Nature 328:830 (1987).
13. P. Walter, Signal recognition. Two receptors act sequentially, Nature 328:763 (1987).
14. R. Gilmore, and G. Blobel, Translocation of secretory proteins across the microsomal membrane occurs through an environment accessible to aqueous perturbants, Cell 42: 497 (1985).
15. G. Blobel, and B. Dobberstein, Transfer of proteins across membranes II. Reconstitution of functional rough microsomes from heterologous components, J. Cell Biol. 67:852 (1975).
16. E. A. Evans, R. Gilmore, and G. Blobel, Purification of microsomal signal peptidase as a complex, Proc. Natl. Acad. Sci. USA 83:581 (1986).
17. R. K. Baker, G. P. Bentivoglio, and M. O. Lively, Partial purification of microsomal signal peptidase from hen oviduct, J. Cellular Biochem. 32:193 (1986).
18. R. K. Baker, and M. O. Lively, Purification and characterization of hen oviduct signal peptidase, Biochem., in press.
19. L. T. Duong, M. P. Caulfield, and M. Rosenblatt, Synthetic signal peptide and analogs display different activities in mammalian and plant in vitro secretion systems, J. Biol. Chem. 262:6328 (1987).
20. P. Walter, and G. Blobel, Preparation of microsomal membranes for cotranslational protein translocation, Methods Enzymol. 96:84 (1983).
21. P. Walter, and G. Blobel, Signal recognition particle: a ribonucleoprotein required for cotranslational translocation of proteins, isolation and properties, Methods Enzymol. 96:682 (1983).
22. J. F. Habener, M. Rosenblatt, B. Kemper, H. M. Kronenberg, A. Rich, and J. T. Potts, Jr., Pre-proparathyroid hormone: amino acid sequence, chemical synthesis, and some biological studies of the precursor region, Proc. Natl. Acad. Sci. USA 75:2616 (1978).
23. M. Rosenblatt, J. F. Habener, G. A. Tyler, G. L. Shepard, and J. T. Potts, Jr., Chemical synthesis of the precursor-specific region of preproparathyroid hormone, J. Biol. Chem. 254:1414 (1979).
24. J. A. Majzoub, M. Rosenblatt, B. Fennick, R. Maunus, H. M. Kronenberg, J. T. Potts, Jr., and J. F. Habener, Synthetic pre-proparathyroid hormone leader sequence inhibits cell-free processing of placental, parathyroid, and pituitary prehormones, J. Biol. Chem. 255:11478 (1980).
25. P. Walter, R. Gilmore, and G. Blobel, Protein translocation across the endoplasmic reticulum, Cell 38:5 (1984).
26. P. Ray, I. Dev, C. MacGregor, and P. Bassford, Jr., Signal peptidases, Current Topics Microbiol. Immunol. 125:75 (1986).
27. C. Zwizinski, and W. Wickner, Purification and characterization of leader (signal) peptidase from Escherichia coli, J. Biol. Chem. 255:7973 (1980).
28. W. Born, M. Freeman, G. N. Hendy, A. Rapoport, A. Rich, J. T. Potts, Jr., And H. M. Kronenberg, Human preproparathyroid hormone synthesized in E. coli is transported to the surface of the bacterial inner membrane but not processed to the mature hormone, Molec. Endocrin. 1:5 (1987).

EFFECTS OF WR-2721 ON PARATHYROID HORMONE SECRETION AND BONE

M.F. Attie, S. Goldfarb, M. Fallon, J. Shaker,
and K. Carmichael

Departments of Medicine and Pathology
University of Pennsylvania School of Medicine
Philadelphia, PA, USA

INTRODUCTION

WR-2721 (S-2(3-aminopropylaminoethyl) phosphorothioic acid) is an organic thiophosphate derivative of cysteamine which was developed under the auspices of the Walter Reed Army Institute of Research in an attempt to develop non-toxic means of introducing thiol-containing compounds into tissues. Thiols are known to protect cells against the toxic effects of ionizing radiation and alkylating agent chemotherapy, however agents with free sulfhydryl groups such as cysteamine are very toxic. To avert the toxicity of this reactive group, several thioester derivatives were synthesized (1). Yuhas (2) found that one of the thiophosphates, WR-2721, is accumulated by, and provides radioprotection to normal tissues, but not certain tumors in experimental animals. The mechanism of this tissue selectivity is unknown. In studies in animals and humans, there are few side effects at doses providing radioprotection (3). During initial trials of its efficacy as a radio- and a chemoprotective agent in patients with malignancies, acute transient hypocalcemia was noted; intravenous WR-2721 produced a 20% fall in the serum calcium concentration at four hours and serum calcium levels remained depressed at 24 hours. Serum concentrations of immunoreactive PTH were reduced after infusion of WR-2721 instead of increasing in response to hypocalcemia suggesting that WR-2721 causes hypocalcemia by reducing secretion of PTH (4).

While these data suggest that WR-2721 reduces serum calcium by producing acute hypoparathyroidism, our more recent studies suggest the mechanism is more complex. The hypocalcemic effect of WR-2721 is, at least in part, independent of its effect on the parathyroid glands since it reduces serum calcium in parathyroidectomized rats (see below).

The effects of WR-2721 on both parathyroid gland and bone imply that this compound affects unique properties in both systems. Further more, WR-2721 may be the prototype of a unique class of pharmacologic agents which alter both bone and parathyroid function. In these studies we describe our experience characterizing the effect of WR-2721 on PTH secretion in vitro and on bone metabolism in vivo and in vitro. In addition, we present preliminary studies showing that WR-2721 reduces bone loss in an animal model with excess bone resorption.

EFFECTS OF WR-2721 ON PTH SECRETION FROM DISPERSED PARATHYROID CELLS

The effect of WR-2721 on PTH secretion was studied using dispersed bovine parathyroid cells prepared from calf glands by a modification of the methods of Brown et al. (5,6). Cell preparations consisted of nearly 100% parathyroid cells with viability consistently greater than 95% as determined by Trypan Blue exclusion. To analyze the time course of the effect of WR-2721 on PTH release, we measured the rate of release of PTH into the cell incubation medium at 30 minute intervals (4).

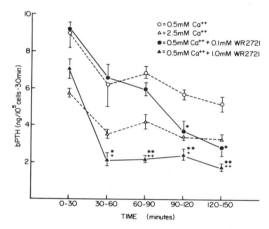

Fig. 1. Effect of WR-2721 on the rate of PTH release from bovine parathyroid cells. Dispersed cells were incubated with 0.5 or 2.5 mM $CaCl_2$. Incubations with 0.5 mM $CaCl_2$ also had either no WR-2721, 0.1 mM WR-2721 or 1.0 mM WR-2721. Release of hormone is shown for the intervals on the abscissa. Points represent triplicate determinations (mean ± S.E.M.), each assayed in duplicate. * and ** indicate a significant difference from incubations with 0.5 mM $CaCl_2$ alone at $P<0.05$ and at $P<0.01$, respectively; + and ++ indicate significant difference from incubations with 2.5 mM $CaCl_2$ alone at $P<0.05$ and $P<0.01$, respectively. (From Glover et al. (ref.4), with permission).

This medium was obtained by gently pelleting the parathyroid cells, removing the medium, and resuspending the cells in fresh medium. Bovine PTH was measured in an assay using goat anti-human PTH antiserum (NG-5 supplied by L. Mallette) using [^{125}I]-bPTH (1-84) as tracer. As shown in figure 1, PTH release from bovine parathyroid cells was inhibited within the first 30 minutes of incubation by high concentration of calcium (2.5 mM) in the incubation medium. WR-2721 inhibited PTH release but this effect did not occur as rapidly as with high concentrations of calcium. After the first 30 minutes of incubation, the amount of hormone release from cells incubated with 1.0 mM WR-2721 in medium with low calcium (0.5 mM) was significantly lower than the amount of released from cells either stimulated with low levels of calcium or inhibited by high levels. The effect of the lower concentration of WR-2721, 0.1 mM, was even more gradual than that of 1 mM; only after 90 minutes of incubation was the rate of PTH release from cells incubated with 0.1 mM WR-2721 significantly lower than that of cells in low-calcium medium without WR-2721 (fig. 1).

WR-2721 also inhibited the release of radiolabeled proteins from parathyroid cells in a dose-dependent manner. As shown in figure 2, concentrations of WR-2721 as low as 0.05 mM inhibited release of trichloroacetic acid-insoluble radioactivity during continuous incubation with [^{3}H]-leucine and this inhibitory effect on labeled protein release was parallel to the effect on release of immunoreactive PTH (not shown).

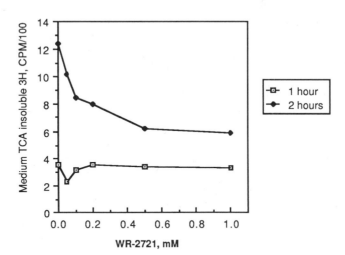

Fig. 2. Effect of WR-2721 on release of TCA-insoluble radioactivity from dispersed bovine parathyroid cells. Cells are incubated for one (□) or two (●) hours in leucine-free medium with 25 mCi/ml ^{3}H-leucine in 0.5 mM Ca and the indicated concentrations of WR-2721. Reactions were terminated and TCA-insoluble radioactivity in medium measured.

When the proteins in the incubation medium were analyzed by SDS-polyacrylamide gel electrophoresis (Fig 3), both exposure to high concentrations of calcium and to WR-2721 inhibited release of two radiolabeled proteins. The more rapidly migrating peak is presumably PTH since it co-migrates with [^{125}I]-bPTH. The other is chromogranin A, a large molecular weight protein secreted by parathyroid cells (and other endocrine tissues); its secretion is known to be inhibited by high concentrations of calcium (7,8).

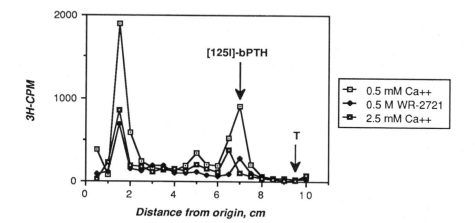

Fig. 3. Effect of WR-2721 and high medium Ca on release of ^{3}H-labeled protein by parathyroid cells: analysis of SDS-polyacrylamide gel electrophoresis. TCA precipitated media from cell incubations from experiment in Fig. 2 in 0.5 mM CaCl$_2$ with or without 0.5 mM WR-2721, or with 2.5 mM CaCl$_2$ were analyzed by SDS-PAGE. The position of the tracking dye and ^{125}I-PTH (run on a parallel gel) are indicated by T and ^{125}I-bPTH, respectively.

The reversibility of the inhibitory effect of WR-2721 was examined measuring PTH release from cells initially exposed to 0.5 mM WR-2721 for one hour and then resuspended in WR-2721-free medium. The rate of PTH release from these cells was compared to: 1) cells resuspended after the first hour in medium containing WR-2721; 2) cells never exposed to WR-2721 incubated in medium with either a low or a high concentration of calcium. Except for the latter group, all incubations were in low medium calcium (0.5 mM). PTH release was linear with time for the five hours in cells not exposed to WR-2721 (Fig 4). The rate of PTH release from cells preincubated with WR-2721 was less than that from cells not exposed to the agent for the first two hours, however, beyond that point, the rate of PTH release from cells in incubations where the agent had been removed accelerated and was indistinguishable from control cells not exposed to WR-2721. At four and five hours, the amount of

PTH released from these cells was significantly greater
(P<.05 and P<.02, respectively) than from cells that were
kept in WR-2721-containing medium (Fig. 4). Thus the effect
of WR-2721 on PTH secretion is reversible with a lag time
similar to the lag time in the onset of the effect.

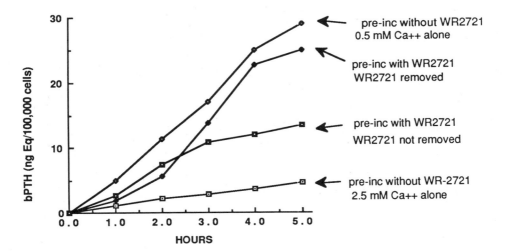

Fig. 4. Reversibility of the inhibitory
effect of WR-2721. Parathyroid cells
were pre-incubated in medium and 0.5 mM
$CaCl_2$ with or without 0.5 mM WR-2721 for
one hour and then washed twice in fresh
medium. Cells exposed to WR-2721 were
incubated in standard medium with 0.5 mM
$CaCl_2$ and no WR-2721, or 0.5 mM WR-2721.
Cells not exposed to WR-2721 were
incubated in medium without WR-2721 and
either 0.5 mM $CaCl_2$ or 2.5 mM $CaCl_2$. At
the indicated times, cells were pelleted
and medium removed for PTH analysis.
Results are means of triplicate
determinations assayed in duplicate.

PTH release from parathyroid cells after one hour of
incubation with 0.5 mM WR-2721 is independent of
extracellular calcium concentration. High concentrations of
calcium in the medium do not further inhibit and low
concentrations do not increase PTH release from these cells
over a two hour period. Even in the virtual absence of
extracellular calcium (medium with EGTA and no added
calcium), there was no increase in the rate of release of
PTH suggesting that WR-2721 does not act by increasing the
sensitivity of the parathyroid cell to inhibition by
extracellular calcium.

A potential mode of action of WR-2721 is by altering cyclic AMP levels. cAMP is an intracellular modulator of PTH secretion; agents such as beta-adrenergic agonists and dopamine stimulate cAMP accumulation with PTH release from bovine parathyroid cells and alpha-adrenergic agents inhibit PTH release and cAMP accumulation (9). To determine whether WR-2721 reduces PTH secretion by reducing cAMP accumulation, we examined the effects of WR-2721 on basal and dopamine-stimulated cAMP accumulation and PTH release. Bovine parathyroid cells were incubated with and without 0.5 mM WR-2721 for 60 minutes and then for a subsequent 30 minutes with 0.01 mM dopamine. cAMP, measured in cell pellets, was 0.28 ± 0.02 pmoles/10^5 cells in WR-2721-treated and 0.27 ± 0.05 in control cells at 60 minutes. Dopamine markedly increased cellular cAMP; 20 ± 3 pmoles/10^5 cells in WR-2721-treated cells and 27 ± 5 in control cells ($P<0.05$). WR-2721, as expected, inhibited PTH release and dopamine did not further stimulate secretion from these cells (in contrast to cells not exposed to WR-2721 which were significantly stimulated by dopamine). Weaver et al. (10) found that WR-2721 significantly reduced baseline cellular cAMP levels and proposed this as its mode of action. However, it seems unlikely that a small reduction in baseline cAMP levels is the sole cause of an inhibition of secretion since even with cellular concentrations that are nearly 100-fold basal levels, PTH release is still inhibited.

By electron microscopy, the ultrastructure of parathyroid cells exposed to 0.5 mM WR-2721 for one hour was not different from cells incubated without WR-2721 (not shown). There were no degenerative features; cytoplasmic and nuclear membranes remained distinct and outlines of mitochondria and secretory granules were sharp.

Several agents have been shown to inhibit PTH secretion in vitro including prostaglandins of the F series (10), sodium nitroprusside (11), aluminum (12), and high ambient magnesium (13,14). Of these, only magnesium has been demonstrated to cause hypocalcemia; however, doses producing a three-fold increase in serum magnesium concentration are required (14). WR-2721 causes hypocalcemia at doses causing few side effects (4). Thus, WR-2721 represents a new and unique hypocalcemic agent which, by virtue of its parathyroid-inhibitory effect, may be important in the therapy of certain hypercalcemic disorders.

These studies with dispersed parathyroid cells show that WR-2721 at concentrations as low as 0.05 mM inhibits the release of newly synthesized radiolabeled PTH from bovine parathyroid cells. This inhibitory effect increases with time. The time lag is consistent with several mechanisms; slow concentration-dependent accumulation of WR-2721, slow metabolism to an active form, or accumulation of depletion of a cellular constituents affecting the secretory process. Yuhas found that uptake of radiolabeled WR-2721 into normal tissue fragments is a slow and concentration-dependent process; after several hours, the tissue is several-fold that in the medium (15). The slow reversal of the inhibitory effect of WR-2721 is also consistent with any of these mechanisms. The in vitro effects of WR-2721 occur at concentrations that are within the range of concentrations occurring after hypocalcemic doses of WR-2721 that are given to humans (16).

Whether the cellular effects of WR-2721 are specific for bone and parathyroid gland is unclear. It suggests that WR-2721 interacts with a unique biochemical system shared by these two tissues. Unfortunately, little information is available regarding cellular effects of WR-2721 on other tissues. In one study, concentrations of WR-2721 as low as 0.1 mM inhibited [^{3}H]-thymidine incorportation by murine T-cells in culture (17). Few immediate side effects have been noted in patients receiving WR-2721; a minority have developed mild hypotension, emesis, somnolence and sneezing (3) suggesting that there are no major toxic effects on the other organ systems. In preliminary studies the humans receiving WR-2721 prior to receiving chemotherapy, we found that serum prolactin, growth hormone and cortisol levels rise after intravenous WR-2721 infusion, while serum levels of glucose, thyroid stimulating hormone, lutenizing hormone and follicle stimulating hormone remain unchanged (K.A. Carmichael, P. Snyder, M. Attie, unpublished observations). The increases in serum prolactin, growth hormone, and cortisol (which may represent a response to stress in patients receiving chemotherapy) and lack of decrease in other hormone levels argues against a general suppressive effect of this agent on hormone secretion.

The mechanism by which WR-2721 inhibits PTH secretion can not be deduced from these studies. WR-2721 is dephosphorylated intracellulary (18, 19). Larson et al. recently found that WR-2721 raised cytoplasmic calcium (measured with Quin2) in parathyroid cells from humans with hyperparathyroidism (22). Cytoplasmic calcium may transduce or may be related to the inhibitory effect of high extracellular calcium (23) and may be a result of changes in cellular metabolism produced by WR-2721. This rise in cytosolic calcium could also represent a non-specific disruption of energy metabolism. One could speculate that the presence of a reactive sulfhydryl group in the cell could alter the redox state of the cell or alter the activity of critical proteins by formation of mixed disulfides. At present there is no information on the effect of WR-2721 on the redox state of the cell. Although the free sulfhydryl could shift cellular constituents to a more reduced state, if WR-2721 is a substrate for flavin-containing monoxygenases (as is cysteamine) it would be oxidized to the disulfide form at the expense of molecular oxygen and then re-reduced at the expense of cellular reducing equivalents; the net effect is oxidation of pyridine nucleotides and glutathione (20). There is indirect evidence that changes in the redox state of cells may alter PTH secretion. Sodium nitoprusside, a drug which oxidizes cellular constituents, inhibits PTH release from bovine parathyroid cells (11). Furthermore, Morrissey and Klahr (21) found that when PTH secretion from bovine cells is inhibited by high medium calcium, there is an increase in the activity of the hexose monophosphate shunt. This increasae in the shunt activity would increase the NADPH/NADP ratio of the cell unless, as they postulate, the increased activity is a response to a decrease in this ratio. These studies together suggests that cellular redox may be important in regulating PTH secretion and agents such as WR-2721 may provide insights into this regulatory process as well as a means to modify it.

MECHANISM OF THE HYPOCALCEMIC ACTION OF WR-2721

WR-2721 could produce hypocalcemia by inhibiting the entry of calcium into serum from pools such as bone or by enhancing its exit form serum into urine or tissues. To distinguish between these potential mechanisms, we analyzed the rate of disappearance of ^{45}Ca given two hours before an intravenous injection of WR-2721 (30 mg/kg) or vehicle in rats (24). If WR-2721 accelerated the exit of calcium from serum then total serum calcium and isotopic calcium would be reduced in the same proportion and the rate of decline of serum ^{45}Ca specific activity would not differ from animals which had not received WR-2721. Although WR-2721 lowered serum calcium, there was no significant increase in the rate of disappearance of ^{45}Ca; the specific activity of ^{45}Ca was significantly greater at 75 and 150 minutes after infusion of WR-2721 (24). Therefore, the major effect of WR-2721 in lowering serum calcium appears to be an inhibition of calcium release into serum. These findings are similar to those which have been obtained with calcitonin (25) and mithramycin (26) which are both believed to cause hypocalcemia by inhibiting bone resorption.

To determine whether WR-2721 produces hypocalcemia by mechanisms which are independent of its effect on the parathyroid gland, we administered WR-2721 to chronically parathyroidectomized rats (PTX) (24). PTX rats and sham-operated controls were kept on a low phosphorus diet to maintain serum calcium within the normal range. Intravenous WR-2721 (30 mg/kg) produced a nearly identical fall in serum calcium in both groups of animals, $20.2 \pm 2\%$ in PTX and $20 \pm 1\%$ in sham-operated rates (Fig. 5). This reduction in serum calcium in the absence of parathyroid glands strongly suggested that WR-2721 has hypercalcemic actions that are independent of its parathyroid-inhibitory effects. In a subsequent similar study, Hirschel-Scholz et al. found that WR-2721 significantly reduced serum calcium in PTX rats but the reduction was only a fraction of that in intact rats (27). This discrepancy may be a result of a higher dietary phosphorus Hirschel-Scholz used; their rats were hypocalcemic during the study suggesting that serum calcium was less dependent on hypophosphatemia-induced release of calcium from bone.

The effect of WR-2721 on radiocalcium kinetics and its effect in PTX rats strongly suggest that it reduces bone resorption (24). Further evidence for a direct effect of WR-2721 on osteoclasts comes from the in vitro studies of Fallon (24,24a). He showed that WR-2721 reduced calcium release from fetal rat bone in organ culture and chick osteoclasts in cell culture. Examination of the cells by electron microscopy revealed that, in contrast to cells not exposed to WR-2721, many of the cells in contact with bone

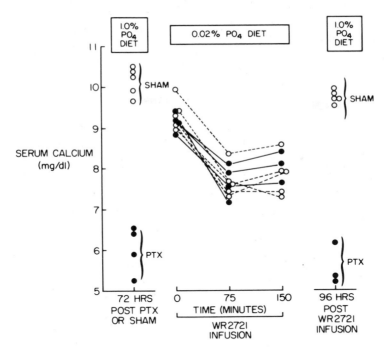

Fig. 5.   Effect of WR-2721 in PTX and sham-
operated   rats.   Serum   calcium
concentration was measured 72 h after
PTX   or   sham   operation while on   a
standard   diet containing 1% phosphorus
(left panel).   Dietary phosphorus was
then decreased to 0.02%.   After 7 days
on this diet, WR-2721 (30 mg/kg) was
infused via tail vein and serum calcium
measured   (middle panel)   immediately
before drug administration (0 time) and
then 75 and 150 minutes later.   After
the infusion, the diet was again changed
to the standard 1% phosphorus diet, and
96 h later serum calcium was measured
(right   panel).   (Reprinted   with
permission from Attie et al. , ref 24).

did not contain well developed ruffled borders,   the
cytoplasmic specializations that characterize osteoclastic
bone resorbing cells.

    In all animals the femoral weights from the intact
limbs were greater than that of immobilized limbs. However,
as shown in figure 6, the percent loss of dry and ashed
weight was significantly lower in the WR-2721-treated group,
but   this did not reach statistical significance
(0.05<P<0.1).   These data indicate that treatment with
WR-2721 reduces the amount of bone loss associated with limb

immobilization. There was also a tendency for the femurs from the intact limbs of WR-2721-treated rats to have higher weights than control animals, but this did not reach statistical significance. Tibias were also examined by histomorphometry three days after tendonotomy (a time when osteoclastic resorption is accelerated) in seven WR-2721-treated and control rats. The number of osteoclasts per unit area in the immobilized tibia from the conrol rats was 2.6±0.5 times that of the non-immobilized tibia from the control rats was 2.6±0.5 times that of the non-immobilized limb while in WR-2721-treated rats the osteoclast number was only 1.7±0.3 (P<0.02).

These data indicate that WR-2721 attenuates the loss of bone mass which occurs after knee tendonotomy. Our data and previous studies with this model (24) suggest that the early bone loss occurs as a result of accelerated bone resorption. The effect on bone loss in this model is not only consistent with our in vitro data demonstrating that WR-2721 inhibits osteoclast activity but also suggests that WR-2721 inhibits formation of osteoclasts and/or enhances their destruction. It should be noted that WR-2721 did not prevent a large component of the bone loss after tendonotomy. This may have occurred because WR-2721 only partly inhibited bone resorption (as suggested above by the histomorphometry data) or, alternatively, the reduced bone formation which occurs is not affected by WR-2721.

REFERENCES

1. Phillips, T.L., Kane, L., and Utley, J.F., 1973, Radioprotection of tumor and normal tissues by thiophosphate compounds, Cancer 32:528.
2. Yuhas, J.M., and Storer, J.B., 1969, Differential chemoprotection of normal and malignant tissues. J. Natl Cancer Inst 42:331.
3. Blumberg, A.L., Nelson, D.F., Gramkowski, M., Glover, D., Glick, J.H., Yuhas, J.M., and Kligerman, M.M., 1982, Clinical trials of WR-27221 with radiation therapy, Int J Radiat Oncology Biol Phys 8:561.
4. Glover, D., Riley, L., Carmichael, K.., Spar, B., Glick, J., Agus, Z., Slatopolsky, E., Attie, M., and Goldfarb, S., 1983, Hypocalcemia and inhibition of parathyroid hormone secretion following administration of WR-2721 (a radio- and chemoprotective agent), N Engl J Med 309:1137.
5. Brown, E.M., Hurwitz, S., and Aurbach, G.D., 1976, Preparation of viable isolated bovine parathyroid cells, Endocrinology 99:1582.
6. MacGregor, R.R., Sarras, M.P., Houle, J.A., and Cohn, D.V., 1983, Primary monolayer cell cultures of bovine parathyroids: effects of calcium, isoproterenol, and growth factors, Mol and Cellular Endocrinol 30:313.
7. Cohn, D.V., Elting, J.J., and Frick, M., 1984, Selective localization of the parathyroid secretory protein I/adrenal medullary chromogranin A protein in a wide variety of endocrine cells of the rat, Endocrinology 114:1963.
8. Kemper, B., Habener, J.F., Rich, A., and Potts, J.T., 1974, Parathyroid secretion: Discovery of a major calcium-dependent protein, Science 184:167.

9.   Brown, E.M., and Aurgach, G.D., 1980, Role of cyclic nucleotides in secretory mechanisms of parathyroid hormone and calcitonin, Vitam Horm 38:205.

10.   Gardner, D.G., Brown, E.M., Windeck, R., and Aurbach, G.D., 1979, Prostaglandin F2 inhibits 3'.5'-adenosine monophosphate accumulation and parathyroid hormone release from dispersed bovine parathyroid cells, Endocrinology 104:1.

10a.   Weaver, M.E., Morrissey, J., McConkey, C. Jr., Goldfarb, S., Slatopolsky, E., and Martin, K.J., 1987, WR-2721 inhibits parathyroid adenylate cyclase, Am J Physiol 252:E197.

11.   Gardner, D.G., Brown, E.M., Windeck, R., and Aurbach, G.D., 1979, Prostaglandin F2 inhibits 3'.5'-adenosine monophosphate accumulation and parathyroid hormone release by sodium nitorprusside, Endocrinology 105:360.

12.   Morrissey, J.M., Rothstein, M., Mayor, G., and Slatopolsky, E., 1983, Suppression of parathyroid hormone secretion by aluminum, Kidney Int 23:699.

13.   Habener, J.F., Potts, J.T., Jr., 1976, Relative effectiveness of magnesium and calcium on the secretion and biosynthesis of parathyroid hormone in vitro, Endocrinology 98:197.

14.   Cholst, I.N., Steinberg, I.N., Tropper, P.J., Fox, H.E., Segre, G.V., and Bilezikian, J.P., 1984, The influence of hypermagnesemia on serum calcium and parathyroid hormone levels in human subjects, N Engl J Med 310:1221.

15.   Yuhas, J.M., 1980, Active versus passive absorption kinetics as the basis for selective protection of normal tissues by S-2(3-aminopropylamino)-ethylphosphorothioic acid, Cancer Research 40:1519.

16.   Shaw, L.M., Turrisi, A.T., Glover, D.J., Bonner, H.S., Norfleet, A.L., Weiler, C., and Kligerman, M.M., 1986, Human pharmacokinetics of WR-2721, Int J Radiat Oncol Biol Phys 12:1501.

17.   Noelle, R.J., and Lawrence, D.A., 1981, Modulation of T-cell function. II Chemical basis for the involvement of cell surface thiol-reactive sites in control of T-cell proliferation, Cell Immunol 60:453.

18.   Mori, T., Watonabe, M., Horikawa, M., Nikaido, D., Kimura, H., Aoyama, T., and Sugahara, T., 1983, WR-2721, its derivatives, and their radioprotective effects on mammalian cells in culture, Int. J. Radiat Biol 44:41.

19.   Purdie, J.W., Inhaber, E.R., Schneider, H., and Labelle, J.L., 1983, Interaction of cultured mammalian cells with WR-2721 and its thiol, WR-1065: implications for mechanisms of radioprotection, Int J Radiat Biol 43:517.

20.   Ziegler, D.M., 1980, Microsomal flavin-containing monoxygenases: oxygenation of nucleophilic nitrogen and sulfur compounds. in "Enzymatic Basis of Detoxification," Vol. I, W.B. Jakoby, ed., pp. 201. Academic Press.

21.   Morrissey, J.J., and Klahr, S., 1983, Roles of hexose monophosphate shunt in parathyroid hormone secretion, Am J Physiol 245:E468.

22.   Larsson, R., Nygren, P., Wallfelt, C., Akerstrom, G., Radstad, J., Ljunghall, S., and Gylfe, E., 1986, Dual effects of a new hypocalcemic agent, WR-2721, on cytoplasmic Ca2+ and parathyroid hormone release of dispersed parathyroid cells from patients with hyperparathyroidism, Biochem Pharmacol 35:4237.

23.   Shoback, D.M., Thatcher, J.G., Leombrano, R., and Brown, E.M., 1983, Effects of extracellular Ca and Mg on cytosolic Ca and PTH in dispersed bovine parathyroid cells, Endocrinology 113:424.

24.   Attie, M.F., Fallon, M.D., Spar, B., Wolf, J.S., Slatopolsky, E., and Goldfarb, S., 1985, Bone and parathyroid inhibitory effects of S-2(3-aminopropylamino)-ethylphophorothiocic acid. Studies in experimental animals and cultured bone cells, J Clin Invest 75:1191.

24a.   Fallon, M.D., 1984, Direct inhibition of osteoclast bone resorbing activity by WR-2721, a new hypocalcemic agent. Calcified Tissue International, 36:481.

25.   Talmage, R.V., Anderson, J.J.B., and Cooper, C.W., 1968, The influence of calcitonins on the disappearance of radiocalcium and radiophosphorus form plasma, Endocrinology 90:1185..pa

26.   Kiang, D.T., Lokenm, M.D., and Kennedy, B.J., 1979, Mechanism of action of mithramycin, J Clin Endocrinol Metab 48:341.

27.   Hirschel-Scholz, S., Caverzasio, J., and Bonjour, J.P., 1985, Inhibition of parathyroid hormone secretion and parathyroid hormone-independent diminution of tubular calcium reabsortion by WR-2721, a unique hypocalcemic agent, J Clin Invest 76:1851.

28.   Thompson, D., personal communication.

NEW APPROACHES TO DETECTION AND

CHARACTERIZATION OF PTH RECEPTORS

J. E. Zull, J. Chuang, I. Yike,
J. Reese, and R. Laethem

Dept. of Biology
Case Western Reserve University
Cleveland, Ohio

INTRODUCTION

PTH receptors have been demonstrated in several cell types and in isolated membranes from these cells. Putative receptors for both the amino terminal (1-10) and carboxy terminal (11,12) domains of the hormone have been reported. While the receptors for the amino terminal portions of PTH are believed to be related to activation of adenylyl cyclase, the function of receptors for carboxy terminal segments of this peptide is unknown.

Recent work has focused on identification of the membrane proteins which may be candidates for PTH receptors. The approach of photoaffinity labeling and chemical cross linking of hormone to receptor has been developed in several laboratories. Three separate groups have reported specific labeling of a 65-70 kDa protein by these methods. In addition, proteins of both higher and lower mass have been found to be cross linked to the hormone. Several proteins with masses ranging from 150 to 28 kDa are presently candidates for PTH receptor, or fragments of receptor. Whether these proteins are all related or whether they are indeed different receptors with different biological functions remains unknown.

Although these approaches have led to significant advances, our knowledge of PTH receptors is very rudimentary when compared to the information now available about other hormone receptors. Indeed, it seems apparent that new tools and approaches to this receptor will be necessary. In particular, there are two aspects of the studies conducted thus far which suggest the importance of development of additional methods for examination of PTH receptors.

First, although photoaffinity and crosslinking methods are very useful, they have drawbacks which may compromise the interpretation of experimental results, and ultimately will limit biochemical characterization. These drawbacks are as follows: (a) photoaffinity labeling methods require utilization of chemically modified forms of the hormone which may not bind some receptors, or which may bind with a different affinity than the native hormone; (b) since crosslinking is usually of low efficiency, and since receptors are thought to be very low abundance proteins, the purification of useful amounts of receptor will be extremely difficult; (c) any protocol developed for isolation of crosslinked species probably will not be applicable to isolation of the receptor itself (i.e., the receptor without attached ligand), and therefore additional studies of such isolated

New Actions of Parathyroid Hormone
Edited by S. G. Massry and T. Fujita
Plenum Press, New York

hormone-receptor complexes will be limited by the fact that the hormone is already bound; (d) the technical aspects of the affinity labeling techniques will probably tend to limit receptor studies to a small number of labs.

A second aspect which should be addressed is the lack of work conducted with native PTH. Almost all published studies have relied on use of the 1-34 fragment, or chemical derivatives thereof. This approach, however, will not provide information about receptors for the C-terminal domain of the hormone, or about receptors which may require a conformation provided only by the intact hormone.

The work described here addresses some of these issues. We have utilized the technology of protein blotting to examine specific binding of native PTH directly to separated membrane proteins. The approach has led to isolation of one PTH-binding protein, which is a candidate for PTH receptor. In addition, these studies have led to a number of unexpected findings which are not yet fully understood, but which appear to be of considerable interest to the PTH receptor field.

SUMMARY OF THE METHOD

The general approach and the theory of the method for detection of putative PTH receptors is outlined in Figure 1. The membrane proteins of a target tissue (we have used bovine kidney) are first separated on denaturing polyacrylamide gels, then blotted onto nitrocellulose paper, and the binding of PTH to the blotted proteins examined by enzyme linked immunoassay methods. The details of the methods for isolation of membranes, electrophoresis, blotting of the gels, and immunostaining the gels have all been presented in prior publications (13,14). As is apparent in Figure 1,

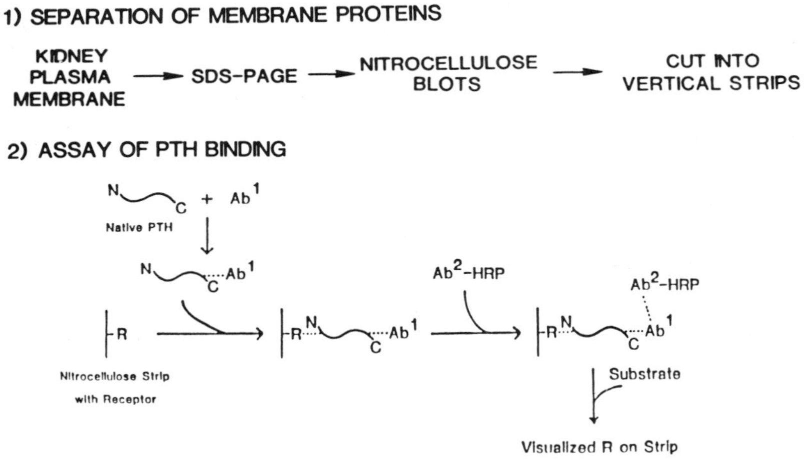

Fig. 1. The detection of PTH binding proteins on nitrocellulose blots of denaturing polyacrylamide gels. Membrane proteins are resolved on the gels and then transferred to the blots, electro-phoretically. The blots are cut into strips corresponding to individual lanes on the gels. These strips are then exposed to PTH which has been previously equilibrated with an antiserum directed against C-terminal segments of the hormone (Ab1). The strips are then washed and exposed to second antibody linked to horseradish peroxidase (HRP). Lastly, the strips are incubated with HRP substrate, which produces a brown band at the position where HRP is present. Control incubations are conducted with normal sera or in the absence of PTH. This assay can also be done by preincubating the strips with PTH alone, washing, and then exposing the blots to PTH antiserum, second antiserum, and the HRP substrate.

the method as originally conceived, relies on the assumption that C-terminal segments of PTH are not involved in receptor binding and will therefore be available to react with the antibodies against the hormone. A similar approach was developed earlier by Hesch and his colleagues (15) for study of PTH binding to isolated membranes, using iodinated antibodies.

The idea of examining PTH binding to blotted proteins was based on reports that receptors and enzymes can renature when transferred from polyacrylamide gels to the nitrocellulose paper (16,17). The method depends on such renaturation, and if some PTH binding proteins do not refold, we will not be able to detect them.

In theory, the only protein bands which will stain are those with bound PTH. However, some cross reactivity of antibodies in the antisera with the bovine kidney membrane proteins is usually found, although the proteins stained in the absence of PTH differ with different antisera. Also, the intensity of staining the bound PTH depends on the antiserum used. In the work described here, we have used three different PTH antisera from rabbits (RSL, RS1, and RSR). The antiserum used is identified in the individual figures.

The method is predominantly qualitative in that we look for a PTH dependent band on the blots. Since the procedure requires several steps wherein dissociation of bound hormone (and presumably antibody) can occur prior to completion of the assay, determination of binding constants is not possible. However, by use of chemically modified forms of PTH, comparisons of the intensity of staining can be made with blots assayed in the same experiment, and the specificity of binding thus evaluated.

IDENTIFICATION AND PURIFICATION OF A PTH BINDING PROTEIN

We have used this method to detect and purify a bovine kidney protein which specifically binds PTH. Figure 2 shows the original identification of this protein with two different PTH antisera. From its migration position on the gels, its mass was determined to be 51 kDa. A concentration of at least 10 nM PTH was required to observe this protein, and normally 100 nM was used. The specificity of binding was determined using oxidized forms of PTH. As indicated in Figure 3, oxidation at position 8 of PTH has a greater effect on binding than does oxidation at position 18. This finding is in agreement with the biological action of these forms of PTH (17). The relationship of the intensity of staining of the blots to the amount of PTH present is logarithmic, and thus the differences observed in staining (Fig. 3) are highly significant. When quantitative comparisons are made of the effects of hormone oxidation on binding to the 51 kDa protein and on biological activity, there is a strong correlation. For example, the Met-8 oxidized form has about 4% of the biological activity of the native hormone and about 2% of the binding to this protein. Similar correlations were found with the other forms (14).

Additional specificity studies showed that fragments of the hormone with amino terminal segments deleted (e.g., 9-84, 19-84, 35-84) do not bind, or only bind very weakly to the 51 kDa protein (See Fig. 4). Thus, the binding of PTH to this blotted protein depends on the integrity of the amino terminal domain, and has the specificity expected of a receptor associated with activation of adenylyl cyclase.

We were able to identify the position of migration of this protein on two dimensional blots using the same PTH-dependent immunostaining method. Once its position was identified, it could subsequently be quickly located on the gels using coomassie blue staining. This allowed purification of about 40 ug of this protein to complete homogeneity. The stained protein was simply excised from multiple two dimensional gels and then electrophoretic-ally eluted. The purified protein retained its PTH binding properties and its specificity when transferred to nitrocellulose blots (14).

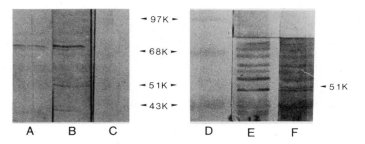

Figure 2. Detection of a PTH-binding protein in bovine kidney membranes, using two different antisera against PTH (RSL, left; RSR, right). Lanes A and E show the proteins stained in the absence of PTH. Lanes B and F show the proteins stained in the presence of PTH. Lane C is a control with no first antibody and Lane D shows the molecular weight markers stained with coomassie blue.

The amount of material obtained by this approach was adequate to undertake microsequencing. However, the purified protein proved refractive to Edman degradation, suggesting that it may be chemically blocked. Clearly, this protein is a candidate for a PTH receptor and further characterization is presently underway.

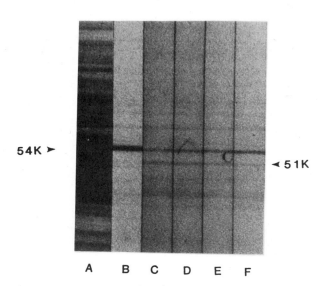

Figure 3. Effect of oxidation of methionine residues of PTH on hormone binding to the 51 kDa protein. Strip A is stained with amido black; strip B is immunostained in the absence of PTH; strip C is incubated with native PTH, strip D with PTH oxidized at Met-18, strip E with PTH oxidized at Met-8; strip F with PTH oxidized at both positions (antiserum used: RS1).

The method described above led to reproducible detection of only one protein whose immunostaining depended on PTH. We did not detect the 70 kDa and 80 kDa species described by others although a 70 kDa species was occasionally noted on the two dimensional blots. These proteins may not renature reproducibly on the blots, or it may be that the method is not sensitive enough for their detection.

However, during the course of these studies, examination of a number of different PTH antisera led to results which were unexpected and of considerable interest. The primary finding was that, depending on the antiserum used, intense staining of certain proteins could be observed which was apparently reduced or even eliminated (rather than enhanced) by the presence of PTH.

One such protein is apparent in Figure 3. The antiserum used for this study produced strong staining of a 54 kDa protein in the isolated membranes. Of importance, antibodies against this protein were not present in the preimmune serum from this animal, and thus they arose as a result of PTH immunization. Furthermore, under certain conditions, it was found that PTH significantly reduced the staining of the 54 kDa protein with this antiserum. This can be observed in Figure 3, but is more clearly shown in Figure 4. Indeed, staining could be prevented by any carboxyl terminal fragments of PTH, while the amino terminal fragment has no apparent impact. (Note that the staining of the 51 kDa protein is also observed with this antiserum, but this staining is PTH-dependent.) This figure also shows the lack of staining of the 54 kDa protein by the preimmune serum and the lack of any effect of PTH with the preimmune serum.

These results raise two related questions: first, how do antibodies against kidney membrane proteins arise upon immunization with PTH; and second, what is the basis for the competition between the antibodies and PTH fragments? Possible answers to these questions are provided by two, significantly different, interpretations. First, the PTH-antibodies in this antiserum may cross react with the 54 kDa protein directly. This would

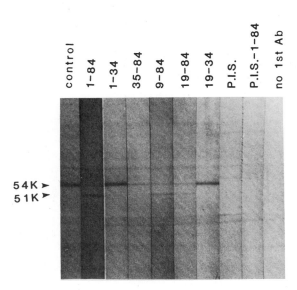

Figure 4. Effect of PTH and related peptides on staining a 54 kDa kidney membrane protein with a PTH antiserum (RS1). The strips were incubated with the indicated peptide and first antibody, as shown in Fig. 1, prior to development. P.I.S. is preimmune serum.

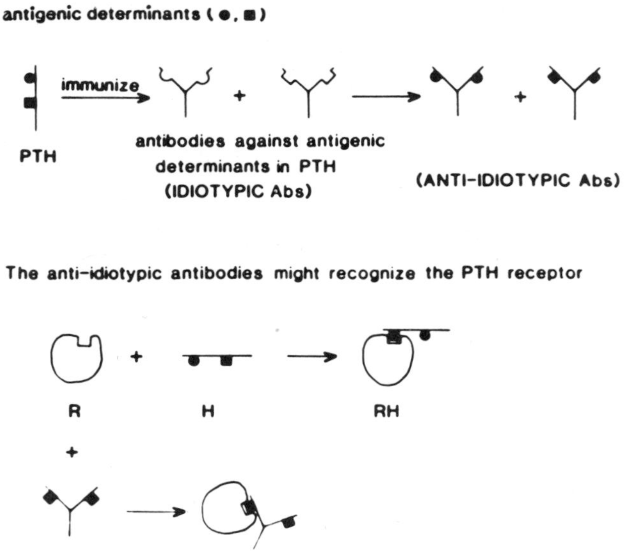

Figure 5. The theory for generation of anti-idiotypic antibodies and their interaction with receptors.

imply that this protein has structural features in common with the hormone. In this case, PTH would eliminate staining of the 54 kDa protein through competition for binding to the antibodies. Since the antibodies in this serum are specific for the carboxy terminal and/or mid-regions of PTH, this would explain the specificity of the competitive phenomenon.

The alternative possibility is that PTH immunization has generated an anti-idiotypic response and that the anti-idiotypic antibodies are binding to the 54kDa protein. In this case it would be expected that the hormone and the antibodies would compete for binding to this protein. This would identify the 54 kDa protein as a putative C-terminal receptor. This possibility is outlined diagrammatically in Figure 5. Anti-idiotypic antibodies with such properties have been observed previously in animals immunized with insulin (18,19) and in several other receptor ligand systems (20).

Presently we cannot distinguish between these two possibilities. However, we have found that removal of the PTH antibodies from this antiserum by adsorption on PTH-Affigel columns also removes the antibodies against the 54 kDa protein. While this may suggest that the two populations of antibody are the same, it is not definitive since anti-idiotypic antibodies crossreact strongly with the first generation antibodies and may, therefore, be difficult to separate by this method.

An interesting observation regarding the 54 kDa protein, regardless of its function, is that it is localized in skeletal and heart muscle. Other than the kidney, this protein stains most strongly in these tissues, which have been proposed to contain PTH receptors. Clearly, additional study of this protein will be of interest.

ADDITIONAL PROTEINS IDENTIFIED BY IMMUNOBLOTTING METHODS

Two other proteins have been found to interact with PTH antisera in a similar fashion as the 54 kDa species. As indicated in Figure 6, these proteins have molecular weights of 90 and 105 kDa. Antibodies against these proteins were found in a different PTH antiserum than used for the prior studies. Again, the presence of PTH prevented immunostaining of the blotted proteins. However, the nature of the competition was somewhat different for these two proteins and they also both differed from the 54 kDa protein described above.

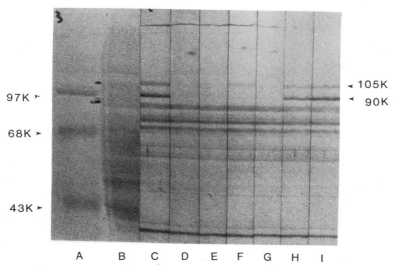

Figure 6. Competition of PTH and related peptides for staining of 90 and 105 kDa proteins in kidney membranes by a PTH antiserum. (RSL) Strip A is MW marker; strip B is total protein staining; strip C is stained in the absence of PTH; strips D-I are stained in the presence of 100 nM concentrations of native PTH (D), oxidized PTH (E), 1-34 (F), 9-84 (G), 19-84 (H), and 35-84 (I).

Staining of the 90 kDa protein was totally prevented by 100 nM concentrations of native PTH, oxidized PTH, 1-34, and 9-84. However, the 19-84 and 35-84 peptides were not effective competitors. The 105 kDa protein was similar but not identical; in this case, 1-34 was not as effective as the native hormone, and some competition with the carboxy terminal fragments was observed. These properties of the 105 kDa protein are somewhat reminiscent of the 54 kDa protein, but less dramatic.

Several interesting features of the competition effect were observed with the 90 kDa protein. First, very low concentrations of native PTH (< 1 nM) were required for significant competition. Second, while 1-34 is a competitor, the concentration of this peptide required to demonstrate competition was about 100-fold greater than with native PTH. Indeed, 1-34 was less effective than the Met-8 oxidized native PTH.

The antiserum used for the studies shown in Figure 6 was specific for C-terminal and/or mid-regions of PTH. Thus, competition between the 90 kDa protein and PTH for binding to the PTH antibodies does not seem likely with these proteins. In that case, one would expect the carboxy-terminal fragments to be good competitors, and the 1-34 fragment to be ineffective; i.e., the opposite of the results shown in Figure 6. Therefore, it is probable that the 90 kDa protein does bind PTH and that this anti-serum contains anti-idiotypic antibodies generated as shown in Figure 5. If so, this protein has a very high affinity for the native hormone.

DISCUSSION

Examination of methods for detection of PTH binding proteins on nitrocellulose blots has proven to be an interesting and intriguing approach to PTH receptors. Although only one PTH binding protein has been identified with certainty, the method has several distinct advantages, and with improved sensitivity may lead to other proteins. Briefly, some advantages are as follows: first, the method does not require any chemical modifications of PTH; second, the method allows detection of unmodified forms of putative receptors rather than cross-linked forms; third, there are technical advantages which could make the method more widely available to investigators interested in examination of PTH receptors; fourth, blots can easily be prepared from small amounts of membrane or cellular protein, and once prepared they retain their PTH binding capability for many months; finally, the method itself can be adapted to purification of proteins of interest.

An obvious drawback is that, to date, we have only been able to detect one PTH binding protein with certainty. This may reflect limits on the sensitivity of the method for proteins present in small amounts. It may also be that renaturation does not occur with all putative PTH receptors. At the present, methods for increasing the sensitivity of the method (e.g., use of biotinylated antibodies) are being examined in efforts to improve sensitivity.

The observation of the 54, 90, and 105 kDa proteins, whose immuno-staining is prevented by PTH, is intriguing. At the present it appears that these proteins either are receptors for this hormone, with very interesting binding properties (such as specificity for the C-terminal domain or the intact hormone), or they have structural features in common with PTH. Certainly the possibility of multiple receptors for this hormone is apparent from the diversity of its functions, and it may well be that several types of receptors are important in the total expression of the biological actions of PTH. On the other hand, the presence of PTH-like sequences or conformation in larger proteins provides new ideas in areas as diverse as evolution of this hormone, its cellular processing, and regulatory aspects of cellular calcium homeostasis. The determination of which of the two possibilities is correct may well require isolation and sequencing of these proteins, which is presently underway.

The function of the 51 kDa protein which specifically binds PTH is not presently known. Proteolytic fragments of PTH receptors with molecular weights of 50-60 kDa have been described (6), and it may be that we have isolated such a fragment. It seems unlikely that a protein with the specificity observed for this molecule would have no biological function related to PTH, but this function remains to be determined. Again, the answer to this question will come as the protein is better characterized biochemically.

In conclusion, examination of protein blotting for detection of PTH binding proteins has proven to be a productive undertaking. Further development of this approach, and combining it with the other methods used for examination of PTH receptors, should lead to significant new insights regarding the biochemical basis for the actions of PTH on cells.

REFERENCES

1. Coltrera, M. D., Potts, J. T., Jr., and Rosenblatt, M. (1981) J. Biol. Chem. 256, 10555-10559.
2. Goldring, S. R., Tyler, G. A., Krane, S. M., Potts, J. T., Jr., and Rosenblatt, M. (1984) Biochemistry 23, 498-502.
3. Draper, M. W., Nissenson, R. A., Winter, J., Ramachandran, J., and Arnaud, C. D. (1982) J. Biol. Chem. 257, 3714-3718.
4. Brennan, D. and Levine, M. A. (1986) J. Bone Miner. Res. 1, Suppl. 1 (Abstr. 320).
5. Wright, B., Tyler, G. A., O'Brien, R., Caporale, L., H., and Rosenblatt, M. (1987) Proc. Natl. Acad. Sci. U.S.A. 84, 26-30.
6. Nissenson, R. A., Karpf, D., Bambino, T., Winer, J., Canga, M., Nyiredy, K., and Arnaud, C. D. (1987) Biochemistry 26, 1874-1878.
7. Weinshank, R. L. and Luben, R. A. (1985) Eur. J. Biochem. 153, 179-188.
8. Weinshank, R. L., Cain, C. D., Vasquez, N. P., and Luben, R. A. (1985) Molecular and Cellular Endocrinology 41, 237-246.

9. Chuang, J., Laethem, R., and Zull, J. E. (1987) J. Bone & Min. Res. 2, Suppl., Abs. 282.

10. Rizzoli, R. E., Murray, T. M., Marx, S. J., and Aurbach, G. D. (1983) Endocrinology 112, 1303-1312.

11. Demay, M., Mitchell, J., and Goltzman, D. (1985) Am. J. Physiol. E437-E446.

12. McKee, M. D., and Murray, T. M. (1985) Endocrinology 117, 1930-1939.

13. Zull, J. E., Chuang, J., and Malbon, C. C. (1977) J. Biol. Chem. 252, 1071-1078.

14. Chuang, J., Yike, I., Reese, J., Laethem, R., and Zull, J. E. (1987) J. Biol. Chem. 262, 10760-10766.

15. McIntosh, C. H. S. and Hesch, R. D. (1976) Biochim. Biophys. Acta 426, 535-546.

16. Oblas, B., Boyd, N. D., and Singer, R. H. (1983) Anal. Biochem. 130, 1-8.

17. Fernandez-Pol, J. A. (1985) J. Biol. Chem. 260, 5003-5011.

18. Shechter, Y., Elias, D., Maron, R., and Cohen, I. R. (1984) J. Biol. Chem. 257, 6411.

19. Shecter, Y, Maron, R., Elias, D., and Cohen, I. R. (1982) Science 316, 542-544.

20. Cleveland, W. L., Wasserman, N. H., Penn, A. S., Ku, H. H., Hill, B. L., Saragnarajan, R., and Erlanger, B. F. (1985) In: "Monoclonal Antibodies and Cancer Therapy." Alan R. Liss, Inc., p. 345.

PULSE AMPLITUDE AND FREQUENCY MODULATION OF PTH AND ITS MODULATION OF PTH RECEPTORS - OSTEOPOROSIS AS AN EXAMPLE OF A DYNAMIC DISEASE

R.D. Hesch, G. Brabant, E.F. Rittinghaus,
M.J. Atkinson and H. Harms

Abteilung Klinische Endokrinologie, Zentrum Innere
Medizin, Medizinische Hochschule Hannover,
300 Hannover 61, Germany

I. BIOLOGICAL INFORMATION IN HORMONES

(1) There is not yet a general or fundamental model to understand the hormone receptor interaction in a way to describe in a holistic approach the transduction of information packed in a hormone molecule into biological action. Actual information theories predict that any information must be encoded and that any code can be reduced to basic informational structures (36). The sequences and dynamics of basic biological information-structures are suspended into complex dynamic networks which have been built up during biological evolution. They offer channeling of thermodynamic reactions in a hierarchy of biological structures and functions.

Encoding is achieved through (1) the conformational structures of a spacefilling molecule hold by electrochemical and physical forces and (2) the pattern of the signal intensity to expose the molecule to the interaction with other molecules during which some of their energy is exchanged in a way to create new conformational states (37). The signal intensity-variation is packed in the dynamic modulation of the concentration pattern of the signal in blood, body compartments and metabolic cellular units.

(1) The conformational structure of a hormone contains a definite information specific for the overall interaction with receptor proteins. The hormone molecule can, however, be the subject of subtle conformational modifications; these can be accomplished within the glands by chemical alteration of the hormone structure (glandular processing). The sequential modifications of steroid hormones in the adrenals or POMC in the pituitary are examples. The modification can also proceed in the periphery (postglandular processing); many peptide hormones like vasopressin, glucagon, atrial natriuretic peptide and parathyroid hormone (PTH) undergo such peripheral processing and there is increasing evidence

New Actions of Parathyroid Hormone
Edited by S. G. Massry and T. Fujita
Plenum Press, New York

that a whole family of peptides with different conformations and biological functions evolves from such fragmentation. The conformational forces of a hormonal ligand determine the overall biological interaction with conformationally prepared spaces and pockets in the receptor molecule. These interactions may determine what is usually referred to as "specificity" of hormone receptor interaction.

(2) The dynamic interaction of a hormone with its receptor is achieved through (I) variation of the concentration of the circulating hormone pool and (II) pulse amplitude and frequency modulation of the hormone concentration on top of the circulating pool in various compartments of body fluids. It is suggested that the slow dynamics of the hormonal pool are related to "receptor status", i.e. "number and concentration of receptors" whereas high dynamic hormonal pulsing (Macro-, micro-, supermicro-pulses and frequency variation) may be associated to information transducing processes by "up- and down regulation of receptors" and modulation of postreceptor intracellular pathways.

Clinical and cellbiological observations suggest that this interaction defines what is usually refered to as "effect and action" as response of the hormone-receptor interaction. Hormones, therefore, deliver biological information through dynamic transduction of conformational energy in a given time and space and may be called "Raum-Zeit-Conformere".

It is our contention that the physiology of the hormone receptor interaction and the biological responses can only be described appropriately by application of biological information theories (36, 38).

We also believe that modulation of hormonal information proceeds in circular hierarchical networks. Most diseases evolve from central to peripheral but like in other non linearly bifurcated systems peripheral derangements may modify the functional architecture of networks up to the center (39).

(2) PTH is a hormone where all these principles can be examined; further, osteoporosis may serve as an example to analyze a "dynamic disease" (40). Such diseases do not originate as the consequence of a single "cause-effect event" (39) but typically result from a multidimensional disturbancy in non linear dynamic networks. Osteoporosis after estrogen withdrawal evolves through several dynamic stages until it ends in the low turnover state where almost more than 50% of the skeleton were lost. Estrogen, hence, modulates a complex system of hypothalamo-pituitary-parathyroid regulations which hold 50% of bone mass. In the following section we will examine one of the components of this system as a first attempt to demonstrate the most forms of osteoporosis develop from the central regulation system to the periphery.

II.   CELL BIOLOGY OF PTH RECEPTOR

Parathyroid hormone (PTH) acts on the bone to modulate

bone turnover (1), but we still do not know how it exerts its action at the organ-specific and cellular niveau. In the last few years we have learned much about the hierarchial order of hypothalamo-pituitary networks which modulate the function of peripheral glands in order to express their biological signals at the organ- and tissue level. In Endocrinology it became obvious that dynamic regulations occur through pulse amplitude and frequency .pa modulation of hormonal signals transporting biological information of the hypothalamus, the pituitary and the peripheral glands. This has been demonstrated for gonadotropins (2), growth hormone (3), TSH (4) and ACTH (5).

It is known since many years that the dynamic up- and down regulation of the hormone receptor unit by the delivery of dynamically encoded hormone signals ("Raum-Zeit-Conformere") to the hormone receptor unit will determine the further signal transduction to the main cellular pathways (6). Two main such pathways will be further discussed. A receptor type I operated pathways acts through Gs- and Gi-proteins to stimulate adenylate cyclase and produces cAMP and subsequent phosphorylation of regulatory cellular proteins by protein kinases (7,11).

A second pathway is operated by type II receptor functions whereby upon binding of the hormone to its receptor a regulatory Gp-protein is activated in a way that inositolphosphates are cleaved by phospholipase-C (PIC) to produce either inositoltriphosphate (IP-3) or diacylglycerol (DG) (8). IP-3 acts to control intracellular free calcium either by intracellular exchange of calcium between various compartments or subsequently by increasing transmembrane transport (9). It is interesting to note that even intracellular Ca++ pulses to encode its messages upon stimulation by the hormone receptor unit (10). Recent research has demonstrated that activation of the type I receptor pathway results in an increase in differentiation and function of a cell whereas stimulation of the type II receptor leads to an increase of mitotic events and ultimately to transformation and cell growth (11,12). This general rule may be subject to tissue specific modifications and other receptor operated pathways have to be considered like exocytosis mediated by a new G-protein and direct hormonal effects on ionic channels.

Spratt et al (13) have recently demonstrated that artificial manipulation of LH and FSH secretion by GnRH pulse amplitude and frequency modulation shifts the testicular function either to preferential hormone secretion (type I receptor pathway). We consider that as an example of human physiology which proves that central package of information determines the cell biological response in far distant organs. Although we will not discuss the feedback circuits of such complex dynamical network regulations it is evident that pulse amplitude and frequency modulation of hormonal signals determines the biological responses of an organism (14,15).

PTH can directly be compared to the pituitary POMC because it acts through a whole peptide family cleaved from the intact hormone at peripheral enzymatic receptors. Like

ACTH it also governs a main steroid synthesis pathway, i.e.
synthesis of 1.25 vitamin D. The reason why the parathyroid
glands have their unique anatomical location outside the
brain is unknown but since it was reported that PTH is also
produced by the brain (41) the phylogenetical similarity to
other neuroendocrine peptides is even more striking (see
also chapter Gennari and chapter Pang, this book).

Harms et al (16) recently demonstrated that PTH is
secreted in a pulsatile fashion analogous to pituitary
hormones. They observed micro- and macropulses with
different frequences which are only partly related to
changes in ionized Ca++. Other pulse generators have to be
considered by future research. In view of our hypothesis of
a predominant central origin of osteoporosis we currently
investigate how estrogen and/or estrogen dependent endocrine
systems influence PTH pulsatile pattern.

The secretory pattern of PTH in our view has the
intrinsic possibility to influence peripheral receptor
pathways by pulse amplitude and frequency modulation as it
has been shown for the gonadotropins. Both type I and type
II PTH receptor functions have recently described in various
cells (17, 18, 19). We do not infer that the PTH receptor
functions are distributed over several proteins. From
experiments of Zull et al (see chapter this book), and
recent work of Numa (personal discussion) it is expected
that the various receptor actions are related to subtypes of
one receptor family like for example the family of
rhodopsin-receptors.

We do, however, up to now not understand how the
secretory pattern of a hormone, particularly PTH, modulates
the various biophysical states of subtypes of receptors and
this will be a key issue for future research. We expect
that like for other hormones the pulse amplitude and
frequency modulation of PTH ultimately governs the
expression of either type I and/or type I PTH receptor
functions and their biological action. Although the
stimulation of cAMP by the PTH receptor type I in
osteoblasts is known since long time the exact mechanism of
interaction with PTH receptor type II was only described
recently. Hruska et al (18, 19) showed in renal tubular
cells that PTH stimulates the production of IP3 and DG and
that this was followed by a dose dependent-rise in
intracellular free calcium. This cascade of intracellular
information-transduction has now been described also in
osteoblasts by Reid et al (20) and Avioli et al (see chapter
this book).

Atkinson et al (17a) reported recently upon the
exclusive expression of type II function in human
lymphocytes and rat thymocytes. PTH-operated stimulation of
a calmodulin dependent Ca++ uptake resulted in cellular
mitosis. The existence of PTH-specific membrane receptors
in lymphocytes was already published before by Bialasievicz
et al (17b). Although Atkinson et al (17a) concluded also
that these events were induced by a PTH mediated increase in
cytosolic Ca++ through activation of C-kinase branch these
conclusions must be interpreted in view of those of Pang et
al (see chapter this book) demonstrating a definite decrease

in Ca++ upon PTH. The tissue and concentration dependent difference of PTH action on intracellular Ca++ awaits further explanation.

In sumarry it is postulated that the secretory pattern of PTH determines the expression of various receptor operated cellular metabolic pathways.

III. RECEPTOR AGONISTS AND ANTAGONISTS?

The pioneering work of Rosenblatt et al (42) has led to the synthesis of numerous PTH receptor agonists and antagonists and has given the appropriate tools for many investigations in the field. The structure-activity relationship between a ligand and receptor is one important aspect to study hormone action. Another way to modulate receptor function is by selecting the mode of application. The biological state of a receptor upon exposure to a ligand can change dramatically from complete desensitization to maximal upsensitization of the system depending of how the ligand interacts with the receptor. Although PTH acts at its receptor identical to GnRH (43) where such principles have been explored in more detail a systematic investigation of dynamic modulation of the PTH receptor(s) in vivo has not been performed. First results have been obtained during the treatment of osteoporosis in animal models (44) and human beings. Although cellbiological experiments could not yet completely differentiate both PTH pathways in osteoblasts (21) they do however exist and appropriate design and planning of dynamic PTH experiments is underway to investigate their biological mechanism of regulation and mode of action.

IV. THE FRAGMENTATION OF PTH

Further to select pathways and to modulate the functional state of the PTH-receptor the PTH secretory pattern may influence the function of the hormone receptor unit in that the sequential peripheral fragmentation of intact PTH or molecules shortened at the C-terminus will generate either N-terminal intact or N-terminal deleted PTH peptides. The regulatory enzyme should be located in the near vicinity of the receptor protein(s). This situation (although different with respect to the substrate) again reminds the analogy to ACTH where the differential activation of the cytochrome P450 enzymes by pulsatile ACTH in the adrenals generates different steroid hormone pattern. The exact nature of how dynamic PTH pattern will influence its own enzymatic fragmentation is, however, still unknown and we are not aware of any investigator who has addressed this question. N-terminal intact hormones can stimulate both receptors whereas N-terminal deleted PTH peptides only stimulate type II receptor function but are antagonistic at type I receptor function (17). An identical pathway for N-terminal intact and deleted peptides acting on receptor type I and type II has recently been demonstrated for glucagon and also for vasopressin (22,23, 24, 25). Pulse amplitude and frequency modulation of hormones might, therefore, govern hormone receptor interaction and in addition local peripheral hormone fragmentation (26) to start, specifically modulate and terminate biological information by hormones.

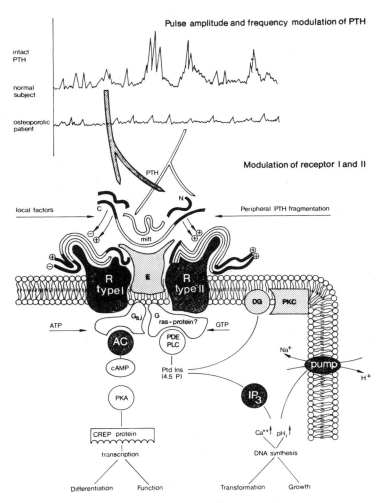

Pulse amplitude and frequency modulation of PTH

intact
PTH

normal
subject

osteoporotic
patient

Modulation of receptor I and II

local factors

Peripheral PTH fragmentation

FIGURE 1

The upper part shows a representative example of pulse and frequency modulation of PTH in a normal subject and in an osteoporotic patient. It is assumed that the dynamic PTH-pattern acts upon PTH operated pathways imbedded in receptor protein(s). In analogy to other receptors this could be an ensemble of membrane bridging proteins which upon hormonal activation change conformation to modulate transduction pathways. The dynamic pattern of intact PTH in various compartments of the circulation will (1.) deliver this hormone to receptor(s), (2.) modulate a receptor associate enzyme producing specific PTH peptides with different affinities for different receptor states and (3.) regulate expression of receptor states. The different receptor states will determine the signal transduction pathways, i.e. activation of adenylate cyclase (type I), activation of c-kinase (type II) or other ion channels.

We do not yet understand how modulation of osteoblastic PTH receptors will affect their functional coupling to osteoclasts but what we know from cell biological experiments (27) suggests that upon incubation with PTH osteoblasts produce a soluble factor that directly stimulates osteoclastic bone resorption. PTH dependent modulation of either type I or type II receptor function in osteoblasts, hence, results in predominant expression of highly differentiated secretion of paracrine ligands by mature osteoblasts (28) or predominant recruitment and proliferation of the osteoblast-line cell (29). Our current views are summarized in Fig.1. Although many experiments need still to be done a more dynamic portray of PTH physiology and pathophysiology emerges and this may lead to a new understanding of many old facts and the design of comprehensive experiments.

V. WHAT DOES ALL THIS NEW INFORMATION ON PTH-SECRETION AND HORMONE RECEPTOR INTERACTION MEAN TO OUR UNDERSTANDING OF OSTEOPOROSIS?

Harms et al (16) recently have shown that osteoporotic subjects exhibit a disturbed pulse amplitude and frequency modulation of PTH with smaller and less pulses. This observation in conjunction with the earlier described peripheral metabolic defect for PTH (30) suggests to us that a disturbed glandular PTH secretory pattern could be involved in the pathogenesis of low turnover osteoporosis. The resulting "low-dynamic functional state" of bone cells is certainly different from hypoparathyroidism due to tissue deficiency. Similar observations have been made with other hormones in various diseased states like amenorrhea, oligospermia, delayed puberty and short stature. They have led to the development of new therapeutic strategies who rational is to reach a new health state by restauration of the physiological hormone receptor modulation (31,32). We have previously discussed the implications of such strategies for osteoporosis (16,33). The administration of N-terminal intact PTH peptides has so far produced the highest gain in bone mineral content in a small number of osteoporotic subjects (34,35) and this encourages us to further pursue our hypotheses.

ACKNOWLEDGEMENT

This work is supported by the DFG He/18-1 and He 593/16-1. Part of the text of this presentation and the figure are published as Editorial in Calc. Tiss. Int.

REFERENCES

1.   Parfitt A.M. (1976) The actions of parathyroid hormone on bone: Relation to bone remodeling and turnover, calcium homeostasis, and metabolic bone disease. Metabolism 25:809-955.

2.   Crowley Jr. W.F., Filicori M., Spratt D., Santoro N. (1985) The physiology of gonadotropin releasing hormone secretion in men and women.   Recent Prog Horm Res   41:473-531.

3.   Ho K.Y., Evans W.S., Blizzard R.M., Vewldhuis J.D., Merriam G.R., Samojlik E., Furlanetto R., Rogol A.D., Kaiser D.L. and Thorner M.O.   (1987) Effects of sex and age on the 24-hour profile of growth hormone secretion in man: Importance of endogenous estradiol concentrations. J Clin Endocrinol Metab 64:51-58.

4.   Brabant G., Brabant A., Ranft U., Owan K., Kohrle J., Hesch R.D. and von zur Muhlen A.   (1987) Circadian and pulsatile thyrotropin secretion in euthyroid man under the influence   of   thyroid   hormone   and   glucocorticoid administration. J Clin Endocrinol Metab 65:83-88.

5.   van Cauter E., Refetoff S.   (1985) Evidence for two subtypes of Cushing's Diseases based on the analysis of piosodic cortisol secretion. N Engl J Med 312:1343-1349.

6.   Zor U. (1983) Role of cytoskeletal organization in the regulation of adenylate cyclase-cyclic AMP by hormones. Endocrine Rev 4:1-21

7.   Montminy M.R. and Bilezikian L.M.   (1987) Binding of a nuclear protein to the cyclic-AMP response element of the somatostatin gene. Nature 328:175-178.

8.   Berridge M.J., and Irvine R.F. (1984) Insositol triphosphate, a novel second messenger in cellular signal transduction. Nature 312:315-321.

9.   Streb H., Irvine R.F., Berridge M.J., Schulz I. (1983) Release of Ca++ from a nonmitochondrial intracellular store in pancreatic acinar cells by inositol-1,4,5 triphosphate. Nature 306:67-69.

10.   Woods N.M., Cuthbertson K.S.R., Cobbold P.H.   (1986) Repetitive transient rises in cytoplasmatic free calcium in hormone-stimulated hepatocytes. Nature 319:600-602.

11.   Cambier J.C., Newell M.K., Justement L.B., McGuire J.C., Leach K.L. and Chen Z.Z. I a binding ligans and cAMP stimulate nuclear translocation of PKC in B lymphocytes. Nature 327:629-632.

12.   Ratan R.R., Shelanski M.L. (1986) Calcium and the regulation of mitotic events. TIBS 11:456-459.

13.   Spratt D.I., Finkelstein J.S., Butler J.P., Badger T.M., and Crowley W.F. Effects of increasing the frequency of low doses of gonadotropin-releasing hormone (GnRH) on gonadotropin secretion in GnRH deficient men. ICEM Vol 64 No. 6, June/87, pp 1179-1186.

14.   Glass L. (1987) Coupled oscillators in health and disease; in temporal disorder in human oscillatory systems (Rensing L., an der Heiden U. and Machey M.C., Editors) Springer Berlin Heidelberg New York London Paris Tokyo 8-14.

15.   Goldbeter A.   (1987) Periodic signaling and receptor densensitization: From cAMP oscillations in Dicostyleum cells to pulsatile patterns of hormone secretion in: Temporal   disorder in human oscillatory systems (see Reference No. 14) 15-23.

16.   Harms H., Kapteina U., Kulpmann T. and Hesch R.D. (1987) The pulse amplitude and frequency modulation of PTH secretion in man.   International Symposium on Osteoporosis, Aalborg, Abstract 232.

17.   Hesch R.D., Herrmann G., Perris A.D. and Atkinson M.J. (1986) Type II PTH receptor-operated calcium channel and its importance for PTH peptide elevations in coronary artery disease. Am J Nephrol 6: suppl a pp 155-161.
(17a)   Atkinson M.J. et al. Parathyroid hormone stimulation of mitosis in rat thymic lymphocytes is independent of cyclic AMP. J Bone and Mineral Research (in press)
(17b)   Bialasiencz A.A., Juppner H., von zur Muhlen A. and Hesch R.D. (1979) Biochem. Biophys. ACTA 584:467-472.
18.   Hruska K.A., Goligorsky M., Scoble J., Tsutsumi M.T., Westbook S., and Moskowitz D. (1986) Effects of parathyroid hormone on cytosolic calcium in renal proximal tubular primary cultures. Am J Physiol 251:F188-F198.
19.   Hruska K.A., Moskowitz D., Esbrit P., Civitelli R. and Huskey M. (1987) Stimulation of inositol triphosphate and diacylglycerol production in renal tubular cells by parathyroid hormone. J Clin Invest 79:230-239.
20.   Reid I.R., Civitelli R., Avioli L.V., Hruska K.A. (1987) Evidence for new second messengers of PTH in osteoblast-like cells. International Symposium in Osteoporosis. Aalborg, Abstract 76.
21.   Yee J.A., Sutton J.K., Shew R.L. and Olansky L. (1986) Parathyroid hormone stimulation of alkaline phosphatase activity in cultured neonatal mouse calvarial bone cells: involvement of cyclic AMP and calcium. J Cell Physiol 128:246-250.
22.   Wakelam M.J.O., Murphy G.J., Hruby V.J., Honsly M.D. (1986) Activation of two signals in hepatocytes by glucagon. Nature 232:68-71.
23.   Mallat A., Pavoine C., Dufour M., Cotersztajn S., Bataille D., Pecker F. (1987) A glucagon fragment is responsible for the inhibition of the liver Ca++ pump by glucagon. Nature 325:620-622.
24.   Burbach J.P.H., Kovacs G.L., de Wied D., van Nipsen J.W., Greven H.M. (1983) A major metabolite of arginine vasopressin in the brain is a highly potent neuropeptide. Science 221:1310-1312.
25.   van Leeuven F.W. (1987) New 3H arginine vasopressin antagonist: A specific and sensitive means to show vasopressin binding in the brain. Biotechnology Update 2:1-2.
26.   Knights E.B., Baylin S.B., Foster G.V. (1973) Control of polypeptide hormones by enzymatic degradation. Lancet II:719-723.
27.   Chambers T.J. (1987) The regulation of osteoclastic function. International Symposium in Osteoporosis, Aalborg, Abstract 290.
28.   Yee J.A. (1985) Stimulation of alkaline phosphatase activity in cultured neonatal mouse calvarial bone cells by parathyroid hormone. Calcif Tissue Int 37:530-538.
29.   Lowik C.W.G.M., van Leeuwen J.P.T.M., van der Meer J.M., van Zeeland J.K., Scheven B.A.A., Herrmann-Erke M.P.M. (1985) A two-receptor model for the interaction of parathyroid hormone on osteoblasts: A role for intracellular free calcium and cAMP. Cell Calcium 6:311-326.
30.   Atkinson M.J., Schettler T., Bodenstein H. and Hesch R.D. (1984) Osteoporosis: A bone turnover defect resulting

from an elevated parathyroid hormone concentration within the bone marrow cavity? Klin Wschr 62:129-132.

31. Santora N., Wirman M.E., Filicori M., Walstreicher J., and Crowley W.F. (1986) Intravenous administration of pulsatile gonadotropin-releasing hormone in hypothalamic amenorrhea: Effects of dosage J Clin Endocrinol Metab 62:129-132.

32. Avgerinos P.C., Schurmeyer T.H., Gold P.W., Tomai T.P., Louriaux D.L., Sherius R.J., Cuther G.B. and Chronsos G.P. (1986) Pulsatile administration of human corticotropin-releasing hormone in patients with secondary adrenal insufficiency: Restoration of the normal cortisol secretory pattern. J Clin Endocrinol Metab 62:816-821.

33. Hesch R.D., Harms H. (1986) Episodic secretion of parathyroid hormone and osteoporosis; in: Episodic hormone secretion: from basic science to clinical application; TM-Verlag 1987 ISBM-3-921936-14-4; Edts: T.O.F. Wagner and M. Filicori.

34. Slovic D.M., Rosenthal D.I., Doppelt S.H., Potts J.T., Daly M.D., Campbell J.A. and Nwe R.M. (1986) Restoration of spinal bone in osteoporotic men by treatment with human parathyroid hormone (1-34) and 1.25 dihydroxy-vitamin D. J Bone Min Res 1:377-381.

35. Rittinghaus E.F., Busch U., Prokop M., Delling G. and Hesch R.D. (1987) Dramatic increase of bone-mass and turnover in osteoporosis by combined (1-38) hPTH and Calcitonin therapy. International Symposium on Osteoporosis, Aalborg, Abstract 365.

36. Kuppers B.O. Der Ursprung biologischer Information. Piper, Munchen-Zurich, 1986.

37. Huber R. and Bennett W.S. Antibody-antigen flexibility. Nature (1987) 326, 334-335.

38. Martiel J.L. and Goldbeter A. (1987) A model based on receptor desensitization for cyclic AMP signaling in dyctostelium cells. Biophys. J. 52, 807-828.

39. Hesch R.D. (1987) Gesundheit und Krankheit. Med. Klin. 82 (1987) 337-341 (Nr. 9).

40. Mackey M.C., and der Heiden U. (1982) Dynamical diseases and bifurcations: Understanding functional disorders in physiological systems. Funkt. Biol. Med. 1:156-164.

41. Balabanova S. (1986) Parathyroid hormone secretion by brain and pituitary of sheep. Klin Woschenschr (1986) 64:173-176.

42. Rosenblatt M. (1981) Parathyroid hormone: Chemistry and structure-activity relationship. Pathobiology Annual II: 53-86.

43. Pavlou S.N., Interlandi J.W., Wakefield G., Isalnd D.P., Rivier J., Vale W. and Kovacs W.J. Gonadotropins and testosterone escape from suppression during prolonged LHRH antagonist administration in normal men. JCEM 64 (1987) 1070-1074.

44. Tam C.S., Heersche J.N.M., Murray T.M. and Parsons J.A. (1982) Parathyroid hormone stimulates the bone apposition rate independently of its resorptive action: Differential effects of intermittent and continous administration. Endocrinology 110:506-512.

NEW DIRECTIONS FOR THE DESIGN OF PARATHYROID HORMONE ANTAGONISTS

Michael Rosenblatt,[1]* Michael Chorev,[1] Ruth F. Nutt,[1] Michael P. Caulfield,[1] Noboru Horiuchi,[2] Thomas L. Clemens,[2] Mark E. Goldman,[1] Roberta L. McKee,[1] Lynn H. Caporale,[1] John E. Fisher,[1] Jay J. Levy,[1] Jane E. Reagan,[1] Thomas Gay,[1] and Patricia DeHaven[1]

[1]Department of Biological Research and Molecular Biology
Merck Sharp and Dohme Research Laboratories
West Point, Pennsylvania 19486
and [2]Regional Bone Center, Helen Hayes Hospital
(New York State Department of Health)
West Haverstraw, New York 10993

INTRODUCTION

Peptide hormone antagonists that are effective in vivo are uniquely precise tools for biomedical research. They can be used to determine how peptide hormones act, what their role is in normal physiological processes, and how they contribute to pathophysiologic states.

In recent years, the potential utility of parathyroid hormone (PTH) antagonists has extended beyond clinical states of PTH excess, such as primary hyperparathyroidism and the persistently increased secretion of PTH that accompanies renal failure and renal transplantation, to the arena of tumor biology (1). PTH antagonists may prove useful in elucidating the mechanism of the humorally-mediated hypercalcemia which accompanies certain cancers, and may eventually offer a new approach to therapy.

In this article we describe two new initiatives that offer insight into structural features which may enhance the binding of PTH to its receptor(s) and which, when incorporated into PTH analogs, may generate more effective PTH antagonists. Substitutions directed at specific secondary structural aspects of the PTH molecule have been used as "reporters" of the conformation of the hormone at the time of receptor-interaction. In an entirely separate approach, the biological activity of a newly discovered factor thought to be responsible for the clinical syndrome of humoral hypercalcemia of malignancy (HHM) has been evaluated (2). The sequence differences and similarities in this peptide compared to PTH highlight promising areas for further PTH antagonist design.

Essential to the design of PTH antagonists is an understanding of hormone-receptor interaction; this interaction may be envisioned as having two components. The first is binding of the hormone to the receptor. Binding to target tissue is necessary but not sufficient for the expression of biological action. Binding must be followed by a

New Actions of Parathyroid Hormone
Edited by S. G. Massry and T. Fujita
Plenum Press, New York

second event induced by the hormone -- a conformational shift within the receptor that leads to transmission of the hormonal signal to an effector system, and ultimately, the expression of biological activity. This fundamental concept of a two-stage process for hormone action provides the foundation for the design of hormone antagonists; an ideal antagonist is a molecule that binds strongly to receptors but is unable to produce the conformational shift that leads to activation of the effector system.

For PTH, we have succeeded in separating the domain of the hormone responsible for binding from that responsible for receptor activation both _in_ _vitro_ and _in_ _vivo_. The analog [Tyr-34]bPTH-(7--34)NH$_2$ can inhibit the PTH-stimulated calcemic response (3), the promotion of phosphaturia and urinary cAMP excretion (4,5), and the generation of 1,25-dihydroxy vitamin D$_3$ by the renal 1α-hydroxylase (5). The analog lacks PTH-like agonist activity. Its potency _in_ _vivo_ is such that a 20- to 100-fold molar excess of antagonist is required to inhibit PTH action by 50%.

PROBING PTH CONFORMATION

To improve the potency of the 7--34 antagonist, we have undertaken structure-conformation-activity analyses. Secondary structural predictions employing the Chou and Fasman algorithm suggest that PTH-(1--34) contains two long α-helical stretches separated by a twin (located at residues 12-15), and a β-sheet comprising the C-terminal region (residues 29-34) (6). A proton nmr study in aqueous solution reveals that PTH-(1--34) is predominantly flexible, excluding the segment 20-24, which contains distinct conformational features (7). This non-random conformation is stabilized by a hydrophobic interaction between the side-chains of Val^{21} and Trp^{23} and a hydrogen bond involving Glu^{22}. The conformation described in this region is closely comparable to a γ-turn. However, other studies claim to find more organized structure within PTH-(1--34) (8).

In our studies, we have probed some of the conformational issues identified within the PTH molecule, namely the β-turn at positions 12 through 15 and the γ-turn at positions 22 through 24, by introducing single residue replacements and assessing their effect on _in_ _vitro_ biological activity. The modifications selected either promote or disrupt these conformations.

Table I summarizes the biological evaluation of the conformationally-substituted analogs in two _in_ _vitro_ assay systems. The activities of the analogs were compared to corresponding PTH reference peptides (I-IV). Under our assay conditions, we demonstrated an excellent correlation between binding and stimulation of adenylate cyclase for the agonist peptides (I-II). For the antagonists (III-IV), there is also a good correspondence between binding and cyclase potencies; however, there is a systematic difference of about 10-fold in potency between the two systems. The binding affinity is about 10-fold greater than the Ki for the inhibition of cyclase for each of the antagonists. The cause of this difference is not known.

As mentioned above, residues 12-15 are predicted by Chou-Fasman analysis to form a β-turn (9). The loss in potency due to substitution of either Pro or Sar for Gly at position 12 cannot be attributed to a major perturbation in the potential for formation of a β-turn. Rather, these imino acids are known to disrupt α-helical structure. These findings, taken together with the retention of potency following substitution with D- or L-Ala, Aib, or β-Ala, and the wide latitude of

Table 1. Biological Activities of PTH Analogs with Substitutions in Positions 12, 22 and 23

Analogs	Binding Ki (nM)	Adenylate Cyclase Km (Agonist) (nM) / Ki (Antagonist) (nM)
I [Tyr^{34}]hPTH(1--34)NH$_2$	0.7 ± 0.3	0.7 ± 0.1
II [Tyr^{34}]bPTH(1--34)NH$_2$	1.1 ± 0.3	1.1 ± 0.4
		<u>Ki (Antagonist) (nM)</u>
III [Tyr^{34}]bPTH(7--34)NH$_2$	75.0 ± 8.3	835 ± 65
IV [Nle^{8,18},Tyr^{34}]bPTH(7--34)NH$_2$	145.0 ± 9.0	1550 ± 33
1 [Ala^{12},Tyr^{34}]hPTH(7--34)NH$_2$	114 ± 32	413 ± 67
2 [D-Ala^{12},Tyr^{34}]hPTH(7--34)NH$_2$	124 ± 12	612 ± 116
3 [Pro^{12},Tyr^{34}]hPTH(7--34)NH$_2$	471 ± 36	6310 ± ?
4 [Sar^{12},Tyr^{34}]bPTH(7--34)NH$_2$	503 ± 91.4	2506 ± 732
5 [Aib^{12},Tyr^{34}]bPTH(7--34)NH$_2$	51.0 ± 8.7	536 ± 144
6 [β-Ala^{12},Tyr^{34}]bPTH(7--34)NH$_2$	137 ± 23	?
7 [D-Trp^{23},Tyr^{34}]bPTH(7--34)NH$_2$	76250 ± 14553	95590 ± 16346
8 [Phe^{23},Tyr^{34}]bPTH(7--34)NH$_2$	476.0 ± 34	2327 ± 827
9 [Nle^{8,18},Leu^{23},Tyr^{34}]bPTH(7--34)NH$_2$	2260 ± 912	7100 ± ?
10 [Nle^{8,18},N-MePhe^{23},Tyr^{34}]bPTH(7--34)NH$_2$	----	----
11 [Nle^{8,18},N-MeGlu^{22},Tyr^{34}] bPTH(7--34)NH$_2$	8000 ± 1500	39800 ± ?

structural tolerance observed for substitution at position 12 in PTH analogs, favor the conclusion that an α–helical conformation, instead of the predicted ß–turn is likely in this region.

Bundi and coworkers identified a conformational motif in position 21–23 of PTH–related peptides, which could be defined as a γ–turn (7,10). Substitution of Glu[22] with N–MeGlu (analog 11) should promote that conformation and yield an active analog. On the other hand, substitution by N–MePhe for Trp[23] (the contributor of hydrogen to the stabilizing hydrogen bond in this 3–>1 intramolecular H–bonded conformation) should eliminate this turn. Indeed, this analog (analog 10) is devoid of bioactivity. As noted in Table I, however, position 23 can accommodate an aromatic residue provided it is of the L–configuration (cf. analogs 7–8). [1]H–nmr studies indicate that the side–chains of residues Val[21] and Trp[23] are in close proximity, allowing a strong hydrophobic interaction which may be the driving force for the formation of the γ–turn. In the series of native PTH homologs, Trp[23] is highly conserved while Val can be replaced by another highly hydrophobic amino acid, namely Met. Replacing Leu for Trp[23] does not provide the essential hydrophobic interaction for stabilizing the γ–turn. Therefore, the evidence from the structure–conformation–activity studies at this position neither supports nor controverts the relevance of the γ–turn to antagonistic activity.

PTH–LIKE FACTOR ASSOCIATED WITH HUMORAL HYPERCALCEMIA OF MALIGNANCY

Recently, three groups isolated and obtained partial amino acid sequence of a peptide derived from several different human tumors (lung squamous carcinoma, renal cell carcinoma, breast carcinoma) (11–14). One group obtained the putative full–length peptide structure (141 amino acids) based on the cDNA nucleotide sequence (12). In each case, within the N–terminal thirteen residues there is considerable homology to the biologically critical N–terminal region of PTH. Thus, a unique structure–activity "experiment" related to PTH has been performed by nature.

In order to 1) determine if this human "humoral hypercalcemic factor" (hHCF) alone can produce hypercalcemia in vivo, 2) further define its actions in vitro, and 3) compare its biological profile and potency to PTH, we chemically synthesized an N–terminal fragment of the factor.

Using a multiparameter, in vivo assay based on the thyroparathyroidectomized rat, we compared the activity of hHCF–(1––34)NH2 to bPTH–(1––84). In this system, hHCF–(1––34)NH2 produces hypercalcemia with an apparent potency 6–10 times greater than bPTH–(1––84) (Fig. 1A) (2). Reductions in serum phosphate and striking elevations in circulating 1,25–dihydroxyvitamin D_3 levels were also observed (Fig. 1B) (2). The action of hHCF–(1––34)NH2 on vitamin D metabolism is particularly pronounced relative to PTH and important with regard to its implication for promoting long–term hypercalcemia clinically.

The hHCF–(1––34)NH2 also exhibited other PTH–like effects on the kidney, increasing urinary excretion of cyclic AMP and phosphate (2). Again, hHCF–(1––34)NH2 was more potent than bPTH–(1––84). At high doses, a white precipitate was observed in the kidneys after 16 h infusion. This was presumed to represent nephrocalcinosis; this pathology was not seen in rats infused with PTH at comparable doses.

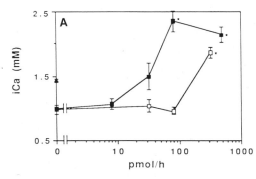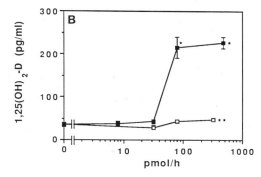

Fig. 1. Effects of bPTH-(1--84) and hHCF-(1--34)NH2 on serum
concentrations of ionized calcium (A), and
1,25-dihydroxyvitamin D3 (B) in thyroparathyroidectomized
rats. bPTH-(1--84) (□); hHCF-(1--34)NH2 (■); and vehicle
(in sham-treated animals) (▲) were continuously infused
(8-480 pmol/h) into rats for 16 h. Values represent the mean ±
S.E.M. for each group (n = 3-5). Values that are significantly
different from control are indicated by * (p <0.001) or ** (p
<0.05). Reprinted with permission from (2).

To determine whether bone is a target organ for hHCF-(1--34)NH2
and if the action on bone per se can produce hypercalcemia, we developed
an animal model in which rats are thyroparathyroidectomized, fed a low
calcium diet, and nephrectomized. In this assay, hypercalcemia is
skeletal in origin (2). The hHCF-(1--34)NH2 produces calcium
elevations comparable to those obtained with bPTH-(1--34), and greater
than that obtained with bPTH-(1--84).

We also evaluated directly the interaction of hHCF-(1--34)NH2 with
PTH receptors in vitro. Binding affinity comparable to PTH for renal
PTH receptors was observed. In an adenylate cyclase assay based on
bovine renal cortical membranes, hHCF-(1--34)NH2 also had a potency
comparable to PTH.

An adenylate cyclase assay based on intact bone-derived osteosarcoma
(ROS 17/2.8) cells was also employed (15). The hHCF-(1--34)NH2,
unlike the PTH peptides, displayed greater potency in stimulating bone
than renal adenylate cyclase, a finding similar to that observed by
others using tumor extracts or conditioned media, or using UMR
bone-derived cells (16). Also, in the bone adenylate cyclase assay, the
peptide was approximately 100 times more potent than hPTH-(1--84).

Although the greatest homology of hHCF-(1--34)NH2 to PTH is
limited to a few amino acids within the N-terminal 13 positions, the
biological profile of the tumor-derived peptide is closely similar to
PTH, implicating the importance of these residues in expression of
calcium metabolism bioactivity. The finding that hHCF-(1--34)NH2 is
more potent than PTH in some systems may be attributable to structural
features which confer increased avidity for receptors or resistance to
degradation and clearance. The synthesis of "hybrid" molecules of hHCF
and PTH and antagonists based on the hHCF sequence is underway.

CONCLUSIONS

Two separate lines of investigation hold the promise of directing
future PTH analog design to selected sites within the hormone molecule

where critical interactions with the receptor take place. Some of the sites have been identified by systematic analysis of conformation-activity relations; others are highlighted by the experiment provided by nature in the sequence of the PTH-like product of tumors, hHCF.

ACKNOWLEDGEMENTS

This work was supported, in part, by NIH grant no. AR36446 and AR39191 (TLC) and Merck Sharp & Dohme Research Laboratories.

REFERENCES

1. M. Rosenblatt, Peptide hormone antagonists that are effective in vivo: lessons from parathyroid hormone, N. Engl. J. Med. 315:1004 (1986).
2. N. Horiuchi, M. P. Caulfield, J. E. Fisher, M. E. Goldman, R. L. McKee, J. E. Reagan, J. J. Levy, R. F. Nutt, S. B. Rodan, T. L. Schofield, T. L. Clemens, and M. Rosenblatt, Similarity of synthetic peptide from human tumor to parathyroid hormone in vivo and in vitro, Science 238:1566 (1987).
3. S. H. Doppelt, R. M Neer, S. R. Nussbaum, P. Federico, J. T. Potts, Jr., and M. Rosenblatt, Inhibition of the in vivo parathyroid hormone-mediated calcemia response in rats by a synthetic hormone antagonist, Proc. Natl. Acad. Sci. USA 83:7557 (1986).
4. N. Horiuchi, M. F. Holick, J. T. Potts, Jr., and M. Rosenblatt, A parathyroid hormone inhibitor in vivo: design and biological evaluation of a hormone analog, Science 220:1053 (1983).
5. N. Horiuchi and M. Rosenblatt, Evaluation of a parathyroid hormone antagonist in an in vivo multiparameter bioassay, Am. J. Phys. 253:E187 (1987).
6. S. R. Nussbaum, N. V. Bendetti, G. D. Fasman, J. T. Potts, Jr., and M. Rosenblatt, Design of analogues of parathyroid hormone: a conformational approach, J. Prot. Chem. 4:391 (1985).
7. A. Bundi, R. Andreatta, W. Rittel, and K. Wuthrich, Conformational studies of the synthetic fragment 1--34 of human parathyroid hormone by NMR techniques, FEBS Lett. 64:126 (1976).
8. L. M. Smith, J. Jentoft, and J. E. Zull, Proton NMR studies of the biologically active 1--34 fragment of bovine parathyroid hormone: examination of a structural model, Arch. Biochem. Biophys. 253:81 (1987).
9. J. E. Zull and N. B. Lev, A theoretical study of the structure of parathyroid hormone, Proc. Natl. Acad. Sci. USA 77:3791 (1980).
10. A. Bundi, R. H. Andreatta, and K. Wuthrich, Characterization of a local structure in the synthetic parathyroid hormone fragment 1--34 by ^{1}H nuclear-magnetic-resonance techniques, Eur. J. Biochem. 91:201 (1978).
11. D. M. Barnes, New tumor factor may disrupt calcium levels, Science 237:363 (1987).
12. L. J. Suva, G. A. Winslow, R. E. H. Wettenhall, R. G. Hammonds, J. M. Moseley, H. Diefenbach-Jagger, C. P. Rodda, B. E. Kemp, H. Rodriguez, E. Y. Chen, P. J. Hudson, T. J. Martin, and W. I. Wood, A parathyroid-hormone-related protein implicated in malignant hypercalcemia: cloning and expression, Science 237:893 (1987).
13. R. A. Nissenson, S. Leung, D. Diep, R. D. Williams, G. J. Strewler, Purification of a low molecular weight form of the tumor-derived parathyroid hormone-like protein, J. Bone & Mineral Research 2: Abstract 388 (1987).

14. A. F. Stewart, T. Wu, D. Goumas, W. J. Burtis, Amino-terminal sequence of a human HHM-associated adenylate cyclase-stimulating protein contains PTH-like and PTH-unlike domains, <u>J. Bone & Mineral Research</u> 2: Abstract 392 (1987).
15. S. B. Rodan, K. L. Insogna, A. M-C Vignery, A. F. Stewart, A. E. Broadus, S. M. D'Souza, D. R. Bertolino, G. R. Mundy, and G. A. Rodan, Factors associated with humoral hypercalcemia of malignancy stimulate adenylate cyclase in osteoblastic cells, <u>J. Clin. Invest.</u> 72:1511 (1983).
16. R. A Nissenson, G. J. Strewler, R. D. Williams, S. C. Leung, Activation of the parathyroid hormone receptor-adenylate cyclase system in osteosarcoma cells by a human renal carcinoma factor, <u>Cancer Res.</u> 45:5358 (1985).

INOSITOL LIPIDS IN CELL SIGNALING BY PARATHYROID HORMONE

Keith Hruska, Michael Goligorsky, Ian Reid, Roberto Civitelli,
Iris Verod, Yasuo Suzuki, and Louis Avioli

Renal Division, The Jewish Hospital of St. Louis, Washington
University School of Medicine, St. Louis, Missouri

Parathyroid hormone has long been thought to activate its target cells through stimulation of cellular calcium.[1,2] However, the evidence in support of this stimulation rested solely on isotopic fluxes.[3,4] Shortly after the Michell review in 1975, suggesting that inositol phospholipids may serve as a mechanism of receptor associated stimulation of cell calcium entry,[5] Lo et al reported that PTH stimulated ^{32}Pi incorporation into phosphatidylinositol (PI).[6] We reported that PTH stimulated an increase in myoinositol turnover in isolated perfused canine kidneys, and we suggested that this may have been related to PTH induced stimulation of inositiol phospholipid turnover.[7] Subsequently, we[8,9,10] reported that PTH stimulated the initial rates of ^{32}Pi incorporation into phosphatidylinositol 4'5-bisphosphate (PIP2), phosphatidylinositol 4-monophosphate (PIP), PI, and phosphatidic acid (PA). At this time, muscarinic-cholinergic stimuli H_1-histamine receptor stimulation, vasopressin, serotonin, and α_1-catecholamines in several different tissues[11,12] had been shown to stimulate phosphoinositide turnover through phosphodiesteratic cleavage of the phosphoinositides, and subsequent resynthesis through PA. This stimulation usually resulted in an initial decrease in the mass levels of the phosphoinositides, and it was associated with an increase in cytosolic Ca^{2+}. The results of Farese et al[9] and ourselves[8] demonstrated that PTH stimulation of phosphoinositide turnover resulted in an increase in the actual mass of the phosphoinositdes in renal proximal tubule segments isolated from PTH treated animals. The PTH effect was specific in that the major plasma membrane phospholipids, phosphatidylethanolamine and phosphatidylcholine, were not affected by PTH treatment. However, our results differed significantly from those of Farese et al in that cyclic nucleotides failed to stimulate phosphoinositide turnover in agreement with the previous publication of Lo et al.[6] In contrast, Bidot-Lopez et al found that cyclic nucleotides were able to mimic the action of PTH on phosphoinositide turnover.[10]

In subsequent studies[13,14], we were able to localize the increase in the mass of the polyphosphoinositides stimulated by PTH to the apical membrane of the proximal tubular cell. There, we found that the basis for this statement is that PTH receptors reside mainly on the basolateral membrane, and the role of these substances in low affinity Ca^{2+} binding/translocation.

In companion studies to those on the apical membrane of proximal tubular epithelial cells, the mass levels of the polyphosphoinositides in the basolateral membrane were found to be less than the apical membrane and their mass levels were not detectably affected by PTH (Hruska et al, unpublished observations). However, the question remained whether PTH produced turnover of the polyphosphoinositides associated with activation of its target cells. Our next attempts to demonstrate the stimulation of the Ca^{2+} messenger system by PTH derived from studies of cytosolic Ca^{2+} in proximal renal tubular cells. We demonstrated that PTH added to primary cultures of canine proximal tubular cells produced an immediate increase in cytosolic Ca^{2+} using the fluorescent Ca^{2+} indicator, quin-2.[15] The rise in cytosolic Ca^{2+} induced by PTH in the primary cultured cells was sustained, dose-dependent, and was not mimicked by cyclic nucleotides. Inhibitors of Ca^{2+} release from the endoplasmic reticulum, 8-(N,N-diethylamino)octyl-3,4,5-trimethoxybenzoate (TMB-8) and dantrolene, blocked the effects of PTH on cytosolic Ca^{2+}. Removal of extra-cellular Ca^{2+} also produced rapid depletion of intracellular Ca^{2+} stores and inhibited the effects of PTH on cytosolic Ca^{2+}. These studies were confirmed in subsequent measurements of cytosolic Ca^{2+} using fura-2 as the Ca^{2+} indicator and studying the fluorescence of individual cells.[16] These studies also demonstrated that homologous desensitization to the PTH response required much shorter time intervals between PTH doses for inhibi-tion of the Ca^{2+} transient than it did for inhibition of cyclic nucleotide stimulation. This latter finding suggest that a separate mechanism of PTH signaling for the increase in cytosolic Ca^{2+} was present. In all of our studies, the effects of PTH on cytosolic Ca^{2+} have not been mimicked by cyclic nucleotides. Recently, we have extended our results on cytosolic Ca^{2+} into clonal cell lines expressing the phenotype of the proximal tubule, opposum kidney cells and osteoblasts (UMR-106 cells, a rodent osteogenic sarcoma cell line). In these cell lines, PTH produces a transient increase in cytosolic Ca^{2+} due to release of Ca^{2+} from the endoplasmic reticulum.[17,18] Cyclic nucleotides failed to mimick the effect of PTH, and the dose response curve for PTH stimulated increase in cytosolic Ca^{2+} was at least as sensitive as that for stimulation of cAMP production. These results in osteoblast-like cells have been confirmed in three other laboratories.[19,20,21]

In our most recent studies, we have demonstrated that PTH produced a dose-dependent immediate stimulation of inositol trisphosphate and diacylglycerol production in the opposum kidney cell line, primary cultures of canine renal proximal tubular cells, and basolateral membranes from proximal tubular segments[18]. Similar results have been observed in the osteoblast-like UMR-106 cell line.[22] The increase in inositol trisphosphate production was as sensitive to PTH stimulation as cAMP production and was inhibited by cyclic nucleotides. Associated with the changes in inositiol trisphosphate and diacylglycerol production, there was an immediate hydrolysis of PIP2. Recent studies have demonstrated that the basolateral membrane of proximal tubular cells and the plasma membrane of of UMR-106 cells possess a PIP2 specific phospholipase C that is stimulated by PTH[23] (Hruska et al-unpublished observations). The effect of PTH on phospholipid hydrolysis was followed by stimulation of phosphorylation of PI 4'-monophosphate and PI.[18] Inositol trisphosphate transiently increased cytoplasmic Ca^{2+} in Saponin-treated opposum kidney and primary opposum kidney cells, UMR-106 cells, and primary culture of proximal tubular cells. Again, these effects were not mimicked by cyclic nucleotides. These results demonstrate that PTH activates renal tubular cells by the production of inositol trisphosphate and diacylglycerol leading to the production of a transient elevation of cytosolic Ca^{2+}. Future studies will be required to understand the relationship between the stimulation of PIP2 hydrolysis and adenylate cyclase. Furthermore, the biologic effects attributable to the activation of the Ca^{2+} messenger system by PTH remain to be clearly determined.

References

1. H. Rasmussen, "Calcium and cAMP as Synarchic Messengers," Wiley, New York (1981).
2. H. Rasmussen, and D.B.P. Goodman, Relationships between calcium and cyclic nucleotides in cell activation, Physiol. Rev. 57:421 (1977).
3. A.B. Borle, and T. Uchikawa, Effects of parathyroid hormone on the distribution and transport of calcium in cultured kidney cells, Endocrinology 102:1725 (1978).
4. A.B. Borle, and T. Uchikawa, Effects of adenosine 3',5'-monophosphate, dibutyryl adenosine 3',5'-monophosphate, aminophylline, and imidazole on renal cellular calcium metabolism, Endocrinology 104:122 (1979).
5. R.H. Michell, Inositol phospholipids and cell surface receptor functions, Biochim. Biophys. Acta. 415:81 (1975).
6. H. Lo, D.C. Lehotay, D. Katz, and G.S. Levey, Parathyroid hormone-mediated incorporation of ^{32}P-orthophosphate into phosphatidic acid and phosphatidylinositol in renal cortical slices, Endocrinol. Res. Commun. 3:377 (1976).
7. B.A. Molitoris, K.A. Hruska, Fishman, N., and W.H. Daughaday, Effects of glucose and parathyroid hormone on the renal handling of myoinositol by isolated perfused dog kidneys, J. Clin. Invest. 63:1110 (1979).
8. V. Meltzer, S. Weinreb, E. Bellorin-font, and K.A. Hruska, Parathyroid hormone stimulation of renal phosphoinositide metabolism is a cyclic nucleotide-independent effect, Biochim. Biophys. Acta 712:258 (1982).
9. R.B. Farese, P. Bidot-Lopez, A. Sabir, J.S. Smith, B. Schinbeckler, and R. Larson, PTH acutely increases polyphosphoinositides of the rabbit kidney cortex by a cycloheximide-sensitive process, J. Clin. Invest. 65:1523 (1980).
10. P. Bidot-Lopez, R.V. Farese, and M.A. Sabir, Parathyroid hormone and adenosine-3',5'-monophosphate acutely increases phospholipids of the phosphatidate-polyphosphoinositide pathway in rabbit kidney cortex tubules in vitro by a cycloheximide-sensitive process, Endocrinology 108:2078 (1981).
11. J.N. Fain, J.A. Garcia-Sainz, Role of phosphatidylinositol turnover in alpha^1 and of adenylate cyclase inhibition in alpha^2 effects of catecholamines, Life Sci. 26:1183 (1980).
12. A.A. Abdel-Latif, R.A. Akhtar, and J.N. Hawthorne, Acetylcholine increases the breakdown of triphosphoinositide of rabbit iris muscle prelabeled with [^{32}P] phosphate. Biochem. J. 162:61 (1977).
13. S. Khalifa, S. Mills, and K.A. Hruska, Stimulation of calcium uptake by parathyroid hormone in renal brush-border membrane vesicles, J. Biol. Chem. 258:14400 (1983).
14. K.A. Hruska, S.C. Mills, S. Khalifa, and M.R. Hammerman, Phosphorylation of renal brush-border membrane vesicles, J. Biol. Chem. 258:2501 (1983).
15. K.A. Hruska, M. Goligorsky, J. Scoble, M. Tsutsumi, S. Westbrook, and D. Moskowitz, Effects of parathyroid hormone on cytosolic calcium in renal proximal tubular primary cultures, Am. J. Physiol. 251:F188 (1986).
16. M.S. Goligorsky, D.J. Loftus, and K.A. Hruska, Cytoplasmic calcium in individual proximal tubular cells in culture, Am. J. Physiol. 251:F938 (1986).

17. I.R. Reid, R. Civitelli, L.R. Halstead, L.V. Avioli, and K.A. Hruska, Parathyroid hormone acutely elevates intracellular calcium in osteoblastlike cells, Am. J. Physiol. 252:E45 (1987).

18. K.A. Hruska, D. Moskowitz, P. Esbrit, R. Civitelli, S. Westbrook, and M. Huskey, Stimulation of inositol trisphosphate and diacylglycerol production in renal tubular cells by parathyroid hormone, J. Clin. Invest. 79:230 (1987).

19. C.W.G.M. Lowik, J.P.T.M. van Leeuwen, J.M. van der Meer, J.K. van Zeeland, B.A.A. Scheven, and M.P.M. Herrmann-Erlee, A two-receptor model for the action of parathyroid hormone on osteoblasts: a role for intracellular free calcium and cAMP, Cell Calcium 6:311 (1985).

20. E.F. Eriksen, M. Fryer, H. Donahue, and H. Heath III, Dose-dependent biphasic effect of parathyroid hormone (PTH) on cytosolic calcium in aequorin-loaded ROS 17/2.8 cells, Clin. Res. 35:622A (1987).

21. D.T. Yamaguchi, T.J. Hahn, A. Iida-Klein, C.R. Kleeman, and S. Muallem, Parathyroid hormone-activated calcium channels in an osteoblast-like clonal osteosarcoma cell line, J. Biol. Chem. 262:7711 (1987).

22. R. Civitelli, I.R. Reid, S. Westbrook, L.V. Avioli, and K.A. Hruska, Parathyroid hormone elevates inositol trisphosphate and diacylglycerol in a rat osteoblast-like cell line, Submitted - Am. J. Physiol. (1987).

23. Y. Suzuki, U. Alvarez, K.A. Hruska, and L.V. Avioli, Guanine nucleotide activated phosphatidylinositol-4,5-diphosphate-specific phospholipase C activity in the plasma membrane of osteoblast-like osteosarcoma cells, Submitted - Mol. Endocrin. (1987).

PARATHYROID HORMONE AND PHOSPHATIDYLINOSITOL METABOLISM IN FETAL RAT LIMB BONES

Paula H. Stern and Victoria M. Stathopoulos

Department of Pharmacology
Northwestern University
Chicago, IL USA

INTRODUCTION

We have previously shown that bPTH-(1-34) stimulates the incorporation of ^{3}H-myo-inositol into phosphatidylinositol in fetal rat limb bones (Rappaport and Stern, 1986). The current studies were undertaken to determine whether the hormone would also show effects on the production of inositol phosphates. We have compared the effects of bPTH-(1-34) with those of Nleu^{8,18}Tyr^{34}-bPTH-(3-34)amide, a PTH analog shown to be without effects on cyclic AMP in renal (Rosenblatt, et al., 1977) or osseous (Goldring, et al., 1985, Hermann-Erlee, et al., 1983) tissue. In addition, we have examined the effects of α-thrombin, which stimulates resorption in fetal rat limb bones (Hoffmann, et al., 1986) and which increases production of inositol phosphates in several tissues (Rendu et al., 1983, Carney, et al. 1985).

METHODS

For studies of resorption, ^{45}Ca-prelabelled fetal rat limb bones were cultured for 3 days according to previously-published techniques (Stern, et al., 1980). For studies of inositol phosphate metabolism, the same techniques as for studies of resorption were used, with the exception that the bones were not labelled with ^{45}Ca. Instead, ^{3}H-myo-inositol, 8 μCi/ml was added to the culture medium. Four 19-day mid-shafts were cultured in 0.5 ml DMEM supplemented with 5% heat-inactivated horse serum. The bones were preincubated with ^{3}H-myo-inositol for 48 hr. Groups of 14-20 bones were then transferred to 25 ml flasks containing 2 ml of medium, either DMEM supplemented with 15% horse serum or BGJ supplemented with 1 mg/ml bovine serum albumin and LiCl. After a 20 min preincubation, hormones were added for times from 30 sec to 30 min. The reaction was stopped by the addition of 0.4 ml of ice-cold 50% TCA. Tissues were homogenized and extracted twice with 0.5 ml of 10% TCA. The extracts were combined and washed five times with 3 ml water-saturated diethyl ether to remove the TCA. Inositol phosphates were separated by Dowex ion exchange chromatography (Berridge, et al. 1983). bPTH-(1-34) was purchased from Bachem. α-Thrombin was from Hoffmann-La Roche, Basle. Nleu^{8,18}Tyr^{34} bPTH-(3-34)amide was a generous gift from Dr. Michael Rosenblatt.

RESULTS

We examined the effects of bPTH-(1-34), Nleu^{8,18}Tyr^{34}-bPTH-(3-34) amide and bovine α-thrombin on resorption and inositol phosphate production in fetal rat limb bones. In DMEM supplemented with 15% serum, bPTH-(1-34) elicited a maximal effect on resorption at a concentration of 10^{-9}M (Figure 1). Nleu^{8,18}Tyr^{34}-bPTH-(3-34) amide was a weak agonist in this medium, producing small but significant effects at 3×10^{-7} and 10^{-6}M (Figure 1). In BGJ supplemented with 1 mg/ml albumin, the responses to bPTH-(1-34) were slower, and a concentration of 10^{-8}M was required to obtain maximal effects by the third day of culture. In this medium, Nleu^{8,18}Tyr^{34}-bPTH-(3-34) amide failed to stimulate resorption and antagonized the effects of bPTH-(1-34) (data not shown). The effects of bPTH-(1-34) and the analog on inositol phosphate metabolism were examined in the DMEM-serum medium. bPTH-(1-34) elicited small and inconsistent effects on inositol phosphates, and no effects were seen at concentrations below 10^{-7}M. In order to elicit this effect, a high concentration of LiCl (100 mM) was required. In contrast, Nleu^{8,18}Tyr^{34}-bPTH-(3-34) amide displayed marked effects on inositol phosphates. The effects of bPTH-(1-34) and Nleu^{8,18}Tyr^{34}-bPTH-(3-34) amide on inositol phosphates are shown in Figure 2.

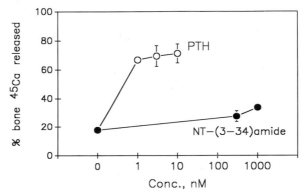

Figure 1. Effects of bPTH-(1-34) and Nleu^{8,18}Tyr^{34}-bPTH-(3-34) amide on resorption of fetal rat limb bones.

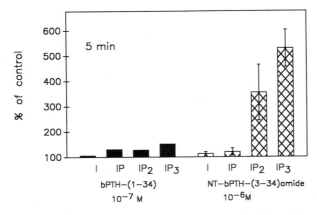

Figure 2. Effects of bPTH-(1-34) and Nleu^{8,18}Tyr^{34} on inositol phosphates in fetal rat limb bones.

α-Thrombin stimulated resorption in BGJ-albumin medium. A significant effect was seen at 100 U/ml but not at 10 U/ml in this system (Figure 3). A 5 min incubation with 100 U/ml α-thrombin in the presence of 20 or 100 mM LiCl markedly stimulated incorporation of ^{3}H-myo-inositol into inositol phosphates (Figure 4). In preliminary studies, more marked effects of α-thrombin on InsP$_3$ were seen at 30 sec and no effect was seen on InsP^3 at 30 min. In contrast, incorporation into InsP was still increasing at 30 min (data not shown).

We have also examined effects of 10^{-7}M bPTH-(1-34) on inositol phosphates in neonatal mouse calvaria and calvarial cells in the presence of 20 mM LiCl and have not detected significant effects. Interestingly, PTH, at concentrations as low as 10^{-9}M, maximally stimulated the incorporation of ^{3}H-arachidonate into DAG in neonatal mouse calvaria (Stewart and Stern, unpublished).

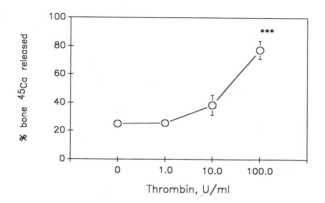

Figure 3. Effect of α-thrombin on resorption of fetal rat limb bones.

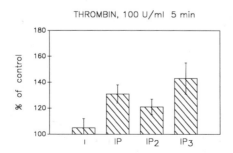

Figure 4. Effect of thrombin on inositol phosphates in fetal rat limb bones.

DISCUSSION

The responses to a large number of hormones and neurotransmitters, including epinephrine, acetylcholine, histamine, vasopressin and glucagon appear to be mediated through both cyclic AMP and calcium-activated mechanisms (Exton, 1985, Abdel-Latif, 1986, Wakelam, et al.,1986). To establish that a hormone acts through a calcium second messenger pathway, evidence should be available to show that the hormone can increase calcium in the target cells, and that increases or decreases in calcium affect the responses in an appropriate manner. Since stimulation of the phosphatidyl inositol pathway seem to provide the crucial second messenger, inositol trisphosphate (InsP$_3$), that leads to increased intracellular calcium as well as diacylglycerol (DAG), an activator of the protein kinase C (Abdel-Latif, 1986), this pathway might be expected to be stimulated by hormone treatment.

Many of these criteria have been satisfied for the effects of PTH on bone resorption. A rapid stimulation of calcium influx into bone was elicited by PTH treatment both in vivo and in vitro (Parsons, et al., 1971, Robinson, et al., 1972). We (Dziak and Stern, 1975a) demonstrated that PTH treatment caused a rapid transient influx of calcium into cells isolated from calvaria of fetal rats. Recently, several groups have shown that PTH increases intracellular calcium in UMR 106 osteosarcoma cells (Lowik, et al., 1985, Reid, et al., 1987, Yamaguchi, et al., 1987). This effect was not seen in ROS 17/2.8 osteosarcoma cells, and only a small inconsistent response was observed in SaOS-2 human osteosarcoma cells (Boland, et al., 1986).

The second criterion, the dependence of PTH effects on changes in ambient calcium concentration, has been demonstrated in a number of ways. In bone organ cultures, Raisz, et al. (1972) showed that exposure of bones to low calcium during a brief treatment with PTH attenuated the response to the hormone. The calcium antagonist verapamil can inhibit bone resorption, and the effect is reversed by increasing the calcium concentration (Herrmann-Erlee et al., 1977). We have also shown that the antagonist neomycin, which interferes with the breakdown of phosphatidylinositol bisphosphate (Carney, et al. 1985) inhibits bone resorption and that this inhibition can be overcome by increasing the medium calcium concentration (Stern, 1984). Divalent cation ionophores can stimulate or potentiate PTH action (Dziak and Stern, 1975b, Hahn, et al., 1980, Lorenzo and Raisz, 1981, Stern, 1985) although this has not been seen in all bone culture systems (Ivey 1976). Cells isolated from rodent bone synthesize greater amounts of hyaluronate (Wong, et al., 1978) and show a greater cAMP response to PTH (Peck, et al. 1981) when calcium concentrations are increased. Evidence for dual receptors for PTH in bone derives from studies with PTH analogs. Herrmann-Erlee, et al. (1983) showed that bPTH-(2-34), bPTH-(3-34), and desamino bPTH-(1-34), which did not increase cAMP in bone, could stimulate resorption. bPTH-(3-34) was also shown to increase intracellular calcium in osteosarcoma cells (Lowik, et al. 1985). The Nleu[8,18]Tyr[34]bPTH(3-34)amide analog did not increase cAMP or stimulate bone resorption of fetal rat calvaria in their studies, and only acted as an antagonist of resorption for the first 4 hr.

Studies of PTH effects on phospholipid metabolism have progressed somewhat more rapidly in kidney than in bone. Lo et al. (1976) and Meltzer et al. (1982) showed that PTH stimulated the incorporation of ^{32}P into phospholipids in renal cortical slices and isolated tubules, respectively. Meltzer et al. also showed increased incorporation of ^{14}C-arachidonic acid into DAG and a net increase in phosphoinositides. These effects were independent of cAMP. Farese, et al. (1980) and Bidot-Lopez, et al. (1981) demonstrated net increases in inositol phospholipids in rabbit renal cortical tubules, an effect apparently secondary to increased cAMP and sensitive to cycloheximide. Recently, Hruska et al. (1987) have shown increases in $InsP_3$ and DAG after stimulation of several renal tissues by PTH. Recent studies by Cole, et al. (1987) indicate that these effects of PTH on renal phosphatidylinositol metabolism are likely to be related to hormone-induced changes in renal phosphate transport.

In 1975, Dirkson, et al. showed that bone tissues sythesize phosphatidylinositol. Studies of PTH effects on phospholipid metabolism in bone include the demonstration in 1971 by Tanaka and Hollander that PTH stimulates ^{32}P incorporation into bone phospholipids. Matsumoto, et al. (1986) examined effects of PTH on UMR 106 osteosarcoma cells and found a decrease in phosphatidylethanolamine synthesis, with no change in phosphatidylserine synthesis. We have found (Rappaport and Stern, 1986) that PTH increases the incorporation of ^{3}H-myo-inositol into phosphatidylinositol in fetal rat limb bones in organ culture. The dose-response curve for the effect paralleled that for stimulation of resorption by PTH. No significant effects were seen before 2 hr with $10^{-9}M$ PTH. However, $10^{-7}M$ PTH elicited significant stimulation at 1 hr. Two brief reports indicate that PTH can stimulate accumulation of individual inositol phosphates in UMR cells (Civitelli, et al. 1987, Lerner et al. 1987). The former study also reported an increase in DAG. Lerner et al. also showed preliminary data (single values) that PTH increases ^{3}H-inositol incorporation in the total inositol phosphate pool in mouse calvarial cells.

The results presented here show that α-thrombin elicits effects on ^{3}-myo-inositol incorporation into inositol phosphates in fetal rat limb bones at concentrations of α-thrombin that elicit resorption. In contrast, the effects of bPTH-(1-34) and Nleu^{8,18}Tyr^{34}-bPTH-(3-34)amide on inositol phosphates do not correlate well with their effects on resorption. The failure to readily elicit PTH effects on inositol phosphates in bone cannot be explained at the present time.

REFERENCES

Abdel-Latif, A. A., 1986, Calcium-mobilizing receptors, polyphosphoinositides, and the generation of second messengers, <u>Pharmacol. Rev.</u>, 38:227.

Berridge, M. J., Dawson, R. M. C., Downes, C. P., Heslop, J. P., and Irvine, R. F., 1983. Change in the levels of inositol phosphates after agonist dependent hydrolysis of membrane phosphoinositides, <u>Biochem. J.</u> 212:473.

Bidot-Lopez, P., Farese, R. V., and Sibir, M. A., 1981, Parathyroid hormone and adenosine-3',5'-monophosphate acutely increase phospholipids of the phosphatidate-polyphosphoinositide pathway in rabbit kidney cortex tubules <u>in vitro</u> by a cycloheximide-sensitive process, <u>Endocrinology</u>, 108:2078.

Boland, C. J., Fried, R. M., and Tashjian, A. H., Jr.,1986, Measurement of cytosolic free Ca^{2+} concentrations in human and rat osteosarcoma cells: actions of bone resorption-stimulating hormones, <u>Endocrinology</u>, 118:980.

Carney, D. H., Scott, D. L., Gordon, E. A., and LaBelle, E. F., 1985, Phosphoinositides in mitogenesis: neomycin inhibits thrombin-stimulated phosphoinositide turnover and initiation of cell proliferation. <u>Cell</u> 42:479.

Civitelli, R., Reid, I. R., Dobre, V., Shen, V., Halstead, L., Avioli, L. V., and Hruska, K., 1987, PTH stimulation of bone resorption: role of Ca^{2+} message system, J. Bone Min. Res. 2:Supp.1, Abs. 233.

Cole, J. A., Eber, S. L., Poelling, R. E., Thorne, P. K. and Forte, L. R., 1987, A dual mechanism for regulation of kidney phosphate transport by parathyroid hormone, Amer. J. Physiol., 253:E221.

Dirkson, T. R., 1975, Incorporation of radioactive bases into calvaria of the newborn rat, Rattus norvegicus. Comp. Biochem. Physiol. 50B:345.

Dziak, R. and Stern, P. H. 1975, Parathyromimetic effects of the ionophore, A23187, on bone cells and organ cultures, Biochem. Biophys. Res. Comm., 65:1343.

Dziak, R. and Stern, P. H. 1975, Calcium transport in isolated bone cells. III. Effects of parathyroid hormone and cyclic 3',5'-AMP, Endocrinology, 97:1281.

Exton, J. H., 1985, Role of calcium and phosphoinositide in the actions of certain hormones and neurotransmitters, J. Clin. Invest. 75:1753.

Farese, R. V., Bidot-Lopez, P., Sabir, A., Smith, J. S., Schinbeckler, B., and Larson, R., 1980, Parathyroid hormone acutely increases polyphosphoinositides of the rabbit kidney cortex by a cycloheximide-sensitive process, J. Clin. Invest., 65:1523.

Goldring, S. R., Roelke, M. S., Bringhurst, F. R., and Rosenblatt, M., 1985, Differential effects of parathyroid hormone responsive cultured human cells on biological activity of parathyroid hormone and parathyroid hormone inhibitory analogs. Biochemistry, 24:513.

Hahn, T. J., DeBartolo, T. F., and Halstead, L. R., 1980, Ouabain effects on hormonally-stimulated bone resorption and cyclic AMP content in cultured fetal rat bones. Endoc. Res. Comm. 7:189.

Herrmann-Erlee, M. P. M., and Gaillard, P. J., Hekkelman, J. W., and Nijweide, P. J., 1977, The effect of verapamil on the action of parathyroid hormone on embryonic bone in vitro, Eur. J. Pharmacol., 46:51.

Herrmann-Erlee, M. P. M., Nijweide, P. J., van der Meer, J. M., and Ooms, M. A. C., 1983, Action of bPTH and bPTH fragments on embryonic bone in vitro: dissociation of the cyclic AMP and bone resorbing response, Calc. Tiss. Int., 35:70.

Hoffmann, O., Klaushofer, K., Koller, K., Peterlik, M. Mavreas, T., and Stern, P., 1986, Indomethacin inhibits thrombin-, but not thyroxin-stimulated resorption of fetal rat limb bones, Prostaglandins 31:601.

Hruska, K. A., Moskowitz, D., Esbrit, P., Civitelli, R., Westbrook, S., Huskey, M., 1987, Stimulation of inositol trisphosphate and diacylglycerol production in renal tubular cells by parathyroid hormone, J. Clin. Invest., 79:230.

Ivey, J. L., Wright, D. R., and Tashjian, A. H., Jr., 1976, Bone resorption in organ culture: inhibition by the divalent cation ionophores A23187 and X-537A. J. Clin. Invest. 58:1327.

Lo, H., Lehotay, D. C., Katz, D., and Levey, G. S., 1976, Parathyroid hormone-mediated incorporation of ^{32}P-orthophosphate into phosphatidic acid and phosphatidylinositol in renal cortical slices, Endoc. Res. Comm., 3:377.

Lerner, U. H., Dewhirst, F. E., Ransjo, M., Sahlberg, K., and Fredholm, B. B., 1987, On the role of cyclic AMP and inositol phosphates as second messenger of the bone resorptive effect of parathyroid hormone, $1\alpha(OH)$ vitamin D_3 and interleukin 1, in: "Calcium Regulation and Bone Metabolism: Basic and Clinical Aspects", vol. 9 D. V., Cohn, T. J. Martin, and P. J. Meunier, eds., Elsevier, Amsterdam.

Lorenzo, J., and Raisz, L. G., 1981, Divalent cation ionophores stimulate resorption and inhibit DNA synthesis in cultured fetal rat bone, Science 212:1157.

Lowik, C. W. G. M., van Leeuwen, J. P. T. M., van der Meer, J. M., van Zeeland, J. K., Scheven, B. A. A., and Herrmann-Erlee, M. P. M., 1985, A two-receptor model for the action of parathyroid hormone on osteoblasts: a role for intracellular free calcium and cAMP, Cell Calcium, 6:311.

Matsumoto, T., Morita, K., Kawanobe, Y., and Ogata, E., 1986, Effect of parathyroid hormone on phospholipid metabolism in osteoblast-like osteogenic sarcoma cells, Biochem J. 236:605.

Meltzer, V., Weinreb, S., Bellorin-Font, E., Hruska, K. A., 1982, Parathyroid hormone stimulation of renal phosphoinositide metabolism is a cyclic nucleotide-independent effect, Biochim. Biophys. Acta, 712:258.

Parsons, J. A., Neer, R. M., and Potts, J. T., Jr., 1971, Initial fall of plasma calcium after intravenous injection of parathyroid hormone, Endocrinology, 89:735.

Peck, W. A., Kohler, G., and Barr, S., 1981, Calcium-mediated enhancement of the cylic AMP response in cultured bone cells, Calc. Tiss. Int. 33:409.

Raisz, L. G., Trummel, C. L., and Simmons, H., 1972, Induction of bone resorption in tissue culture: prolonged response after brief exposure to parathyroid hormone or 25-hydroxycholecalciferol, Endocrinology, 90:744.

Rappaport, M. S., and Stern, P. H., 1986, Parathyroid hormone and calcitonin modify inositol phospholipid metabolism in fetal rat limb bones, J. Bone Min. Res., 1:173.

Reid, I. R., Civitelli, R., Halstead, L. R., Avioli, L. V., and Hruska, K. A., 1987, Parathyroid hormone acutely elevates intracellular calcium in osteoblastlike cells, Amer. J. Physiol., 252:E45.

Rendu, F., Marche, R., MacLouf, J., Birard, A. and Ley-Toledano, S., 1983, Triphosphoinositide breakdown and dense body release as the earliest events in thrombin-induced activation of human platelets, Biochem. Biophys. Res. Comm. 116:513

Robinson, C. J., Rafferty, B., and Parsons, J. A., 1972, Calcium shift into bone: a calcitonin-resistant primary action of parathyroid hormone, studied in rats, Clin. Sci., 42:235.

Rosenblatt, M., Callahan, E. N., Mahaffey, J. E., Pont, A., and Potts, J. T., Jr., 1977, Parathyroid hormone inhibitors. Design, synthesis, and biologic evaluation of hormone analogues. J. Biol. Chem. 252:5847.

Stern, P. H., Phillips, T. E., and Mavreas, T., 1980, Bioassay of 1,25-dihydroxyvitamin D in human plasma purified by partition, alkaline extraction, and high-pressure chromatography, Anal. Biochem. 102:22.

Stern, P. H., 1984, Role of calcium in the initiation of hormonal effects on bone, in: Epithelial Calcium and Phosphate Transport: Molecular and Cellular Aspects, M. Peterlik and F. Bronner, eds. Alan R. Liss, Inc. New York, p. 159.

Stern, P. H. 1985, Interactions of calcemic hormones and divalent cation ionophores on fetal rat bone in vitro, in: Calcium in Biological Systems, R. P. Rubin, G. B. Weiss, and J. W. Putney, Jr., eds. Plenum, New York, p. 541.

Stewart, P. J. and Stern, P. H., 1987, Calcium/phosphatidylserine-stimulated protein phosphorylation in bone: effect of parathyroid hormone, J. Bone Min. Res., 2:281.

Tanaka, T. and Hollander, V. P., 1971, Effect of parathyroid extract on bone phospholipid. Proc. Soc. Exp. Biol. Med., 136:174.

Wakelam, M. J. O., Murphy, G. J., Hruby, V. J., and Houslay, M. D., 1986, Activation of two signal-transduction systems in hepatocytes by glucagon, Nature, 323:68.

Wong, G. L., Kent, G. N., Ku, K. Y., and Cohn, D. V., 1978, The interaction of parathormone and calcium on the hormone-regulated synthesis of hyaluronic acid and citrate decarboxylation in isolated bone cells, Endocrinology, 103:2274.

Yamaguchi, D. T., Hahn, T. H., Iida-Klein, A., Kleeman, C. T., Muallem, S., 1987, Parathyroid hormone-activated calcium channels in an osteoblast-like clonal osteosarcoma cell line, J. Biol Chem., 262:7711.

PARATHYROID HORMONE-ACTION AND DEGRADATION

Takuo Fujita, Hisamitsu Baba, Toru Yamaguchi,
Masashi Nishikawa, and Mariko Sase

Third Division, Department of Medicine
Kobe University School of Medicine, Kobe

Masafumi Fukushima and Yasuho Nishii

Research Laboratories of Chugai Pharmaceutical Company, Tokyo

INTRODUCTION

Peptide hormone hydrolysis has two main purposes. One is processing, and the other is degradation. In most of the hormones, these two processes are clearly distinguished, because the former takes place in the secretory gland and the latter in the target organ. The former is a metabolically controlled limited hydrolysis yielding certain active fragment, whereas the latter is a random hydrolysis to generate small, inactive fragments with no other purpose but getting rid of the biological effect of the hormone. While the processing and generation of active fragment is directly connected with the action of the hormone, degradation into small fragments may be involved only indirectly in the control of hormone action, by controlling its rate of disappearance and consequently, the half-life of the hormone in blood. Parathyroid hormone is unique in its inhibition of secretion by calcium ion along with renin, and this was explained by calcium stimulation of its degradation already in the secretory gland, from which only inactive fragments are secreted during hypercalcemia, because of the augmentation of PTH degradation in the parathyroid glands. It is thus difficult to separate processing and degradation of PTH. In the target cells of PTH, both processing and degradation may take place. It was the purpose of the present study to explore the possibility of PTH processing along with degradation in the classical target tissue of PTH, the the kidney and bone, in order to find a chain connecting the action and degradation of this hormone. In the case of PTH, processing and degradation may be coherent.

MEASUREMENT OF PTH DEGRADATION

Utilizing ready precipitation of intact PTH in 10 % trichloroacetic acid in contrast to a very high solubility of its fragment, PTH degradation has been measured. Use of ^{125}I-PTH facilitated such measurement, since ^{125}I radioactivity measurement in the TCA supernatant is sufficient to assess the degradation.[1] Although ^{125}I-labeled hormone has been used extensively to study the fate and degradation, a possibility a ^{125}I-labeling changing the configuration of the hormone as the enzyme substrate cannot be excluded. In our hand, moreover, native PTH failed to suppress ^{125}I-PTH hydrolysis by rat kidney supernatant, indicating a different behavior of native and ^{125}I-PTH against enzymic hydrolysis.

New Actions of Parathyroid Hormone
Edited by S. G. Massry and T. Fujita
Plenum Press, New York

A new method of measurement of PTH hydrolysis by using native unlabeled PTH was therefore developed. The method essentially consists of radioimmuno-assay of the TCA supernatant to quantify the fragments still retaining the structure recognized by the antibody after removal of TCA with ether.

Results of preliminary experiments indicating a predominance of in-tact PTH–hydrolyzing activity in the cytosolic fraction prompted us to search for a specific and limited PTH–hydrolyzing activity in the 100,000 × g supernatant of rat kidney. After exanguination, the kidney was re-moved and the cortex separated, minced and homogenized with 8 volumes of 0.45 M sucrose solution containing 0.68 m MEDA, pH 7.0, in a teflon homogenizer at a speed of less than 1000 r.p.m. The mixture was then centrifuged at 3000 r.p.m. for 10 minutes at 4°C. The supernatant was then centrifuged at 35000 r.p.m. (100,000 × g) at 4°C for 60 minutes, and used as the enzyme sample.[2]

PROPERTIES OF RAT RENAL CYTOSOLIC PTHase

The optimum pH for the native PTH–degrading enzyme activity of the supernatant fraction of rat renal cortical homogenate was predominant at pH 7.25, along with minor peaks at pH 4.5, 6.0 and 8.5. The pH optimum of ^{125}–PTH hydrolyzing activity, on the other hand, was mainly seen at pH 4.5, with a minor peak at the neutral range.

On ammonium sulfate fractionation, the PTH–hydrolyzing activity at pH 7.25 was mainly precipitated between 45 – 60 % saturation unlike the activity at pH 9 precipitated between 0 – 45 % saturation as shown in Fig 1. All enzyme activities were inhibited by citrate except for the one at pH 4.5. At pH 7.25, the activity was more distinctly inhibited by $(NH_4)_2SO_4$, while K_2SO_4 mainly inhibited the activity at pH 9.

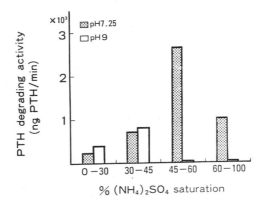

Fig 1.

Ammonium sulfate fractionation of PTH hydrolyzing activity at pH 7.25 (neutral) and at pH 9.0 (alkaline). Neutral PTH–hydrolyzing activity is mainly precipitated at 45 – 60 % saturation, whereas alkaline PTH–hydroly-zing activity at 0 – 45 % saturation, making a separation possible.

Since the neutral PTHase activity appeared to be predominant in the cytosolic fraction of rat renal cortical homogenate, attempts were made to further characterize this enzyme. ATP, Ca ion and glutathione appeared to inhibit the activity as shown in Fig 2. Enzyme inhibitors such as trypsin inhibitor, PMSF, E64, chymostatin, leupeptin and pepstatin did not, ruling out the possibility that this neutral PTHase belongs to groups of serine proteinase, cysteine proteinase and aspartic proteinase. Gel filtration over sephadex G-200 revealed that all PTH-hydrolyzing activities at pH 7.25 and 9 eluted around the position of blue dextran, suggesting a high molecular weight, at least several hundred thousand.

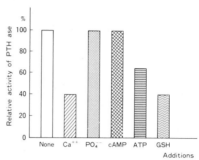

Fig 2.

Effect of Ca^{++}, PO_4^{--}, cAMP, ATP and glutathione on neutral PTHase activity. Ca^{++}, ATP and glutathione significantly inhibited the activity, whereas PO_4^{--} and cAMP did not.

Elution by stepwise method of neutral PTHase from DEAE cellulose column with 0.1, 0.2 and 0.5M NaCl gave rise to at least 3 fractions, neutral PTHase P - I, P - II and P - III. On rechromatography on DEAE cellulose, they were found to be interchangeable possibly due to changes of molecular configuration. The peak II enzyme also hydrolyzed A-Phe-Arg-MCA, but this activity was activated by ATP and GSH. Leu-MCA hydrolyzing activity was also distinguished from PTHase activity.

When cytosolic fraction was isolated from rats placed on vitamin D deficient diet for 3 weeks, a definite rise of neutral PTHase activity was noted as shown in Fig 3. This tended to normalize in rats treated with $1\alpha25(OH)_2$ vitamin D_3 during the third week, with partial restoration from vitamin D deficiency. Inhibition of PTHase in vitro by addition of calcium persisted regardless of vitamin D depletion or repletion, as shown in Fig 3. Vitamin D deficiency, on the contrary, tended to decrease ^{125}I-PTHase as reported previously.[3]

Fig 3.

Effect of vitamin D deficiency and supplement on neutral PTHase activity from renal cortical cytosolic fraction in rats. In rats maintained on vitamin D deficient diet for 3 weeks, neutral PTHase activity significantly rose. Supplementation with $1\alpha25(OH)_2$ vitamin D_3 in the 3rd week partially restored the animal from vitamin D deficiency along with concomitant fall of neutral PTHase activity.

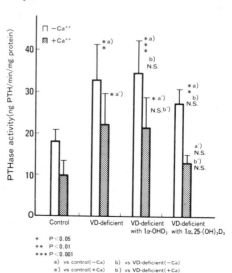

Since the isolated cell lines with receptor for PTH appears to provide a much better tool for the study on the action-degradation interrelationship of PTH, as well as the characterization of PTHase, PTH hydrolyzing activities of UMR-106, rat osteosarcoma cell line with osteoblast-like properties, and those OK cells, opossum kidney cells with proximal tubular cell-like properties were tested. These two cell lines represented PTH-responsive cells in two major target tissue for PTH, the bone and kidney.[4]

UMR 106 cells, a kind gift from Dr. T.J. Martin, were grown in Dulbecco's modified Eagle medium (DMEM) containing 10 % fetal calf serum in a humidified 95 % air 5 % CO_2 at 37°C. After reaching confluence, the monolayers of UMR 106 cells (4.0×10^6 cells per 9.6 cm^2 dish) were incubated in 1.5 ml serum free DMEM containing 50 ng/ml hPTH 1-84. After an appropriate incubation period, immunoreactive PTH fragments produced from PTH 1-84 by degradation in 1 ml medium was separated from intact PTH by adding 1 ml 10 % trichloroacetic acid and 50 µl 10 % bovine serum albumin. After centrifugation at 1870 ×g for 10 minutes, 1 ml supernatant was washed with diethylether to remove TCA. After evaporating diethylether in vacuo for 2 hours at 4°C, PTH fragments were measured by radioimmunoassay. Similar method was employed for OK cells, kind gift of Dr. L.R. Forte.

Both in UMR-106 cells and OK cells, PTH was degraded into several large immunoreactive fragments, suggesting limited hydrolysis. Km for UMR cells was 5.1×10^{-7}M, whereas that for OK cells was 9.2×10^{-9} M. Participation of C-kinase was suggested in the PTH degradation by UMR-106 cells, through augmentation by diacylglycerol and phorbol ester (TPA).[5]

UMR-106 produced peak A and B, fragments distinct from intact PTH, PTH 53-84 and PTH 39-84, indicating a limited hydrolysis. Longer retention times of these fragments on HPLC might suggest high hydrophobicity expected in C-terminal fragments.

SUMMARY

1. I^{125}-PTH and native PTH behave differently against enzymic hydrolysis.
2. Rat renal cortical cytosolic fraction contains a high molecular weight neutral PTHase for limited and specific PTH hydrolysis, inhibited by Ca^{++}, ATP and glutathione. Vitamin D deficiency increases the activity of this enzyme.
3. Osteoblast-like rat osteosarcoma cell line (UMR-106) and opssum proximal tubular cell line (OK) with PTH receptors contain PTHase. Protein kinase C is involved in PTH degradation as a part of signal transduction mechanism.

CONCLUSION

PTH degradation may be important not only for controling the level of available hormone, but also in the mechanism of PTH action through steps of signal transduction.

REFERENCES

1. T. Fujita, M. Ohata, M. Yoshikawa, M. Maruyama, Enzymatic hydrolysis of ^{125}I-labeled Parathyroid Hormone, Endocrinol. Japan. 16:383 (1969).

2. T. Fujita, H. Baba, M. Sase, M. Fukushima, Y. Nishii, Parathyroid hormone-degrading enzyme of high molecular weight in the cytosol of rat renal cortical cells, Bone & Mineral, 1: 457 (1986).
3. T. Fujita, H. Baba, Y. Yoshimoto, M. Fukase, M. Kishihawa, M. Tomon, T. Fukami, Y. Imai, Y. Nishii, M. Fukushima, Physiological significance of PTH degradation through limited hydrolysis by rat kidney cytosolic enzymes, Endocrine Control of Bone & Calcium Metabolism Ed. D.V. Cohn, T. Fujita, J.T. Potts, Jr., Elsevier p 238 (1984).
4. T. Yamaguchi, H. Baba, M. Fukase, Y. Kinoshita, T. Fujimoto, T. Fujita, Degrading activity for human parathyroid hormone (hPTH 1-84) in rat osteoblast-like osteosarcoma cell line UMR 106, Biochem. Biophys. Research Comm. 141: 762 (1986).
5. T. Yamaguchi, H. Baba, M. Fukase, Y. Kinoshita, T. Fujimi, T. Fujita, Possible involvement of protein kinase C in parathyroid hormone degradation by osteoblast-like rat osteosarcoma cell line UMR-106.

PARATHYROID HORMONE-RELATED PROTEIN OF CANCER: A NOVEL GENE PRODUCT

WITH A PTH PROTOPE

T.J. Martin*, B.E. Kemp*, J.M. Moseley*† L.G. Raisz**,
L.J. Suva, and W.I. Wood***

*University of Melbourne, Dept. of Medicine, Repatriation
 General Hospital, Heidelberg, Vic. Australia
**University of Conn., Health Center, Conn.
***Genentech Inc., So. San Francisco

The term humoral hypercalcemia of malignancy (HHM)
describes patients with certain cancers in whom the blood
calcium level is elevated, due to production
by the cancer of some substance which acts generally upon
the skeleton to increase bone resorption and upon the kidney
to reduce calcium excretion (1). The condition is
associated with a low plasma level of phosphorus and
increased renal production of cyclic AMP (2). The tumors
most commonly associated with this syndrome are squamous
cell carcinoma of the lung, renal cortical carcinoma, other
squamous cell cancers and some miscellaneous tumors.

Parathyroid hormone (PTH) is known to act on bone to
promote bone resorption and upon the kidney to decrease
calcium excretion, increase phosphorus excretion and promote
renal generation and excretion of cyclic AMP. Since the
1920's the biochemical features of primary
hyperparathyroidism have been recognized as a high plasma
calcium and low plasma phosphorus. In 1941, when discussing
a case of hypercalcemia in a patient with cancer, Dr.
Fuller Albright proposed that the hypercalcemia might be due
to production by the cancer of PTH. In succeeding years
this idea gained acceptance, and the "ectopic PTH" syndrome
was widely used to apply to patients with cancer who had a
high plasma calcium, low phosphorus, and minimal or no bone
metastases. Support for this came in 1966 when Berson and
Yalow published results with the first radioimmunoassay for
PTH, in which they found significant elevations of the PTH
level in a number of unselected patients with lung cancer
(3). Over the next several years until the early 1970's,
several reports were published of measurable PTH (by
radioimmunoassay) in extracts of cancers from such patients
(reviewed in 1). Throughout this time it was evident,
however, that the radioimmunoassay of PTH presented
technical problems, and in no instance were circulating
levels of PTH convincingly very high – certainly not at the
levels frequently found with corresponding levels of plasma
calcium in patients with primary hyperparathyroidism.

New Actions of Parathyroid Hormone
Edited by S. G. Massry and T. Fujita
Plenum Press, New York

Two groups of workers in the early 1970's published results indicating that the circulating immunoreactive PTH in the cancer patients differed from "authentic" PTH (4,5). The levels in plasma were in both cases lower than in primary hyperparathyroidism, in one series the cancer immunoreactivity was significantly non-parallel to PTH standards, and in the other it was of higher molecular weight than PTH. Thus the early 1970's saw some doubt arising that PTH itself was a major contributor to the clinical and biochemical features of this cancer syndrome. This doubt became more firmly based when Powell et al (6) showed in studies of several patients with humoral hypercalcemia that PTH could not be detected in plasma or in tumor extracts, despite their use of a wide range of PTH antisera directed against different parts of the molecule. Other studies, including our own (7), showed that tumors could produce bone resorbing activity in vitro which was clearly due to something other than PTH. In 1979 (8) we reviewed current evidence of the nature of this syndrome, concluding that these cancers caused hypercalcemia by producing a factor which was not PTH, but which produced PTH-like effects.

In careful clinical studies of several such patients, three groups of investigators (2,9,10) identified a substantial group of patients with HHM who, in addition to their hypercalcemia and hypophosphatemia, exhibited increased nephrogenous cyclic AMP. In all these respects therefore, they resemble patients with primary hyperparathyroidism, but differed in that their plasma PTH level were low, as were their $1,25(OH)_2$ vitamin D_3 levels, the plasma chloride levels were elevated and bicarbonate levels low. Thus the real prospect developed that these tumors are producing something which has a PTH-like effect, but which is not PTH itself, and further, that some subtle differences from PTH action existed in the tumor material.

Evidence entirely consistent with this possibility came from the demonstration that extracts of tumors from such patients, although they contained no immunoassayable PTH, were able to activate adenylate cyclase in kidney membranes and increase cyclic AMP production in osteoblast-like bone cells (11,12). Each of these is a standard response to PTH itself. The tumor activity was found to be inhibited by peptide antagonists of PTH, but not by pre-incubation with antibody to PTH which was capable of completely obliterating the PTH response in these systems. Some such tumor extracts were also tested in a very sensitive cytochemical biological assay for PTH, the glucose-6-phosphate dehydrogenase response guinea-pig kidney, and found to possess activity (11) which was inhibited by antagonists but not by anti-PTH antisera. All of this was strong evidence for the production by the cancers of a substance chemically distinct from PTH, which acts upon PTH target cells through the PTH receptor or closely associated with it. Production of such activity was also shown to occur in certain animal tumors associated with humoral hypercalcemia (12), in cell cultures established from them, and in a cell culture established from a renal cortical carcinoma removed originally from a hypercalcemic patient (13).

We discovered that a human lung cancer cell line (BEN) which we had been studying for several years, produced substantial amounts of this PTH-like adenylate cyclase-stimulating activity. It could be detected in dilutions of medium sometimes as much as 1/500, and activity was unimpaired by prior incubation with a goat antiserum against human PTH(1-34), which completely blocked the activity of hPTH(1-34). Purification of the active component from BEN cell medium was achieved by processing large batches of conditioned medium through cation exchange chromatography and several reversed phase high pressure liquid chromatography steps. Purification was monitored at all stages by the use of a sensitive assay, measuring cyclic AMP generation in the PTH responsive clonal osteogenic sarcoma cell line, UMR 106-01. The final two steps in purification are shown in Figs 1 and 2. A protein of molecular weight 17-18,000 daltons on SDS-PAGE was purified in this way, and in the late stages of purification the only active material eluted from SDS gels was at that molecular weight. At early stages of purification we consistently obtained evidence for the production of a slightly higher molecular weight activity (21-24K$_D$), which appeared to differ in no other way from the smaller protein (14).

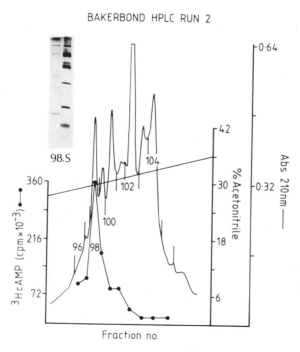

BAKERBOND HPLC RUN 2

Figure 1. HPLC (Bakerbond column) of partially purified PTHrP from BEN cell medium. Inset: SDS-PAGE of tube 98, and of molecular weight standards.

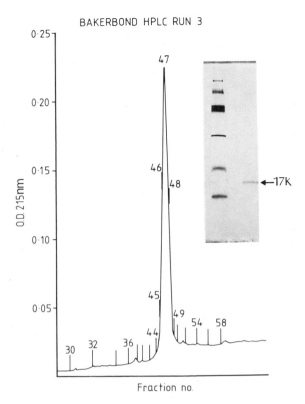

Figure 2. HPLC (Bakerbond column) of four samples of pooled material
equivalent to tube 98 of Fig. 1. Inset shows single 17 K
band on SDS-PAGE, compared with molecular weight standards.

Amino-terminal sequence of purified material was
obtained on three occasions. The first sequence data
consisted of 14 residues (14), obtained with 5 pmols of pure
protein, and pointed to significant homology with PTH about
the amino-terminus. A subsequent analysis of 20 pmols
yielded the first 24 amino acids of sequence and this was
used to prepare synthetic oligonucleotides for cloning (15).
Finally a preparation of 100 pmols yielded sequence to
residue 50 by a combination of amino-terminal sequencing and
an overlapping peptide (15). As part of the same study,
sequence from a tryptic peptide was also obtained from
residue 68 to 79. By preparing a cDNA library in λ gt 10 and
screening with oligonucleotides based on the first 24
residues of amino-terminal sequence, cDNA clones were
isolated and found to encode a prepro peptide of 36 amino
acids and a mature protein of 141 amino acids (Fig. 3,).
The cloned DNA was used to express active material in
mammalian cells (15).

```
hPTH    - - - - - M I P A K D M A K V M I V M L A I C F L T K S D G K S V K K R S V S E I Q L M H N L G K H
PTHrP   M Q R R L V Q Q W S V A V F L L S Y A V P S C G R S V E G L S R R L K R A V S E H Q L L H D K G K S


hPTH    L N S M E R V E W L R K K L Q D V H N F V A L G A P L A P R D A G S Q R P R K K E D N V L V E S H E
PTHrP   I Q D L R R R F F L H H L I A E I H T A E I R A T S E V S P N - S K P S P N T K N H P V R F G S D D


hPTH    K S L G A E D K A D V D V L T K A K S Q
PTHrP   E G R Y L T Q E T N K V E T Y K E Q P L K T P G K K K K G K P G K R K E Q E K K K R R T R S A W L D


PTHrP   S G V T G S G L E G D H L S D T S T T S L E L D S R R H
```

Figure 3. Sequence of PTHrP(15) compared with human PTH. Residues of identity are boxed.

The striking homology with PTH about the amino terminal region (8 of the first 13 residues of the secreted protein identical) is not maintained in the remainder of the molecule, which therefore represents a previously unrecognized hormone, possibly having arisen from the PTH gene by a process of gene duplication. The amino-terminal functional segment, or "prototope" (16), similar in sequence to the corresponding PTH prototope, can explain the interaction of the PTH-related protein (PTHrP) with PTH receptors. Indeed, PTHrP purified from BEN cell medium has at least 6 times the potency of human or bovine PTH(1-34) in stimulating cyclic AMP formation in osteogenic sarcoma cells (14). Furthermore the synthetic peptide PTHrP(1-34) is approximately four times more potent than hPTH(1-34) in the same intact cell cyclic AMP assay (17). Of very great interest, however, is the fact that, despite this greater potency in the adenylate cyclase response, PTHrP(1-34) was found to be appreciably less effective than PTH(1-34) in promoting resorption of fetal rat long bones in organ culture (17, Table 1). This leads to questions regarding the significance for bone resorption responses of the cyclic AMP response to PTH in osteoblasts.

The discovery of PTHrP opens new avenues of investigation. It is very clear that this molecular has several actions in common with PTH, but already certain differences are emerging. First, PTHrP(1-34) is more potent in stimulating adenylate cyclase activity both in bone and kidney (17). Second, it is less potent in promoting bone-resorption (17). It has PTH-like actions in promoting cyclic AMP and phosphorus excretion and reducing calcium excretion (17), but it remains to be seen whether PTH and PTHrP share the many actions attributed to PTH in other tissues and outlined in this Proceedings. These include the vasodilating and hypotensive actions of PTH (18), the relaxing effects in uterine (19), gastrointestinal (20), tracheal (21) and vas deferens tissues (22), and the positive chronotropic and inotropic effects (23).

TABLE 1. EFFECTS OF PTHrP(1-34) AND BOVINE PTH(1-34) ON ^{45}Ca RELEASE FROM CULTURED FETAL RAT LONG BONE

| Treatment | | N | % OF TOTAL ^{45}Ca RELEASED | |
			2 Days	5 Days
Control		24	19 ± 1	31 ± 1
PTHrP(1-34)	100 ng/ml	10	50 ± 4**	94 ± 3**
	25 ng/ml	10	32 ± 5*	66 ± 9**
	6.25 ng/ml	6	19 ± 1	34 ± 4
bPTH(1-34)	6.25 ng/ml	6	53 ± 4**	87 ± 3**
	1.56 ng/ml	12	31 ± 6*	44 ± 8
	0.4 ng/ml	6	19 ± 1	24 ± 1

Culture of fetal rat long bones was carried out as previously described (25).

*$p < 0.05$, **$p < 0.001$.

Certainly the tissue distribution of PTHrP will differ somewhat from that of PTH in that it has already been shown to be produced by keratinocytes in culture (24) and to be very commonly produced by squamous cell cancers. It will be of very great interest to know whether it has a role in keratinocyte differentiation.

REFERENCES

1. Martin, T.J. and Mundy, G.R. (1987) Malignant hypercalcemia. In: "Clinical Endocrinology of Calcium Metabolism" eds. T.J. Martin and L.A. Raisz. Marcel Dekker, New York, pp. 171-200.
2. Stewart, A.F., Hast, R., Deftos, L.J., Cadman, E.C., Lang, R. and Broadus, A.E. (1980). N. Engl. J. Med. 303: 1377-1383.
3. Berson, S.A. & Yalow, R.S. (1966). Science 154:907-909. 4. Roof, B.S. Carpenter, B., Fink, D.J. and Gordan, G.S. (1971). Am. J. Med. 50:686-692.
5. Benson, R.C. Jr., Riggs, B.L., Pickard, B.M. and Arnaud, C.D. (1974). Am. J. Med. 56:821-826.
6. Powell, D., Singer, F.R., Murray, T.M., Minkin, C. and Potts, J.T. Jr. (1973). New Engl. J. Med. 289:176-181.
7. Atkins, D., Ibbotson, K., Hillier, J., Hunt, N.H., Hammonds, J.C. and Martin, T.J. (1977). Brit. J. Cancer, 36:601-607.
8. Martin, T.J. and Atkins, D. (1979). Essays in Med. Biochem. 4:49-82.
9. Kukreja, S.C., Shemerdiak, W.P., Lad, T.E. and Johnson, P.A. (1980). J. Clin. Endocrinol. Metab. 51:167-169.
10. Rude, R.K., Sharp, C.F. Jr., Fredericks, R.S. Oldham, S.B., Elbaum, N., Link, J., Irvin, L. and Singer, F.R. (1981). J. Clin. Invest. 57:765-771.
11. Stewart, A.F., Insogna, K.L., Goltzman, D. and Broadus, A.E. (1983). Proc. Natl. Acad. Sci. USA 80:1454-1458.
12. Radeke, M.N., Musko, T.P., Hsu, C., Hersenberg, L.A. and Shooter, E.M. (1987). Nature 325:593-597.
13. Strewler, G.J., Williams, R.D. and Nissenson, R.A. (1983). J. Clin. Invest. 71:769-774.
14. Moseley, J.M., Kubota, M., Diefenbach-Jagger, H., Wettenhall, R.E.H., Kemp, B.E., Suva, L.J., Rodda, C.P., Ebeling, P.R., Hudson, P.J., Zajac, J.D. and Martin, T.J. (1987). Proc. Natl. Acad. Sci. USA 84:5048-5052.
15. Suva, L.J., Winslow, G.A., Wettenhall, R.E.H., Hammonds, R.G., Mosely, J.M., Diefenbach-Jagger, H., Rodda, C.P., Kemp, B.E., Rodriguez, H., Chen, E.Y., Hudson, P.J., Martin, T.J. and Wood, W.I. (1987). Science 237:893-896.
16. House, C.R. and Kemp, B.E. (1987). Science (in press).
17. Kemp, B.E., Mosely, J.M., Rodda, C.P., Ebeling, P.R., Wettenhall, R.E.H., Stapleton, D., Diefenbach-Jagger, H., Ure, F., Michelangell, V.P., Simmons, H.A., Raisz, L.G. and Martin, T.J. (1987). Manuscript submitted.
18. Pang, P.K.T., Yang, M.C.M., Shew, R. and Tenner, T.E. Jr. (1985). Blood Vessels. 22:57-64.
19. Pang, P.K.T., Shew, R.L. and Sawyer, W.H. (1981). Life Sci. 28:1317-1321.
20. Yang, M.C.M., Kenny, A.D. and Pang, P.K.T. In Current Trends in Comparative Endocrinology, eds. Lofts, B. and Holmes, W.N. Vol. 2., pp 1029-1030, Hong Kong University Press.

21. Yen, Y.C., Yang, M.C.M., Kenny, A.D. and Pang, P.K.T. (1983). Can. J. Physiol. Pharmacol. 62:1324-1328.
22. Zhang, R.H., Yang, M.C.M. and Pang, P.K.T. (1985). Fed. Proc. 44:1650.
23. Katch, Y., Klein, K.L., Kaplan, R.A., Sanborn, W.W. and Kurokawa, K. (1981). Endocrinology 109:2252-2254.
24. Merendino, J.J., Insogna, K.L., Miestone, L.M., Broadus, A.E. and Stewart, A.F. (1986). Science 231:388-399.
25. Raisz, L.G. and Niemann, J. (1969). Endocrinology 85:446-453.

PTH-LIKE TUMOR HYPERCALCEMIA FACTOR

Gideon A. Rodan, Mark Thiede, David D. Thompson,
Masaki Noda, Sevgi B. Rodan, and Michael Rosenblatt

Department of Biological Research
Merck Sharp and Dohme Research Laboratories

INTRODUCTION

Hypercalcemia is frequently a serious complication of malignancy. Since in certain patients this condition resembles hyperparathyroidism, a PTH-like factor secreted by the tumor was implicated in this syndrome. Indeed, it was found that several tumors produce a peptide which has PTH-like activity: it stimulates renal and bone adenylate cyclase (Rodan et al., 1983; Stewart et al., 1983), produces bone resorption in vitro and inhibits phosphate uptake in kidney cells (Strewler et al., 1987). Most recently several tumor-derived peptides were partially sequenced and were found to have sequence similarity to PTH (Moseley et al., 1987; Stewart et al., 1987; Strewler et al., 1987). A complementary DNA sequence cloned from a lung carcinoma cell line (BEN) confirmed the similarity of the deduced N-terminal amino acid sequence to that of PTH, and showed very little similarity to the rest of the molecule (Suva et al., 1987).

The object of these studies was to examine if various tumors produce the same PTH-like peptides (PLPs), if PLPs produce hypercalcemia in vivo, if they act directly on bone, if osteoblasts are their target cells, and if their potency is similar to that of PTH.

To address these questions we cloned the cDNA of the PTH-like peptide purified by Drs. Strewler and Nissenson from a renal carcinoma cell line, and used the (1-34) peptide deduced from the cDNA sequence of the lung PTH-related peptide (Suva et al., 1987) to study its effect on bone and bone-derived cells. The major findings are briefly reviewed below.

CLONING OF A COMPLEMENTARY DNA to mRNA OF A PTH-LIKE PEPTIDE PRODUCED BY THE RENAL CARCINOMA CELL LINE 786-0

A lambda-gt10 library was constructed using poly A (+) RNA extracted from these cells. The library was screened with an oligonucleotide synthesized according to the sequence published by Suva et al. (1987). Several clones were isolated, sequenced and a nearly full-length clone

New Actions of Parathyroid Hormone
Edited by S. G. Massry and T. Fujita
Plenum Press, New York

as well as fragments and oligonucleotides derived from PLP cDNA sequences were used in Northern and Southern blots to further characterize the expression of this gene.

Northern blot analysis revealed that the renal carcinoma cell line makes equal amounts of two major PLP messages of approximately 1800 and 1550 nucleotides and a small amount of a larger message of approximately 2400 bases. The 1550 nucleotide message seems to be complementary to the cDNA reported for the lung carcinoma peptide whereas the 1800 nucleotide message diverges just prior to the end of the coding sequence and contains a different 3' untranslated sequence. The deduced peptide is truncated by two amino acids. The 3' untranslated sequence of the larger message shows significant similarity to the corresponding sequence in the c-myc oncogene. Detailed analysis revealed that the two PLP mRNAs are produced by alternate splicing and that transcription of these messages starts at two very closely positioned initiation sites. Southern blot analysis with the full-length PLP cDNA and with fragments representing the 5' and 3' ends indicates that a single copy gene codes for this peptide. Alternate splicing of coding as well as non coding sequences, plays an important role in the developmental and tissue specific expression of a variety of genes (Leff et al., 1986). Further studies will show if this pattern of PLP-mRNA expression is tissue-specific, if the difference in the C-terminus translates into differences in the action or metabolism of this peptide, and if the similarity to the c-myc sequence is related to the expression of this gene in tumors.

COMPARISON OF THE EFFECTS OF (1-34) PLP AND (1-34) PTH ON RAT OSTEOSARCOMA/OSTEOBLASTIC CELLS (ROS 17/2.8)

A synthetic peptide having the 1-34 amino acid sequence deduced from the cDNA of the lung carcinoma (BEN) was used to compare the effects of PLP to those of human (1-34) PTH on the osteoblastic ROS 17/2.8 osteosarcoma cells. (1-34) PLP stimulated ROS 17/2.8 adenylate cyclase with an EC_{50} of 0.5-1 nM. In repeated experiments (1-34) PLP was about 2-5 fold more potent in this assay (based on the calculated EC_{50}) than (1-34) PTH. This difference was however considerably reduced by treating the ROS 17/2.8 cells with dexamethasone for 3 days. Dexamethasone treatment increases PTH stimulation of adenylate cyclase in these cells by a mechanism which involves an increase in the number of receptors and in the abundance of G_s, estimated by cholera toxin-stimulated NAD-dependent ADP ribosylation (Rodan and Rodan, 1986).

The major object was to assess post-receptor effects of (1-34) PLP in this system. Previous studies showed that PTH modulates the growth of these cells and inhibits alkaline phosphatase activity (Majeska et al., 1985). We found that both (1-34) PLP and (1-34) PTH had a small growth stimulatory effect at concentrations below 100 pM. Similar effects were previously observed for PTH in UMR 106 cells (Partridge et al., 1985) and ROS 17/2.8 cells (Majeska and Rodan, 1985), and could be related to the reported effects of PTH on bone formation (Tam et al., 1982). In ROS 17/2.8 cells treated with dexamethasone both, (1-34) PLP and (1-34) PTH had a pronounced growth inhibitory effect, with an EC_{50} of about 100 pM. It is of interest that these effects were only observed following dexamethasone treatment, which was shown to promote PTH stimulation of type I cAMP dependent protein kinase in these cells (Zajac et al., 1986). Activation of this enzyme has been implicated in the control of proliferation (Ng et al., 1983). These findings are consistent with the observed activation of protein kinase isoenzyme I in UMR 106 cells and the associated inhibition of growth (Livesey et al., 1982).

Both (1-34) PLP and (1-34) PTH had a pronounced dose-dependent inhibitory effect on cellular alkaline phosphatase with an EC_{50} of 30 pM. Unlike the effect on growth, this effect was not dependent on dexamethasone treatment. In cells treated with dexamethasone, which enhanced alkaline phosphatase levels by 4-5 fold, saturating doses of (1-34) PLP or (1-34) PTH inhibited alkaline phosphatase activity by about 80%. In non-treated cells the inhibition was about 70%. The reduction in alkaline phosphatase activity was accompanied in both cases by a decrease of about 80% in alkaline phosphatase mRNA, suggesting control at the level of enzyme abundance. These findings show that complex biological effects of (1-34) PTH on osteoblastic cells, which most likely involve regulation of gene expression, are closely mimicked by (1-34) PLP, which has similar potency in this system.

COMPARISON OF THE EFFECTS OF (1-34) PLP AND (1-34) PTH ON CALCIUM HOMEOSTASIS AND BONE RESORPTION IN VIVO

To examine the ability of the tumor-derived peptide to mobilize calcium from bone during malignancy hypercalcemia, we used the following animal model. Rats weighing around 200 gm were thyroparathyrodectomized and one femoral vein was cannulated with a catheter which was guided subcutaneously to the neck where it was led through a tether connected to a Harvard pump. This arrangement permits continous infusion in unrestrained animals. Twelve hours after surgery the animals were put on a calcium-deficient diet. Twelve hours later animals with blood calcium levels below 6 mg/dl started receiving a constant infusion of 0.01-0.1 nmole/hr (1-34) PTH or (1-34) PLP. Blood calcium levels were measured 24 and 48 hrs later, when the animals were sacrificed and bones were examined histologically. We found that animals receiving 0.01 nmole/hr (1-34) PLP or (1-34) PTH survived for 48 hrs with the same calcium levels of around 5 mg/dl. In animals receiving 0.06 or 0.1 nmole/hr of either peptide serum calcium levels rose to normocalcemic levels, which were sustained until sacrifice at 48 hrs. Animals receiving the intermediate dose of the 0.03 nmole/hr had low calcium concentrations at 24 hrs but reached normocalcemic levels at 48 hrs. The infusion of (1-34) PLP or (1-34) PTH thus showed a dose-dependent ability to maintain circulating calcium levels in these thyroparathyroidectimized rats on calcium deficient diets, presumably by stimulating bone resorption. Indeed histological examination of the tibiae showed a dose dependent increase in osteoclast number, from $3-5/mm^2$ at 0.01 nmol/hr to $32/mm^2$ at 0.1 nmole/hr. For each concentration examined there was no significant difference between the effects of (1-34) PLP and (1-34) PTH on calcium levels or on osteoclast number. The two synthetic peptides used in this study seemed to be equipotent in their ability to mobilize calcium from bone in this experimental model.

DISCUSSION

The studies summarized above examined the possibility that a PTH-like peptide secreted by tumors may suffice to produce the hypercalcemia of malignancy syndrome seen in certain patients. We found that a single gene codes for the PTH-like peptide and, although alternate splicing may generate several peptides, the N-terminal region, which is similar to PTH, does not seem to be affected by this process.

All peptides coded by this gene should thus share the 1-34 sequence used in this study. The synthetic 1-34 fragment infused at the relatively slow rate of 60 pmole/hr into 200 gm rats raised the calcium concentration in the plasma by >5 mg/dl. Since the animals were on the Toverud calcium-deficient diet most of the calcium should have originated from bone. This conclusion was strongly supported by the histomorphometric evidence for active bone resorption, which was proportional to the dose of PLP. If one can extrapolate from rat to man, the parallel and quantitatively similar effects of (1-34) PTH would explain the clinical picture of hyperparathyroidism observed in patients with the hypercalcemia of malignancy syndrome. These findings also support the assumption that the PLP effects are mediated by PTH receptors. This hypothesis was further supported by the in vitro effects of PLP on the osteoblast-like osteosarcoma cells. In addition to stimulation of adenylate cyclase, an assay which had been used to purify PLP, this peptide produced post-receptor effects identical to those caused by (1-34) PTH, with similar dose-response curves. The enhanced adenylate cyclase activation produced by dexamethasone treatment, which causes an increase in receptor number and in the abundance of G_s, was equally observed for (1-34) PLP and (1-34) PTH. Subtle effects of PTH, such as a small stimulation of growth at 30 pM was also observed for PLP at the same concentration. The small differences in EC_{50} between inhibition of growth (100 pM) and inhibition of alkaline phosphatase (30 pM) were again observed for both peptides. These findings are all consistent with similar interaction of the two peptides with a common receptor and point to the osteoblastic-lineage cells as target cells for PLP in bone. It has been speculated that the effects of PTH may be mediated by different classes of receptors (Lowik et al., 1985) which could be functionally differentiated by separate ligands. The studies reviewed here did not address that question, but there is no need to assume differences in receptor-ligand interaction between (1-34) PLP and (1-34) PTH to explain the data obtained. The simplest interpretation of the findings is that PLP can elevate serum calcium levels and produce other effects which resemble hyperparathyroidism through interaction with the PTH receptors.

REFERENCES

Leff, S. E., Rosenfeld, M. G., and Evans R. M., 1986, Complex transcriptional units: Diversity in gene expression by alternative RNA processing, Ann. Rev. Biochem., 55:1091.
Livesey, S. A., Kemo, B. E., Re, C. A., Partridge, N. A., and Martin, T. J., 1982, Selective hormonal activation of cyclic AMP-dependent protein kinase isoenzymes in normal and malignant osteoblasts, J. Biol. Chem., 257:14983.
Lowik, C. W. G. M., van Leuwen, J. P. T. M., vander Meer, J. M., van Zeeland, J. K., Scheven, B. A. A., and Herrmann-Erlee, M. P. M., 1985, A two receptor model for the action of parathyroid hormone on osteoblasts: A role for intracellular free calcium and cAMP, Cell Calcium, 6:311.
Majeska, R. J., and Rodan, G. A., 1981, Low concentrations of parathyroid hormone enhance growth of clonal osteoblast like cells in vitro, Calcif. tissue Int., 33:323.
Majeska, R. J., Nair, B. C., and Rodan, G. A., 1985, Glucocorticoid regulation of alkaline phosphatase in the osteoblastic osteosarcoma cell line ROS 17/2.8, Endocrinology, 116:170.

Moseley, J. M., Kubota, M., Diefenbach-Jagger, H. D., Wettenhall, R. E. H., Kemp, B. E., Suva, L. J., Rodda, C. P., Ebeling, P. R., Hudson, P. J., Zajac, J. D., and Martin, T. J., 1987, Parathyroid hormone-related protein purified from a human lung cancer cell line, Proc. Natl. Acad. Sci., 84:5048.

Ng, K. W., Livesey, S. A., Larkins, R. G., and Martin, T. J., 1983, Calcitonin effects on growth and on selective activation of type II isoenzyme on cyclic adenosine 3':5'-monophosphate-dependent protein kinase in T47D human breast cancer cells, Cancer Res., 43:794.

Partridge, N. C., Opie, A. L., Opie, R. T., and Martin, T. J., 1985, Inhibitory effects of parathyroid hormone on growth of osteogenic sarcoma cells, Calcif. Tissue Int., 37:519.

Rodan, S. B., Insogna, K. L., Vignery, A.M-C., Stewart, A. F., Broadus, A. E., D'Souza, S. M., Bertolini, D. R., Mundy, G. R., and Rodan, G. A., 1983, Factors associated with humoral hypercalcemia of malignancy stimulate adenylate cyclase in osteoblastic cells, J. Clin. Invest., 72:1511.

Rodan, S. B., and Rodan, G. A., 1986, Dexamethasone effects on β-adrenergic receptors and adenylate cyclase regulatory proteins G_s and G_i in ROS 17/2.8 cells, Endocrinology, 118:2510.

Stewart, A. F., Insogna, K. L., Goltzman, D., and Broadus, A. E., 1983, Identification of adenylate cyclase-stimulating activity and cytochemical glucose-6-phosphate dehydrogenase-stimulating activity in extracts of tumors from patients with humoral hypercalcemia of malignancy, Proc. Natl. Acad. Sci., 80:1454.

Stewart, A. F., Wu, T., Goumas, D., Burtis, W. J., and Broadus, A. E., 1987, N-Terminal amino acid sequence of two novel tumor-derived adenylate cyclase-stimulating proteins: Identification of parathyroid hormone-like and parathyroid hormone unlike domains, Biochem. Biophys. Res. Commun., 146:672.

Strewler, G. J., Stern, P. H., Jacobs, J. W., Eveloff, J., Klein, R. F. Leung, S. C., Rosenblatt, M., and Nissenson, R. A., 1987, Parathyroid hormone-like protein from human renal carcinoma cells: Structural and functional homology with parathyroid hormone, J. Clin. Invest., In Press.

Suva, L. J., Winslow, G. A., Wettenhall, R. E. H., Hammonds, R. G., Moseley, J. M., Dienfenbach-Jagger, H., Rodda, C. P., Kemp, B. E., Rodriguez, H., Chen, E. Y., Hudson, P. J., Martin, T. J., and Wood, W. I., 1987, A Parathyroid hormone-related protein implicated in malignant hypercalcemia: cloning and expression, Science, 237:893.

Tam, C. S., Heersche, J. N., Murray, T. M., and Parsons, J. A., 1982, Parathyroid hormone stimulates the bone appositional rate independently of its resorptive actions: Differential effects of intermittent and continous administration, Endocrinology, 110:506.

Zajac, J. D., Livesey, S. A., Michelangeli, V. P., Rodan, S. B., Rodan, G. A., and Martin, T. J., 1986, Glucocorticoid treatment facilitates cyclic adenosine 3',5'-monophosphate-dependent protein kinase response in parathyroid hormone-responsive osteogenic sarcoma cells, Endocrinology, 118:2059.

THE VASCULAR ACTION OF PARATHYROID HORMONE

PARATHYROID HORMONE RECEPTORS IN CULTURED RAT VASCULAR SMOOTH MUSCLE AND

BOVINE ENDOTHELIAL CELLS

Yukio Hirata[1,2], Yasuyuki Takagi[1,2] and Takuo Fujita[2]

[1]Hypertension Division, National Cardiovascular Center
Research Institute, Osaka 565, and [2]Department of Medicine
Kobe University School of Medicine, Kobe 650, Japan

INTRODUCTION

It has been reported that parathyroid hormone (PTH) causes a marked decrease in blood pressure in a variety of species[1,2] and relaxes precontracted vascular strips from conduit- to resistance-type vessels[3,4,5]. Therefore, PTH may have direct action on the vascular tissues other than kidney and bone. However, little is known about the cellular mechanism of vascular action by PTH. To elucidate the mechanism of PTH action in the vasculature, we have attempted to identify and characterize vascular receptors for PTH in cultured rat vascular smooth muscle cells (VSMC) and bovine endothelial cells (EC) using ^{125}I-labeled-synthetic amino-terminal fragment of human (h) PTH as radioligand.

METHODS AND MATERIALS

VSMC from rat aorta and EC from bovine aorta were prepared by collagenase digestion and cultured in Dulbecco's modified Eagle's medium containing 10% fetal calf serum. Subcultured cells from 5-15th passages were used in the experiments.

Synthetic [Nle^{8,18}, Tyr^{34}]hPTH$^{1-34}$ (Peptide Institute, Osaka) was iodinated by lactoperoxidase and purified by adsorption to Quso G-32 and elution with 0.1N HCl/80% acetone[6]. ^{125}I-Tyr^{34}-hPTH (specific activity: 100-120 μCi/μg) was used as radioligand.

The binding experiment was performed essentially in the same manner as described elsewhere[6]. Briefly, confluent cells were usually incubated with 10^{-8}M ^{125}I-hPTH at 4° for 120 min in one-ml Hanks' balanced salt solution containing 0.1% bovine serum albumin unless otherwise stated. After completion, the cells were washed, solubilized in 0.5N NaOH, and the cell-bound radioactivity was measured. Specific binding was defined as total binding minus nonspecific binding in the presence of excess (2.4×10^{-6}M) unlabeled hPTH$^{1-34}$ analog.

To study the degradation of ^{125}I-hPTH, VSMCs were preincubated with ^{125}I-hPTH at 4°C for 2 hrs, rinsed and incubated in fresh medium at 37°C or 4°C; the cell-bound radioactivity was determined and aliquots of the used medium was analysed for its TCA-precipitability and capability of rebinding to fresh VSMC.

For measurement of cyclic AMP, VSMCs were incubated with or without hPTH$^{1-34}$ in medium containing 0.5 mM methylisobutylxanthine at 37° for 10 min; intracellular cAMP content was determined by RIA as reported[7].

New Actions of Parathyroid Hormone
Edited by S. G. Massry and T. Fujita
Plenum Press, New York

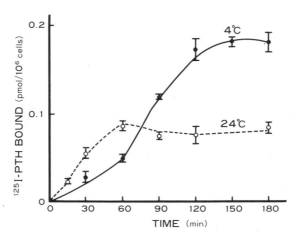

Fig. 1. Effect of temperature on specific binding of ^{125}I-hPTH to rat VSMC. Confluent VSMCs were incubated with 10 nM ^{125}I-hPTH at 4°C (●) or 24°C (O) for indicated times. Each point is the mean ± SE of triplicate dishes.

For determination of prostaglandin (PG) I_2, ECs were incubated with or without hPTH[1-34] at 37° for 60 min; medium was assayed for 6-keto-$PGF_{1\alpha}$, a stable metabolite of PGI_2, by RIA as reported[8].
To assess molecular size of vascular PTH receptors, cells were detacted by a rubber policeman, homogenized in 50 mM phosphate-buffered saline (PBS), pH 7.4, containing 10 mM EDTA, 1 mM phenylmethylsulfonyl fluoride (PMSF), 1 μg/ml each of leupeptin and pepstatin, and centrifuged at 10,000 g for 30 min. Cell membrane preparations (0.5 mg) were incubated with 10^{-7}M ^{125}I-hPTH in 1 ml PBS containing aforementioned protease inhibitors in the presence and absence of excess unlabeled hPTH (5×10^{-6}M) at 4°C for 120 min and the bound ^{125}I-hPTH was covalently cross-linked to the receptor with 0.5 mM discuccimidyl suberate (DSS) as described elsewhere[9]. The affinity-labeled products were subjected to sodium dodecyl sulfate-polyacrylamide gel electrophoresis (SDS-PAGE) and autoradiography.

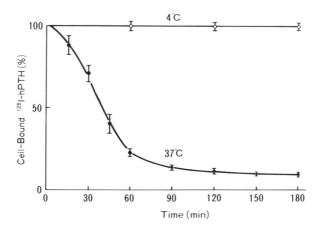

Fig. 2. Temperature-dependent decrease of cell-bound ^{125}I-hPTH in rat VSMC. After binding with ^{125}I-hPTH at 4°C for 2 hrs, VSMCs were further incubated in fresh medium at 37°C (●) and 4°C (O) for indicated times. Each point as expressed % of the initial binding is the mean ± SE of triplicate dishes.

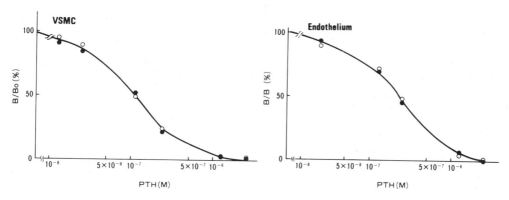

Fig. 3. Competitive binding of ^{125}I-hPTH by unlabeled hPTH analogs to cultured vascular cells. Rat VSMC (left) and bovine EC (right) were incubated with 10 nM ^{125}I-hPTH in the absence (Bo) and presence of hPTH$^{1-34}$ (●) or [Nle^{8,18}, Tyr^{34}]hPTH$^{1-34}$ (O) in concentrations as indicated.

RESULTS

An apparent equilibrium binding of ^{125}I-hPTH to rat VSMC at 4°C reached after 120 min, while at 24°C the maximal binding at 60 min was only a half that of 4°C (Fig. 1); specific binding at 4°C and 24°C was 50-60% and 20-30% of total binding, respectively. Similar time- and temperature-dependent binding of ^{125}I-hPTH was observed in bovine EC. The prebound radioactivity of ^{125}I-hPTH at 4°C, after washing, decreased very rapidly (t$_{1/2}$: 40 min) upon warming the cells at 37°C, whereas there was little, if any, decrease of cell-bound radioactivity upon subsequent incubation at 4°C (Fig. 2): most radioactive material released into medium at 37°C was TCA-soluble and unable to rebind to the fresh cells. The temperature-dependent decrease of cell-bound radioactivity was partially inhibited by pretreatment with 1 mM PMSF and 1 mM chloroquin.

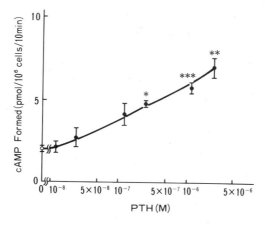

Fig. 4. Effect of hPTH on cAMP formation in rat VSMC. Confluent VSMCs were incubated with (●) or without (O) hPTH$^{1-34}$ at 37°C for 10 min in the presence of methylisobutylxanthine. Intracellular cAMP formed is shown. Each point is the mean ± SE of triplicate dishes: *p<0.01, **p<0.005, ***p<0.001.

Therefore, subsequent binding study was performed at 4°C for 120 min.

As shown in Fig. 3, $hPTH^{1-34}$ and $[Nle^{8,18}, Tyr^{34}]$ $hPTH^{1-34}$ were almost equipotent in inhibiting competitively the binding to both cells; the IC_{50} in VSMC and EC were $\sim 10^{-7}$ M and $\sim 2.5 \times 10^{-7}$ M, respectively. Neither angiotensin II, arginine-vasopressin, vasoactive intestinal peptide, atrial natriuretic peptide, nor calcitonin affected the binding.

$hPTH^{1-34}$ dose-dependently stimulated intracellular cAMP formation in VSMC with the ED_{50} of $\sim 2.5 \times 10^{-7}$ M (Fig. 4), of which effect was not inhibited by 10^{-5} M propranolol. $hPTH^{1-34}$, however, failed to stimulate synthesis of 6-keto-$PGF_{1\alpha}$ and cAMP generation in EC.

Autoradiograph of affinity-labeled membranes revealed that ^{125}I-hPTH interacts with ~ 50-kDa component in both VSMC and EC (Fig. 5); the labeled bands disappeared in the presence of excess unlabeled hPTH, indicating the specificity of affinity labeling. The apparent molecular size of the labeled components in both cells was unaltered by treatment with 2-mercaptoethanol.

DISCUSSION

Using ^{125}I-labeled-$[Nle^{8,18}, Tyr^{34}]$ $hPTH^{1-34}$ as radioligand, the present study first demonstrates the presence of specific binding sites for PTH in cultured rat VSMC as well as in bovine EC. Time- and temperature-dependent binding of ^{125}I-hPTH to both cells appear to be similar at 24-37°C, the binding was rapid but labile, whereas at 4°C an apparent equilibrium binding was attained after longer incubation. The temperature dependent decrease of cell-bound ^{125}I-hPTH and the reciprocal increase of nonspecific binding is most likely due to cell-mediated degradation of PTH during incubation because of the following reasons; 1) radioactive material(s) released into medium after 37°C incubation was mostly TCA-soluble and devoid of binding activity; 2) the temperature-dependent decrease of cell-bound radioactivity was blocked by serine protease inhibitor and lysosomotrophic drug. Therefore, it is suggested that PTH initially bound to the cell-surface receptor is largely degraded by membrane-bound serine protease(s) and/or by lysosomal hydrolase(s) after internalization. In fact, autoradiographic study using electron microscopy revealed that grains of ^{125}I-hPTH were localized not only on the cell-

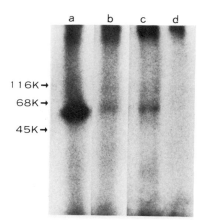

Fig. 5. Autoradiograph after SDS-PAGE of affinity-labeled vascular PTH receptors. Affinity-labeling of ^{125}I-hPTH to membranes of rat VSMC (a,b) and bovine EC (c,d) with DSS is shown in the absence (a,c) or presence (b,d) of excess unlabeled hPTH analog. Arrows: molecular size marker (Da).

membrane, but also within lysosome-like structures of VSMC at 37°C (unpublished observation).

Competitive binding study shows that $hTPH^{1-34}$ and $[Nle^{8,18}, Tyr^{34}]hPTH$ analogs have similar binding affinity in both cells. Although we cannot estimate the exact values of K_d or B_{max} from the present result due to relatively greater nonspecific binding even at 4°C, the binding affinity (10^{-7} M) from the competitive binding study appears to be comparable to the ED_{50} (1.2×10^{-7} M) of bovine PTH^{1-34} to relax rat aorta precontracted by phenylephrine[10]. However, the binding affinity is far greater than the ED_{50} ($2-14 \times 10^{-9}$ M) for relaxation of smaller blood vessels including rat tail artery[3], rat mesenteric artery[4] and cerebral arteries from various species[5]. The discrepancy may be accounted for by differences in species, blood vessels used (conduit- vs. resistance-type) or experimental systems employed (vascular strips vs. cells).

The present study further shows the stimulatory effect of $hPTH^{1-34}$ on intracellular cAMP formation with the ED_{50} comparable to that of binding affinity and the lack of β-blocker in inhibiting PTH-induced cAMP accumulation. Our results are in agreement with those of previous study[16]. Taken together, it is strongly suggested that PTH interacts with its specific vascular receptors distinct from β-adrenergic receptors that are functionally coupled to adenylate cyclase system. Since cAMP has been suggested to play an intracellular mediator role of vasorelaxation by β-adrenergic agonist, the same mechanism may be responsible for PTH-induced vasorelaxation.

In this study, PTH has no effect on synthesis of PGI_2, a potent vasodilator PG by bovine EC. Furthermore, PTH does not require an intact EC for vasorelaxation[3,10], suggesting that PTH-induced relaxation is not dependent on the release of endothelium-derived relaxing factor (EDRF). Therefore, the physiological significance of PTH receptors in EC remains to be answered.

Analysis of the affinity-labeled products by autoradiography after SDS-PAGE clearly demonstrates that ^{125}I-hPTH interacts with a similar 50-kDa membrane component in both VSMC and EC under reducing and nonreducing condition, suggesting that vascular PTH receptors exist in nonsulfide-linked form of almost identical size. While heterogeneity of PTH receptors with different molecular weights (28-, 51-, 60-, 70-, 80- and 90-kDa species) has been reported in plasma membranes of kidney and bone[11-15], recent study has suggested that smaller molecular sized component(s) may be proteolytic products of the predominant 85-kDa component[13-15]. However, we could not observe any PTH binding components larger than 50-kDa species in vascular cell membranes prepared and incubated even in the presence of various protease inhibitors. The questions as to whether the 50-kDa binding component as demonstrated in the vascular tissues is identical to a PTH receptor or its proteolytic fragment in other tissues and whether vascular PTH binding component is coupled to stimulatory guanine nucleotide regulatory protein (N_s) should be clarified.

In conclusion, PTH directly acts on vascular smooth muscle by initial binding to its specific membrane receptor to stimulate adenylate cyclase, thereby generating cAMP and finally leading to vasorelaxation. PTH, after binding to its receptor, is rapidly degraded by proteolytic enzyme(s). However, the physiological function of PTH action on endothelium remains unknown. The physiological role of PTH or PTH-like substance(s) in the regulation of regional blood flow, peripheral vascular resistance and/or blood pressure needs to be studied.

ACKNOWLEDGMENT

This study was supported in part by Research Grants from the Ministry of Health and Welfare, and the Ministry of Education, Science and Culture, Japan.

107

REFERENCES

1. P.K.T. Pang, T.E. Tenner, Jr., J.A. Yee, M. Yang, and H.F. Janssen, Hypotensive action of parathyroid hormone preparations on rats and dogs, Proc Natl Acad Sci USA 77: 675 (1980).
2. H.H. Wang, E.D. Drugge, Y.C. Yen, M.R. Blumenthal, and P.K.T. Pang, Effects of synthetic parathyroid hormone on hemodynamics and regional blood flows, Eur J Pharmacol 97: 209 (1984).
3. P.K.T. Pang, M.C.M. Yang, R. Shew, and T.E. Tenner, Jr., The vosorelaxant action of parathyroid hormone fragments on isolated rat tail artery, Blood Vessels 22: 57 (1985).
4. G.A. Nikols, M.A. Metz, and W.H. Chine, Jr., Vasodilation of the rat mesenteric vasculature by parathyroid hormone, J. Pharmacol Exp Ther 236: 419 (1986).
5. Y. Suzuki, K. Lederis, M. Huang, F.E. LeBlanc, and O.P. Rostad, Relaxation of bovine, porcine and human brain arteries by parathyroid hormone, Life Sci 33: 2497 (1983).
6. Y. Hirata, M. Tomita, H. Yoshimi, and M. Ikeda, Specific receptors for atrial natriuretic factor (ANF) in cultured vascular smooth muscle cells of rat aorta, Biochem Biophys Res Commun 125: 562 (1984).
7. Y. Hirata, M. Tomita, S. Takata, and T. Fujita, Functional receptors for vasoactive intestinal peptide in cultured vascular smooth muscle cells from rat aorta, Biochem Biophys Res Commun 132: 1079 (1985).
8. Y. Hirata, M. Tomita, S. Takata, and I. Inoue, Specific binding of atrial natriuretic peptide (ANP) in cultured mesenchymal non-myocardial cells from rat heart, Biochem Biophys Res Commun 131: 222 (1985).
9. M. Shinjo, Y. Hirata, H. Hagiwara, F. Akiyama, K. Murakami, S. Kojima, M. Shimonaka, Y. Inada, and S. Hirose, Characterization of atrial natriuretic factor receptors in adrenal cortex, vascular smooth muscle and endothelial cells by affinity labeling, Biomed Res 7: 35 (1986).
10. G.A. Nickols, M.A. Metz, and W.H. Cline, Jr., Endothelium-independent linkage of parathyroid hormone receptors of rat vascular tissues with increased adenosine 3',5'-monophosphate and relaxation of vascular smooth muscle, Endocrinology 119: 349 (1986).
11. M.D. Coltrera, J.T. Potts, Jr., and M. Rosenblatt, Identification of a renal receptor for parathyroid hormone by photoaffinity radio-labeling using a synthetic analogue, J Biol Chem 256: 10555 (1981).
12. M.W. Draper, R.A. Nissenson, J. Winer, J. Ramachandran, and C.D. Arnaud, Photoaffinity labeling of the canine renal receptor for parathyroid hormone, J Biol Chem 257: 3714 (1982).
13. B.S. Wright, G.A. Tyler, R. O'Brien, L.H. Caporale, and M. Rosenblatt, Immunoprecipitation of the parathyroid hormone receptor, Proc Natl Acad Sci USA 84: 26 (1987).
14. R.A. Nissenson, D. Karpf, T. Bambino, J. Winner, M. Canga, K. Nyiredy, and C.D. Arnaud, Covalent labeling of a high-affinity, guanyl nucleotide sensitive parathyroid hormone receptor in canine renal cortex, Biochemistry 26: 1874, 1987.
15. J. Chuang, I. Yike, J.H. Reese, R. Laethem, and J.E. Zull, Identification and purification of a kidney membrane protein which specifically binds the amino-terminal domain of native parathyroid hormone, J Biol Chem 262: 10760 (1987).

1,25-DIHYDROXYVITAMIN D RECEPTOR AND ITS BIOLOGICAL ROLE IN VASCULAR

SMOOTH MUSCLE CELL FUNCTIONS

Hiroyuki Kawashima

Department of Pharmacology
Jichi Medical School
Minamikawachi-machi
Kawachi-gun, Tochigi-ken 329-04
Japan

INTRODUCTION

It is well established that 1,25-dihydroxyvitamin D_3 ($1,25(OH)_2 D_3$) has a major role in the regulation of calcium homeostasis. To achieve this, $1,25(OH)_2 D_3$ binds to its receptor followed by activating gene expression, which in turn, induce new protein synthesis such as calcium binding protein leading to cellular functions. The series of event have been established in the intestine, kidney and bone, which are principal tissues responsible for maintaining calcium homeostasis (1).

In addition to these well-known classical effects of $1,25(OH)_2 D_3$ in the regulation of the extra-cellular calcium metabolism, accumulating evidence suggests that $1,25(OH)_2 D_3$ has a variety of cellular functions in different types of tissues including cell differentiation, immunomodulation, and so on (2,3). Calcium is one of the most important factors not only in cellular functions but also in the signal transduction of many hormones and agents. Disturbances in both intra-cellular and extra-cellular calcium homeostasis has been known in the hypertension in animals as well as humans (4-6). However, the exact mechanism which lead to the hypertension is not known. The favorable effect of oral calcium supplement to hypertension has been seemingly controversial. However, since calcium, per se, can not be attributable to the effect of calcium supplement, other factors may possibly be responsible for the effect. These can be any factors, but calcium regulating hormones are most probable. We have demonstrated recently that vitamin D metabolism is impaired in the spontaneously hypertensive rat (SHR), the genetic model of the essential hypertension (7). We have also found that $1,25(OH)_2 D_3$ receptor in the kidney was reduced in the SHR, which may at least in part, explain the reported calcium leak in this animal model as well as in the essential hypertension (8). In addition, Kowarski et al., recently demonstrated that the integrated membrane calcium binding protein (IMCAL), which is vitamin D dependent, is reduced in various tissues in the SHR, and this is in parallel with the reduced calcium binding capacity of cell membrane in this animal model of hypertension (9). These data strongly suggest that vitamin D dependent process may be also involved in the cellular calcium handling, and disturbances in this function may lead to the development or exaggeration of hypertension, since intracellular calcium is the most

New Actions of Parathyroid Hormone
Edited by S. G. Massry and T. Fujita
Plenum Press, New York

probable cause of increased vascular tone. If vitamin D is involved in the cellular calcium regulation, it is natural that vitamin D-related parameters may appear abnormal. Since a receptor mediated event has been always the way this hormone functions, it is reasonable to assume that any target tissue must have receptor for $1,25(OH)_2D_3$. This led us to search for $1,25(OH)_2D_3$ receptor in a vascular smooth muscle cell. Here I report in the present paper that a vascular smooth muscle cell line, A_7r_5, which is derived from fetal rat aorta, has receptors for $1,25(OH)_2D_3$. I will also discuss possible functions of the receptor in the regulation of intracellular calcium in relation to hypertension.

MATERIALS AND METHODS

Tissue culture: A cell line, A_7r_5, was purchased from the American Type Culture Collection, and incubated in DMEM containing 10% fetal calf serum at $37^\circ C$ in the atmosphere of 95% O_2 and 5% CO_2. At subconfluence, cells were detached by the treatment with trypsin EDTA (Gibco) for 3 minutes. Cells were collected, washed three times with Hanks' solution, and homogenized in the KTED buffer (50 mM Tris-HCl, 300 mM KCl, 1.5 mM EDTA, and 5.0 mM dithiothreitol, pH 7.4) by three bursts of sonicator. The homogenates were centrifuged for 60 min at 105,000 x g and $4^\circ C$ to prepare cytosol. The cytosol was stored at $-70^\circ C$ until use.

Equilibrium binding studies: Aliquots of cytosol (0.5 mg protein/0.5 ml) was incubated for 18 hr at $4^\circ C$ with graded amount of $1,25(OH)_2[26,27-methyl-^3H]D_3$ (specific activity: 160 Ci/mmol, Amersham, Arlington Heights, IL, U.S.A.) in the presence or absence of excess amount (200-fold) $1,25(OH)_2D_3$ (generously given by Dr. Uskokovic of Hoffman-La Roche, Nuttley, NJ, U.S.A.). Each tube received 200 µl of dextran-coated charcoal, incubated for additional 10 min, and centrifuged for 10 min at $4^\circ C$ and 2000 x g. The supernatant was transferred to a vial and radioactivity was determined by means of liquid scintillation counter. Specific binding was obtained by subtracting non-specific binding from the total binding. Binding data were obtained by the Scatchard analysis.

Sucrose density gradient analysis: Aliquots of receptor (1 mg protein/ml) were incubated at $4^\circ C$ for 3 hr with $1,25(OH)_2[^3H]D_3$ in the presence or absence of excess (100-fold) amount of $1,25(OH)_2D_3$. Alternatively, a 100-fold excess of unlabeled 24,25-dihydroxyvitamin D3 ($24,25(OH)_2D_3$)(a gift from Dr. Uskokovic of Hoffman-La Roche) or 25-hydroxyvitamin D_3 ($25-(OH)D_3$)(kindly provided by the Upjohn Co., Kalamazoo, MI, U.S.A.) were incubated with $1,25(OH)_2[^3H]D_3$ to test specificity of the binding. Bound hormones were separated from free by absorption of free hormones to dextran-coated charcoal as described above and 0.2 ml aliquots were put on the top layer of the discontinuous sucrose gradient (4-20%sucrose in KTED buffer) and centrifuged for 20 hr at 260,000 x g and $4^\circ C$. Fractions (0.2 ml each) were collected from the bottom and counted for the radioactivity. As a molecular size marker, ^{14}C-ovalbumin was added to each tube.

DNA cellulose chromatography: Cytosol was prepared in KTED buffer. DNA-cellulose was purchased from Sigma Chemicals. Cytosol was labeled with 1 nM $1,25(OH)_2[^3H]D_3$ at $4^\circ C$ for 3 hr, and bound hormone was separated from free as described above. The labeled cytosol was then diluted 6-fold in TED buffer (50 mM Tris-HCl, 1.5 mM EDTA, 5.0 mM dithiothreitol, pH 7.4). One milliliter of cytosol was incubated for 30 min at $0^\circ C$ with a 2-ml packed volume of DNA-cellulose in a batch technique. Then the DNA-cellulose slurry was packed into 3-ml plastic syringe, and the column was rinsed with 20 ml of TED buffer and eluted with a 40-ml 0.05-0.5 M KCl gradient.

RESULTS AND DISCUSSION

$1,25(OH)_2D_3$ bound to the cytosol prepared from the vascular smooth muscle cells and the binding was saturable at 1nM. Scatchard analysis revealed that dissociation constant (K_d) and number of binding site were 3.02x10 M and 33.9 fmole/mg protein. Sucrose density gradient analysis yielded 3.2S for the sedimentation constant. DNA cellulose chromatography also resulted in demonstrating a typical profile of receptor for $1,25-(OH)_2D$. When $24,25(OH)_2D_3$ or $25(OH)D_3$ was incubated with $H-1,25(OH)_2D_3$ in the presence of the receptor the displacement curve shifted to the right and three orders of magnitude higher concentration were needed for these metabolites to displace the bound $1,25(OH)_2D_3$, demonstrating that the binding site is specific for $1,25(OH)_2D_3$. These results indicate that vascular smooth muscle cell has receptors for $1,25(OH)_2D_3$.

To test possible roles of $1,25(OH)_2D_3$ receptor in smooth muscle cells, we first examined metabolism of $H-25(OH)_2D_3$. It is found that the cells metabolize $^3H-25(OH)D_3$ to at least 5 metabolites including $24,25(OH)_2D_3$ and a major metabolite, designated peak A. Production of the peak A was suppressed by $1,25(OH)_2D_3$ in a dose dependent manner suggesting that this seemingly new metabolite may have some role in maintaining the cell function intact.

To investigate a possibility that $1,25(OH)_2D_3$ may directly regulate cellular calcium metabolism, Ca-ATPase activity was determined. $1,25-(OH)_2D_3$ stimulated Ca-ATPase in a dose dependent manner at 0.1-1nM. By contrast, either $24,25(OH)_2D_3$ or $25(OH)D_3$ had a much less effect, namely, approximately three orders of magnitude higher concentration was necessary for the stimulation of the enzyme for these two metabolites, respectively. These findings indicate that the stimulation by $1,25(OH)_2D_3$ of Ca-ATPase is mediated through binding to the receptor followed by a genetic activation leading to the new synthesis of Ca-ATPase enzyme itself. When cells were incubated with $1,25(OH)_2D_3$ for 30 and 60 minutes, the activity of Ca-ATPase was not affected. Furthermore, when the cells were incubated with $1,25(OH)_2D_3$ in the presence of cycloheximide, the effect of $1,25(OH)_2D_3$ was abolished. These results strongly indicate that the effect of $1,25-(OH)_2D_3$ is mediated by a genomic activation followed by the synthesis of Ca-ATPase itself. To further define the effect of $1,25(OH)_2D_3$ on the cellular calcium, Ca-uptake by the cells was determined. Incubation of the cells with $1,25(OH)_2D_3$ increased calcium uptake in a dose dependent manner at 0.1-3nM. The highest stimulation was obtained at 3nM, in which the Ca-uptake increased by 50%. When cells were incubated with 10nM $1,25-(OH)_2D_3$ the increase in calcium uptake was only 20%. The bell-shaped effect like this has been known in the differentiation-inducing action of $1,25(OH)_2D_3$. The Ca-uptake by the cells was also time dependent, reaching to a plateau at 30 min at $27^\circ C$. Similar stimulative effect of $1,25(OH)_2D_3$ on the calcium uptake by primary cell culture of rat has recently been reported by others (10). Whether or not the effect of Ca-ATPase is secondary to the increased Ca-uptake by the cell remains to be studied in the future.

In summary, present data clearly demonstrate the receptor mediated regulation by $1,25(OH)_2D_3$ of cellular calcium, and possible involvement of some abnormalities in this function in the development and maintenance of hypertension.

ACKNOWLEDGMENT

This work was supported, in part, by a Grant-in-Aid from Mochida memorial foundation and by Grants-in-Aid for Scientific Research from Ministry of Education, Science and Culture of Japan (6121509, 62105002 and 62870103).

REFERENCES

1. Norman, A. W. (1979). Vitamin D : The calcium Homeostatic Steroid Hormone. Academic Press, New York

2. Abe, E., Miyaura, C., Sakagami, H., Takeda, M., Konno, K., Yamazaki, T., Yoshiki, S., and Suda, T. (1981) Proc. Natl. Acad. Sci. **78,**4990-4994.

3. Lemire, J. M., Adams, J. S., Sakai, R. and Jordan, S. C. (1984) J. Clin. Invest. **74,** 657-661.

4. McCarron, D. A. (1985) Hypertension **7,** 607-627.

5. Postnov, Y. V. and Orlov, S. N. (1984) J. Hypertens. **2,** 1-6.

6. Robinson, B. F. (1984) J. Hypertens. **2,** 453-460

7. Kawashima, H. (1986) Biochem. J. **237,** 893-897.

8. Kawashima, H. (1987) In Calcium Regulation and Bone Metabolism. Basic and Clinical Aspects. vol.IX, pp602, Elsevier Science Publishers B.U., Amsterdam.

9. Kowarski, S., Cowen, L. A. and Schachter, D. (1986) Proc. Natl. Acad. Sci. **83,** 1097-1100.

10. Bukoski, R. D., Sue, H. and McCarron, D. A. (1987) Biochem. Biophys. Res. Commun. **146,** 1330-1335.

Correspondence should be addressed to the present address :

Central Research Laboratories
Yamanouchi Pharmaceutical Co., Ltd.
1-8 Azusawa 1-chome,
Itabashi-ku, Tokyo 174, Japan

ROLE OF CALCIUM UPTAKE AND CYCLIC AMP IN THE VASCULAR EFFECTS OF PTH

R. Schleiffer, C. Bergmann, P. Schoeffter, F. Pernot and
A. Gairard

Fac. Pharmacie, Lab. Physiologie, Univ.Louis Pasteur
CNRS UA 600, BP 10, 67048 Strasbourg Cedex France

INTRODUCTION

There is experimental evidence for a cardiovascular effect of parathyroid hormone (PTH). A rapid positive inotropic and chronotropic
action of PTH has been described in different animal species in both in
vivo and in vitro conditions (Lhoste et al., 1980; Bogin et al., 1981;
Hashimoto et al., 1981; Katoh et al., 1984). Evidence has also been
accumulated showing that PTH is hypotensive and is a vasodilator
(Charbon, 1968; Charbon and Hustaert, 1974; Schleiffer et al., 1979; Pang
et al., 1980; Ellison and Mc Carron, 1984; Saglikes et al., 1985). These
latter effects seem to be a direct relaxation of vascular smooth muscle
(Suzuki et al., 1983; Pang et al., 1984; Nickols et al., 1987). The
mechanisms responsible for this effect have not been clearly defined
although recent reports have described a stimulation of vascular adenylate cyclase activity (Huang et al., 1983; Helwig et al., 1984; Pang et
al., 1985; Nickols et al., 1986; Nickols and Cline, 1987; Bergmann et
al., 1987). It is generally accepted that cyclic adenosine monophosphate
(cAMP) as well as the cytosolic Ca^{++} concentration modulate vascular
smooth muscle tone. To gain more information on the mechanisms of
vascular effect of PTH we have studied the effects of PTH on contractile
responses, transmembrane Ca^{++} fluxes and cAMP content in rat vascular
preparations.

MATERIAL AND METHODS

The studies were performed in male Wistar and Sprague Dawley adult
rats. We used a synthetic bovine PTH analog containing the 34 first N-
terminal aminoacids [bPTH-(1-34)] obtained from Peninsula and Bachem
Laboratories. Blood pressure measurements were made in pentobarbital-
anesthetized animals by cannulated carotid artery. bPTH-(1-34) and
solvent were administrated intravenously through a jugular vein.

Mechanical responses were recorded in vitro in aortic rings. The
inhibitory contractile effects of bPTH-(1-34) were studied on contractions induced by noradrenaline (NA). The amplitudes of the phasic and
tonic components and maximum of the contraction were measured (see Fig.
1, left). Relaxing responses to bPTH-(1-34) were measured in tissues
precontracted with either NA or prostaglandin $F_{2\alpha}$ (PGF$_{2\alpha}$).

New Actions of Parathyroid Hormone
Edited by S. G. Massry and T. Fujita
Plenum Press, New York

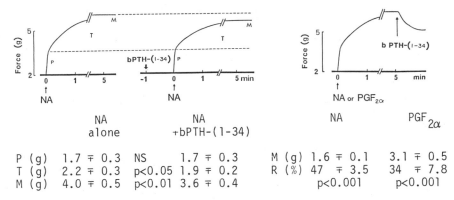

	NA alone		NA +bPTH-(1-34)		NA	PGF$_{2\alpha}$
P (g)	1.7 ∓ 0.3	NS	1.7 ∓ 0.3	M (g)	1.6 ∓ 0.1	3.1 ∓ 0.5
T (g)	2.2 ∓ 0.3	p<0.05	1.9 ∓ 0.2	R (%)	47 ∓ 3.5	34 ∓ 7.8
M (g)	4.0 ∓ 0.5	p<0.01	3.6 ∓ 0.4		p<0.001	p<0.001

Fig. 1. Mechanical responses of isolated aorta. Left: Effect of bPTH-(1-34) 10^{-7}M on the phasic (P) and tonic (T) components and maximum (M = P+T) of the contraction induced by noradrenaline (NA, 10^{-6}M). Values are means $\mp$ SEM of 6 observations. Right : Relaxing effect (R) of bPTH-(1-34) 10^{-7}M. Contractions were induced by NA (10^{-6}M) and prostaglandins (PGF$_{2\alpha}$, 3×10^{-7}M). Values are means $\mp$ SEM of 4-10 observations and expressed as percent reduction of maximal force (M).

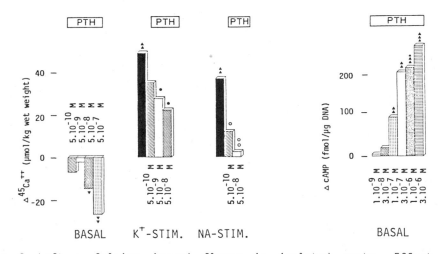

Fig. 2. Left : Calcium inward fluxes in isolated aorta. Effect of increasing concentrations (5.10^{-10}M to 5.10^{-8}M) of bPTH-(1-34) with or without depolarization (K^{+}) - or noradrenaline (NA) - stimulated Ca^{++} inward fluxes. Ca^{++} fluxes across the cell membrane were estimated by measuring the rate of uptake of Ca^{++} into the La^{3+}-resistant Ca^{++} fraction. Changes of $^{45}Ca^{++}$ were measured for 2 min and expressed as the difference between experimental and control (without PTH and agonist) levels. Significance of change from control : ▲ p<0.05, ▲▲ p<0.01 ; from K^{+} (10^{-1}M) alone : ● p<0.05 and from NA (10^{-6}M) alone : o p<0.01, oo p<0.01, (n>6). Right : Cyclic AMP levels of isolated aorta. Effect of a 2 min exposure to increasing concentrations (10^{-9}M to 3.10^{-6}M) of bPTH-(1-34) on cAMP levels of rat aorta. The results are expressed as the difference between experimental and control (without PTH) levels. Significance of change from control : ▲▲ p<0.01, ▲▲▲ p<0.001, (n>6).

Calcium fluxes were performed in isolated aortic strips. Ca^{++} inward fluxes were estimated by measuring the changes in the $^{45}Ca^{++}$ contents by means of the lanthanum method as previously described (Godfraind, 1976). Ca^{++} outward fluxes were measured in isolated aortic strips (Deth and Casteels, 1977) and in primary cultured aortic myocytes (Lassègue and Stoclet, 1986).

The effects of bPTH-(1-34) on vascular adenylate cyclase activity were determined by measurement of aortic cAMP levels (Cailla et al., 1973) in the presence of IBMX (5×10^{-4}M).

RESULTS

Both preparations of bPTH-(1-34) used in this study produced similar dose-related (4×10^{-10} to 6.7×10^{-9} mol/kg) decreases in mean arterial pressure (-5.3 to - 34.8 mmHg). This hypotensive action reaches a maximum 1 to 2 min after injection.

Fig. 1, shows that bPTH-(1-34) did not alter the phasic component of the contraction of isolated aorta induced by NA, but significantly decreased the tonic component. This decrease is sufficient to explain the reduction of the maximum mechanical response. bPTH-(1-34) also produced a consistent (48 and 34 %) relaxation of aortic rings precontracted with either NA or $PGF_{2\alpha}$.

There was no significant modification of Ca^{++} outward fluxes neither in aortic strips nor in cultured myocytes for any concentration of bPTH-(1-34) tested (4×10^{-10} to 4×10^{-8} M) [data not shown]. In contrast, Ca^{++} inward fluxes were significantly affected (Fig. 2). bPTH-(1-34) in a concentration-dependent fashion decreased basal Ca^{++} inward flux and partially inhibited Ca^{++} inward fluxes stimulated by NA or K^{+}-depolarizing solution. On the other hand, bPTH-(1-34) produced a concentration-dependent rise in aortic cAMP production (Fig. 2).

DISCUSSION

Results obtained in the present studies demonstrate that vascular effects (inhibition of contraction and relaxation) of bPTH-(1-34) involve changes in Ca^{++} fluxes and adenylate cyclase activity. Firstly, bPTH-(1-34) decreases the tonic component of NA-induced vascular contraction, a response which is associated with increased Ca^{++} entry. Secondly, it reduces both basal and stimulated Ca^{++} inward fluxes in isolated vessels, without affecting Ca^{++} outward fluxes. Thirdly, vascular adenylate cyclase activity, determined by cAMP measurements, increased in the presence of bPTH-(1-34). Experimental data suggest that bPTH-(1-34) has direct action on vascular smooth muscle cells. It has been shown that bPTH-(1-34) induced vasorelaxation is endothelium-independent (Pang et al., 1985; Nickols, 1985), inhibits NA induced contraction and relaxes NA precontracted cultured rat aortic myocytes (Bodin et al., unpublished data) and increases cAMP levels in cultured vascular smooth muscle cells from bovine, rabbit (Nickols, 1985) and rat (Bergmann et al., 1987). Based on these observations, we propose a schematic model of possible mechanisms whereby bPTH-(1-34) might act on vascular smooth muscle cells (Fig. 3). This simplified model does not exclude other events or factors that can influence the contractile state of the smooth muscle (e.g. calmodulin, Na,K-ATPase, the phosphoinositide cycle, cGMP, etc...).

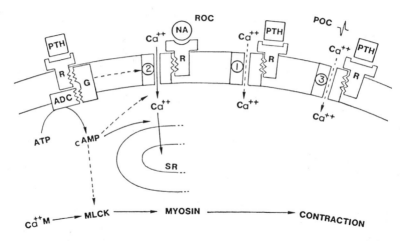

Fig.3. Schematic drawing of possible mechanisms whereby PTH might act on vascular smooth muscle. Cell action begins with receptor (R) binding. The hormone-receptor complex (PTH-R) stimulates adenylate cyclase (ADC) activity and the production of cAMP which inhibits the myosin light chain kinase (MLCK) and stimulates Ca^{++} flux into sarcoplasmic reticulum (SR) which would contribute to a decrease in cytosolic Ca^{++} concentration and induce relaxation. PTH-R also leads to a decrease in Ca^{++} inward fluxes via an inhibition of basal influx (1) and of receptor- (ROC) (2) and potential-(POC) (3) operated channels. Full arrows indicate activatory actions and interrupted arrows inhibitory actions.

ACKNOWLEDGMENTS

We gratefully acknowledge the collaboration of S. Toupozis and B. Lassègue.

REFERENCES

Bergmann, C. ; Schoeffter, P., Stoclet, J.C. and Gairard, A., 1987, Effect of parathyroid hormone and antagonist on aortic cAMP levels. Can. J. Physiol. Pharmacol., in press.

Bogin, E., Massry, S.G., and Harary, I., 1981, Effect of parathyroid hormone on rat heart cells. J. Clin. Invest. 67 : 1215-1227.

Cailla, H.L., Racine-Weisbuch, M.S. and Delaage, M.A., 1973, Adenosine 3',5'-cyclic monophosphate assay at 10^{-15} mole level. Anal. Biochem. 56 : 394-407.

Charbon, G.A., 1968, A diuretic and hypotensive action of a parathyroid extract. Acta Physiol. Pharmacol. Neerl. 14 : 52-53.

Charbon, G., and Hulstaert, R.F., 1974. Augmentation of arterial and renal flow by extracted and synthetic parathyroid hormone. Endocrinoloy 96 : 621-626.

Deth, R.C., and Casteels, R., 1977, A study of releasable Ca fractions in smooth muscle cells of the rabbit aorta. J. Gen. Physiol. 69 : 401-416.

Ellison, D.H., and Mc Carron, D.A., 1984, Structure preriquisites for the hypotensive action of parathyroid hormone. Am. J. Physiol. 246 : (Renal Fluid Electrolyte Physiol. 15) : F 551-F 556.

Godfraind, T., 1976, Calcium exchange in vascular smooth muscle, action of noradrenaline and lanthanum. J. Physiol. (London) 260 : 21-35.

Hashimoto, K., Nakagawa, Y., Shibuya, T., Satoh, H., Ushijuima, T., and Imai, S., 1981, Effect of parathyroid hormone and related polypeptides on the heart and coronary circulation of dogs. J. Cardiovasc. Pharmacol. 3 : 668-676.

Helwig, J.J., Schleiffer, R., Judes, C., and Gairard, A., 1984, Distribution of parathyroid hormone-sensitive adenylate cyclase in isolated rabbit renal cortex microvessels and glomeruli. Life Sci. 35 : 2649-2657.

Huang, M., Hanley, D.A., and Rorstad, O.P., 1983, Parathyroid hormone stimulates adenylate cyclase in rat cerebral microvessels. Life Sci. 32 : 1009-1014.

Katoh, Y., Klein, K.L., Kaplan, R.A., Sandborn, W.G., and Kurokawa, K., 1984, Parathyroid hormone has a positive inotropic action in the rat. Endocrinology 109 : 2252-2254.

Lassègue, B., and Stoclet, J.C., 1986, Phorbol ester inhibition of vasopressin-induced calcium efflux from cultured rat aortic myocytes. FEBS Letters 205 : 251-254.

Lhoste, F.T., Drueke, S.L., and Boissier, J.R., 1980, Cardiac interaction between parathyroid hormone, α-adrenoreceptor, and verapamil in the guinea pig in vitro. Clin. Exp. Pharmacol. Physiol. 7 : 377-385.

Nickols, G.A., 1985. Increased cyclic AMP in cultured vascular smooth muscle cells and relaxation of aortic strips by parathyroid hormone. Eur. J. Pharmacol. 116 : 137-144.

Nickols, A., and Cline, W.H., 1987, Parathyroid hormone-induced changes in cyclic nucleotide levels during relaxation on the rat aorta. Life Sci. 40 : 2351-2359.

Nickols, G.A., Metz, M.A., and Cline W.H., 1986, Endothelium-independent linkage of parathyroid hormone receptors of rat vascular tissue with increased adenosine 3',5'-monophosphate and relaxation of vascular smooth muscle. Endocrinology 119 : 349-356.

Pang, P.K.T., Hong, B., Yen, L., and Yang, M.C.M., 1984, Parathyroid hormone, a specific potent vasodilator in : Contr. Nephrol., Cardiocirculatory Function in Renal Disease, pp. 137-145, H. Jahn, S.G. Massry, E. Ritz, P. Weidmann, eds., Karger, Basel.

Pang, P.K.T., Janssen, H.F., and Yee, J.A., 1980, Effects of synthetic parathyroid hormone on vascular beds of dog. Pharmacology 21 : 213-222.

Pang, P.K.T., and Yang, M.C.M., 1985, The vasorelaxant action of parathyroid hormone fragments on isolated rat tail artery. Blood Vessels 22 : 57-64.

Pang, P.K.T., Yang, M.C., Tenner, T.E., Kenny, A.D., and Cooper, C.W., 1985, Cyclic AMP and the vascular action of parathyroid hormone. Can. J. Physiol. Pharmacol. 64 : 1543-1547.

Saglikes, Y., Massry, S.G., Iseki, K., Nadler, J.L., and Campese, V.M., 1985, Effect of PTH on blood pressure and response to vasoconstrictor agonists. Am. J. Physiol. 248 (Renal Fluid Electrolyte Physiol. 17) : F 674-F 681.

Schleiffer, R., Berthelot, A., and Gairard A., 1979, Action of parathyroid extract on arterial blood pressure and on contraction and [45]Ca exchange in isolated aorta of the rat. Eur. J. Pharmacol. 58 : 163-167.

Suzuki, Y., Lederis, K., Huang, M., Leblanc, F.E., and Rorstad, O.P., 1983, Relaxation of bovine, porcine and human brain arteries by parathyroid hormone. Life Sci. 33 : 2497-2503.

CORONARY VASODILATORY AND CARDIOTONIC EFFECTS OF PARATHYROID HORMONE IN

THE DOG

Keitaro Hashimoto

Department of Pharmacology
Yamanashi Medical College
Tamaho-cho, Japan

INTRODUCTION

Since Crass and Pang (1) reported coronary vasodilator and positive inotropic effects of parathyroid hormone (PTH), it has become clear that PTH definitely increased the coronary blood flow in dogs and decreased the blood pressure of rats (2-4). We also reported soon after Crass and Pang cardiovascular effects of PTH in the dog (2). However questions relating to those effects of PTH, such as on the species difference, selectivity on vascular muscle or cardiac muscle, cellular mechanisms of action, physiological role or its possible clinical implications are still open for discussion. This paper deals with the analysis of our previous paper (2) with a review of recently published papers.

PTH is a polypeptide containing 84 amino acids, the first 34 of which are necessary for its main biological action of raising serum Ca levels. Bovine, porcine, and human PTH differ slightly in the first 34 amino acid residues of the sequence. Crass and Pang demonstrated effects of the synthetic bovine polypeptide with 34 amino acids, PTH-(1-34), on the canine coronary artery of the in situ heart preparation, but the precise modes of action on the coronary vasculature have not been documented (1). We wanted to examine (a) whether the coronary vasodilatory effect of synthetic bovine PTH-(1-34) reported by Crass and Pang (1) is an indirect one resulting from the increase in O_2 consumption due to its positive inotropic and chronotropic effects, (b) whether natural PTH has similar vasodilatory action, (c) whether changes in the serum Ca level accompany the coronary dilator action, and (d) whether smaller fragments of PTH also have coronary vasodilator action. We examined five polypeptides: natural bovine PTH-(1-84) and synthetic bovine PTH-(24-28) containing 5 amino acids, and synthetic PTH-(25-27) containing 3 amino acids for their coronary and cardiac action using the canine heart-lung preparation.

METHODS

We used canine heart-lung preparation supported by a donor, and this allowed us to examine specifically the effects of PTH on coronary vasculature and cardiac functions. Mongrel dogs of either sex, weighing 7-12 kg were anesthetized with pentobarbital sodium (35 mg/kg, i.p.). Heart-lung preparations were prepared as described previously. Coronary sinus outflow was drawn out by a Morawitz cannula and sent to the donor via the femoral vein. The donor dogs, weighing 20-30 kg, were anesthetized with intravenous chloralose (45 mg/kg) and urethane (450 mg/kg) after premedication with morphine (1.5 mg/kg, s.c.). A cannulating-type probe (2 mm i.d.) of an electromagnetic flowmeter (Nihon Kohden MF-26) was placed between the Morawitz cannula and the donor to record the coronary blood flow. By using the donor the coronary vascular tone could be maintained in the heart-lung preparation long enough to compare several drugs in one preparation. The level of the venous reservoir of the heart-lung preparation was kept constant by overflowing, and the excess blood was returned to the larger reservoir by gravity. Systemic output was measured using an electromagnetic flowmeter probe (Nihon Kohden MF-26, 1 cm i.d.) placed at the tubing from the aorta. Myocardial contractility was assessed from recordings of the right atrial pressure and the first differential (dP/dt) of the left intraventricular pressure, which was recorded by inserting a polyethylene cannula at the apex. The heart rate was recorded with a cardiotachometer (Nihon Kohden RT-5) triggered by R waves of the electrocardiogram. The oxygen consumption of the myocardium was calculated by multiplying the coronary-arteriovenous O_2 difference of the blood (vol. %) by the corresponding coronary flow (ml/min/100g heart). The arteriovenous O_2 content difference was continuously and automatically recorded using an Avox Systems, which gave O_2 saturation (%) x hemoglobin content (g/dl) x 0.0136 (O_2 capacity of the hemoglobin, ml/g).

Plasma Ca and inorganic P (P_i) was assayed using the method of Trinder (5), and P_i was assayed by the method of Delsal and Manhouri (6), but there were no significant changes during the experiment.

RESULTS

Effects of PTH-(1-34) on the heart and coronary circulation

PTH-(1-34) introduced into the left atrium (hereafter referred to as intra-arterial injection) increased the coronary flow, decreased the arteriovenous O_2 difference and slightly increased the heart rate (Fig. 1). These prominent coronary vasodilatory effects were produced by a dose of 100 U (10 μg) PTH-(1-34), but these actions could also be observed after the low dose of 10 U (1 μg). The positive inotropic effect of PTH-(1-34) was observed as the decrease in the right atrial pressure and by the increase in the dP/dt of the intraventricular pressure, however it was not as prominent as the coronary vasodilatory effect. This was confirmed by a later paper of Crass et al. (4), that at least in the dog PTH has a prominent coronary vasodilator effect, but has only a weak positive inotropic effect.

Figure 2 shows summarized data of the effects of 100 U PTH-(1-34) from six experiments. PTH-(1-34) almost doubled the coronary blood flow, decreased the right atrial pressure, and only slightly increased the heart rate. This increase in the coronary flow was approximately two thirds of the maximal increase in the coronary flow inducible by adenosine. O_2 consumption increased 30 sec after injection but soon returned to the control value.

The responses to intravenous and intra-arterial injection of PTH-(1-34) were compared in two experiments, and there were no quantitative or qualitative differences. This suggests that there was no inactivation of PTH-(1-34) by the lung. It is interesting that effects of many physiologically important mediators of vascular smooth muscle tone are known to be enhanced or decreased by the passage through the pulmonary circulation.

Figure 3 shows the relationship between the percentage increase in the O_2 consumption and the percentage increase in the coronary blood flow observed 5 min after intra-arterial injection of PTH-(1-34), 30-300 U.

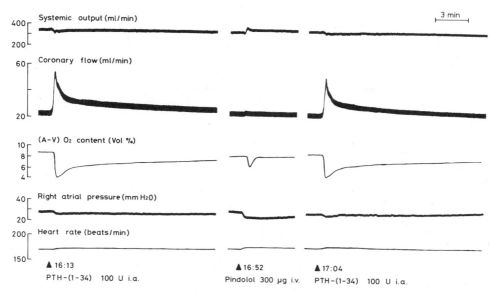

Fig. 1. Effects of PTH-(1-34). Pindolol did not modify the positive inotropic and chronotropic effects.

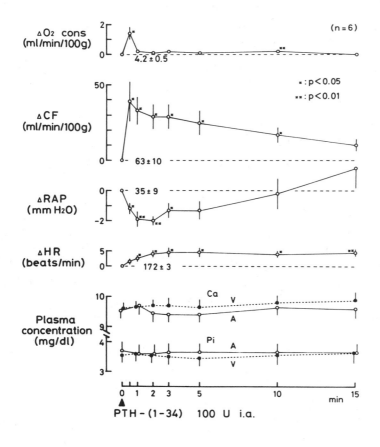

Fig. 2. Summary of effects of PTH-(1-34), 100 U, i.a. O_2 cons: myocardial O_2 consumption; CF: coronary flow; RAP: right atrial pressure; HR: heart rate. Bar represents SEM. * indicates statistically significant change from the control value.

PTH-(1-34) increased coronary flow without a great increase in the O_2 consumption, suggesting a specific vasodilatory effect of PTH-(1-34) on the coronary vasculature than on the positive inotropic and chronotropic effects.

PTH-(1-34) did not modify the transient vasodilatory effect of intravenous adenosine (1-3 mg).

The effects of pindolol, 300 g, i.v., on the actions of PTH-(1-34) were examined. As shown in Fig. 1, neither the cardiac nor coronary effects of PTH-(1-34) were influenced by pindolol. The direct effect of PTH on the cardiovascular system was further confirmed by using alpha blocking, antimuscarinic, anti H_1 and H_2 receptor blocking drugs (4).

Effects of PTH-(1-84)

PTH-(1-84) showed coronary vasodilatory and positive chronotropic and inotropic effects qualitatively similar to those of PTH-(1-34). It increased the coronary flow without significantly increasing O_2 consumption. The effects of PTH-(1-84) were unchanged by pindolol and were not accompanied by changes in serum Ca and P_i concentrations.

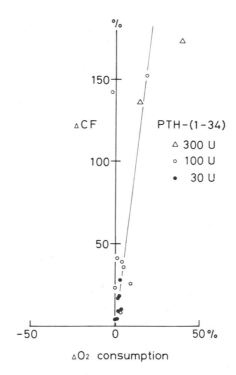

Fig. 3. Effects of PTH-(1-34) on the relationship between the changes in the myocardial oxygen consumption and the changes in the coronary flow.

Effects of synthetic fragments of PTH, PTH-(24-34), PTH-(24-28), and PTH-(25-27)

A high dose of PTH-(24-34), 1 mg, i.a., produced a transient increase in the coronary blood flow. This effect disappeared 1 min after injection, and there were no cardiac stimulatory effects. Fragments containing a smaller number of amino acids, PTH-(24-28) and PTH-(25-27), also had similar effects, but the coronary dilatory effects were much smaller (Fig. 4). In a high dose of 1 mg, there was also a transient coronary vasodilatory effect of the solvent. Thus the responses shown in Fig. 4 were plotted as the actual drug response, subtracting the effects of the solvent from the drug responses.

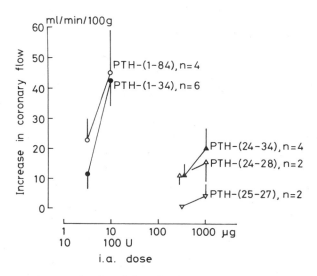

Fig. 4. Dose-response relationships in increasing coronary flow. The dose of PTH-(1-84) and PTH-(1-34) are expressed as units, where 10 U of PTH-(1-34) is 1 μg. The doses of PTH-(24-34), PTH-(24-28), and PTH-(25-27) are expressed in μg. Bar represents SEM.

DISCUSSION

Our previous study using the dog heart-lung preparation showed a coronary vasodilatory effect of PTH-(1-34), which in a dose range of 30-300 U, increased the coronary blood flow for about 15 min with no significant change in O_2 consumption. This direct coronary dilating action was accompanied by slight positive chronotropic and inotropic effects, which were not blocked by the beta blocker pindolol. Later studies further showed that the effect was not produced by muscarinic or H_1 and H_2 histamine receptors (4). The predominant coronary vasodilator effect was at least proved in dogs, but it is still controversial whether the vasodilator effect of PTH is specific to coronary vasculature.

Because of the difficulty in measuring the coronary blood flow of the rat, coronary selectivity has not yet been proven in rats, but as the previous rat studies showed dose-related hypotensive effects (7,8), there may exist some species difference in the vascular effect. Similar, but slightly stronger and longer-lasting effects were observed for the natural bovine PTH-(1-84). However, fragments of PTH containing a smaller number of amino acids showed only transient (less than 1 min duration) coronary dilating action and did not show any cardiac stimulatory effect. These results indicate that the active portions of amino acids eliciting coronary and cardiac actions are found in the first 34 amino acids of the total sequence of 84. Since the smaller fragments between residues 24-34 were almost inactive, the amino acid 1-23 or the whole sequence of 34 amino acids may be important in eliciting coronary and cardiac actions. These results must have decreased the opportunity of PTH fragments to be developed as a therapeutic coronary vasodilator, especially after successful introduction of various Ca antagonists, but it raised a further question as to the physiological role of PTH in the blood flow regulation. As far as judging from the paper of Crass et al. (4) and Nichols (3), it may have some role because of the possible presence of natural PTH in the circulation and also the low dose range of the PTH to cause vasodilation.

As for the mechanism of the weak cardiac stimulating action of PTH-(1-34) and PTH-(1-84), they are not due to beta receptor stimulation. As a coronary vasodilator, PTH-(1-34) did not potentiate the response to intravenous adenosine, showing that PTH is quite different from coronary dilators such as dipyridamole and dilazep (9).

The precise cellular mechanism of coronary vasodilatation has been postulated that PTH inhibit cyclic nucleotide phosphodiesterase and accumulation of intracellular cyclic AMP occurs (3,10), but it needs to be further clarified. As for the clinical implication of the use of PTH in coronary vascular diseases, Feola and Crass recently showed that PTH reduces infarct size of the dog acute myocardial infarction model (11). However there have been many reports relating efficacy in reducing infarct size by various drugs with different mechanism of action (see reference of Hashimoto (12)), so some comparative study is needed to extend this observation to clinical application.

In the present paper, we can conclude that PTH has specific vasodilator effects, and possible clinical usage may be suggested, but the role of PTH in the physiological regulation of coronary blood flow and also in the pathological processes of cardiovascular diseases must be studied in the future.

REFERENCES

1. M.F. Crass III, and P.K.T. Pang, Parathyroid hormone: A coronary artery vasodilator, Science 207:1087 (1980)
2. K. Hashimoto, Y. Nakagawa, T. Shibuya, H. Satoh, T. Ushijima, and S. Imai, Effects of parathyroid hormone and related polypeptides on the heart and coronary circulation of dogs, J. Cardiovasc. Pharmacol. 3:668 (1981)
3. G.A. Nickols, Actions of parathyroid hormone in the cardiovascular system, Blood Vessels 24:120 (1987)
4. M.F. Crass III, P.L. Moore, M.L. Strickland, P.K.T. Pang, and M.S. Citak, Cardiovascular responses to parathyroid hormone, Am. J. Physiol. 249:E187, (1985)

5. P. Trinder, Colorimetric micro-determination of calcium in serum, Analyst 85:889 (1960)

6. J-L. Delsal, and H. Manhouri, Etude comparative des dosages colorimetriques du phosphore. IV. Dosage de l'orthophosphate en presence d'esters phosphoriques (nouvelles methodes), Bull Soc Chim Biol 40:1623 (1958)

7. R. Nakamura, H. Sokabe, T. Kimura, and S. Sakakibara, Action of fragments of human parathyroid hormone on blood pressure in rats, Endocrinol. Japon. 28:547 (1981)

8. P.K.T. Pang, T. E. Tenner Jr, Y. A. Yee, M. Yang, and H.F. Janssen, Hypotensive action of parathyroid hormone preparations on rats and dogs, Proc Natl Acad Sci USA 77:675 (1980)

9. Y. Katano, K. Takeda, T. Otorii, D. Horii, and S. Imai, Effects of dilazep, dipyridamole and hexobendine on the heart and coronary circulation, Fol. Pharmacol Jpn 70:305 (1974)

10. E. Bogin, S.G. Massry, and I. Harary, Effect of parathyroid hormone on rat heart cells, J. Clin. Invest. 67:1215 (1981)

11. M. Feola, and M.F. Crass III, Parathyroid hormone reduces acute ischemic injury of the myocardium, Surg. Gyne. Obst. 163: 523 (1986)

12. K. Hashimoto, H. Mitsuhashi, T. Nakamura, and K. Akiyama, Antiarrhythmic effects of possible anti-ischemic drugs, in "Proc. 4th Cong. Hung. Pharmacol. Soc. Budapest 1985 Vol. 1. Sec. 1. Pharmacological protection of the myocardium", L. Szekeres, and J.Gy. Papp, ed., Akademiai Kiado, Budapest (1985)

RECENT ADVANCES IN THE STUDY OF THE VASCULAR ACTION OF PARATHYROID HORMONE

Peter K.T. Pang

Department of Physiology
University of Alberta
Edmonton, Alberta, Canada
T6G 2H7

INTRODUCTION

Parathyroid hormone (PTH) has been demonstrated to be an important hormone in the maintenance of calcium and phosphate homeostasis in the vertebrate body. It keeps the plasma calcium and phosphate levels within a narrow range by regulating bone, intestinal and renal handling of these electrolytes. Many recent reports have described some "new" actions of PTH in target tissues, including a variety of smooth muscles, hepatic, adipose and juxtaglomerular (JG) cells. The effects on vascular smooth muscle tissue have probably been the most extensively investigated. However, the vascular or hypotensive action is, in fact, not so "new" as one thinks. It is as "old" as the discovery of PTH itself. When Collip and Clark (1925) first extracted PTH from the parathyroid glands, it was tested on dog blood pressure and a hypotensive effect was reported. Since then, there have been a number of reports on the vasodilating action of PTH extracts or synthetic fragments containing the amino terminal 1-34 [PTH-(1-34)] (Handler & Cohn, 1952; Charbon, 1966; Charbon & Hulstaert, 1974; Berthelot & Gairard, 1975; Nickols et al., 1986). There is, however, considerable scepticism about these new actions of PTH because the concentration of PTH needed to produce such effects often exceeds that reasonably expected to be found in the circulation. The physiological meaning of such pharmacological actions therefore remains doubtful. Nevertheless, many of these actions are probably receptor mediated. Why do these target organs have PTH receptors and why are they capable of responding to PTH if these actions are physiologically irrelevant? These questions lead to several interesting aspects of these new actions of PTH which require further investigation. For example, 1) What is the mechanism of these new actions? Do these newly defined target cells respond with cellular events similar to those found in the more classical target organs such as the bone and kidney? 2) What are the structural requirements in the PTH molecule for the production of these new actions? How do these structure-activity relationships compare to those for the maintenance of calcium and phosphate homeo-

New Actions of Parathyroid Hormone
Edited by S. G. Massry and T. Fujita
Plenum Press, New York

stasis? 3) How can one study the physiological significance of these new actions? We have carried out many studies in an attempt to answer some of these questions. In the present paper, not all aspects of these new actions will be covered. Instead, the discussion will concentrate on two areas: the involvement of cellular calcium balance in the action of PTH on smooth muscle, especially vascular smooth muscle, and the demonstration of an extraparathyroid gland origin of PTH or a PTH-like substance. Hopefully, these findings will enhance our understanding of these new actions of PTH.

MECHANISM OF PTH ACTION ON SMOOTH MUSCLES

The discussion here will be mainly on vascular smooth muscle, which was studied most extensively. The hypotensive or vasorelaxing action of PTH is well established in *in vivo* (Charbon, 1966), *in situ* (Crass & Pang, 1980, Dowe & Joshua, 1987) and *in vitro* systems (Huang & Rorstad, 1984; Pang *et al*., 1985). The two cellular messengers that have been investigated in relation to the vascular action of PTH are cyclic adenosine monophosphate (cAMP) and calcium (Ca^{++}). Of the two, the involvement of cAMP has been more extensively reported. PTH has been shown to stimulate the adenylate cyclase of many target organs, especially those involved in plasma Ca^{++} regulation (Chase & Auerbach, 1968; Chase *et al*., 1969; Neuman & Schneider, 1980). Also, cAMP has been recognized to be involved in vascular tissue relaxation (Hardman, 1981). It is therefore not surprising that considerable emphasis has been placed on the involvement of adenylate cyclase and the vascular action of PTH. The supporting evidence comes from several approaches. The involvement of cAMP has been studied with *in vitro* vascular strip tension assays. It has been shown that a phosphodiesterase inhibitor and stimulator potentiated and decreased the vasorelaxing action of PTH, respectively (Pang *et al*., 1986a). The ability of PTH to increase vascular cAMP content has also been reported in vascular strips (Pang *et al*., 1986a) and cultured vascular smooth muscle cells (Nickols, 1985). Several investigators observed stimulation of adenylate cyclase in vascular tissues (Linder *et al*., 1978; Rambausek *et al*., 1982; Huang *et al*., 1983; Helwig *et al*., 1984). However, Stanton *et al*. (1985) observed a decrease in vascular smooth muscle cAMP 1 min after exposure to PTH. On the other hand, in intact rat tail artery and cultured vascular smooth muscle, an increase in tissue cAMP level was demonstrated 1 min after treatment with PTH (Pang *et al*., 1984; Nickols, 1985). The reason for such a discrepancy is not clear. Recently, Helwig *et al*. (1987) compared the effects of PTH on the adenylate cyclase system of rabbit renal microvessels and tubules and observed substantial differences in these two target tissues. First, the presence of GTP substantially potentiated the PTH responses in microvessels but only minimally in tubules. Second, oxidized PTH, which has little or no vasorelaxing effect (Pang *et al*., 1983; Hong *et al*., 1986), had little or no effect on renal microvessel adenylate cyclase but remained rather active in renal tubules. Third, PTH fragments [PTH-(3-34) and bPTH-(7-34)], which antagonized the vascular action of PTH (Daugirdis *et al*., 1987), inhibited the renal microvascular but not renal cyclase responses to PTH. These data indicate that, although cyclase stimulation by PTH may be present in many PTH target organs, there may be substantial differences between the PTH intracellular Ca^{++}. Both PTH and D600 had an insignificant effect on this intracellular Ca^{++}-dependent vasoconstriction. On the other hand, sodium nitroprusside, which can block intracellular Ca^{++} release, was effective in inhibiting such a vasoconstriction. The above three series of tension studies provide strong indications that the effect of PTH is related to extracellular and not intracellular Ca^{++} (Yang *et al*., 1983; unpublished data).

To measure the effect on Ca^{++} entry more directly, the low-affinity lanthanum- (La^{+++}) resistant pool of Ca^{++} was determined in rat tail artery strips. It is generally accepted that this pool of Ca^{++} represents Ca^{++} movement from outside to inside the cell. KCl (60 mM) significantly increased this Ca^{++} pool, suggesting an increase in Ca^{++} entry (Hester et al., 1979). PTH inhibited this increase in a dose-dependent manner. Such an effect was observed in rat tail artery and rabbit renal artery. A dose of BAY-K-8644 effective in producing vasoconstriction in the presence of 15 mM KCl also produces a substantial increase in Ca^{++} entry, as measured by this method. PTH significantly reduced such an increase in entry. In another project, we observed that arginine vasopressin (AVP) produced vasoconstriction in rat tail artery helical strips mainly by stimulating Ca^{++} entry (Mitchell et al., 1985). We tested the effect of PTH on this constricted tissue and found it to be even more effective than in tissues constricted with KCl. The determination of the low-affinity La^{+++}-resistant Ca^{++} pool revealed that indeed AVP stimulated Ca^{++} entry and PTH inhibited such an increase in a dose-dependent manner. These results (Pang et al., 1987a; Yang & Pang, unpublished data) give further support to our hypothesis that PTH relaxes blood vessels by blocking Ca^{++} entry into vascular smooth muscle.

To provide more definitive proof, we recently started a series of studies in which we attempted to measure calcium channel activities with a whole cell voltage clamp method. We began with cultured neuroblastoma cells (NIE-115) which are much easier to patch onto. Using the established criterion (Narahashi et al., 1987), we succeeded in identifying and measuring the T and L channels which are known to be present in vascular smooth muscle cells (Spedding, 1987). In our experiments, BAY-K-8644 significantly increased the activity of the L channel, which could be inhibited by the known calcium entry blocker, D600 (Wang, Karpinski & Pang, unpublished data). PTH also decreased the L channel in a dose-related manner. Subsequent addition of BAY-K-8644 to the same PTH-treated cells resulted in the reopening of the L channel, indicating the involvement of similar channels. At the end of all experiments, La^{+++} was used to show that the channels could be totally blocked by the nonspecific La^{+++}. As reported earlier, oxidized PTH has no vascular effect. It is therefore important that in our experiments, oxidized PTH also had no effect on the L channels. We have recently discovered an analog of PTH which is antagonistic to the vascular action of PTH. When tested in the voltage clamp experiment, this analog also antagonized the action of PTH on the L channel. These PTH studies on the neuroblastoma cells clearly show that PTH can block specific calcium channels (Pang, Karpinski & Wang, unpublished data). However, although the L channels in neuroblastoma cells are similar to those in vascular smooth muscle cells, it is still possible that the effect of PTH on these two cell types may be different. There are only a few patch clamp studies on vascular smooth muscle cells, partly because of the difficulty in holding the channel for a long enough period for manipulation and challenges. When we first started on vascular smooth muscle studies, we could observe L channels, but for only a few minutes. By modifying the microelectrode solution, we can now hold the L current for as long as 30 min. This is indeed most encouraging. In some preliminary studies, we investigated cultured rat tail artery smooth muscle cells which contracted in vitro to high calcium. The L channel in such cells was also inhibited by PTH (Wang, Karpinski & Pang, unpublished data). We are now confident that PTH can block calcium channels.

The tension, calcium flux and channel studies together provide very strong evidence that PTH produces vasorelaxation by blocking the calcium channel, thus inhibiting calcium entry from outside the vascular smooth muscle cell. Presumably intracellular free Ca^{++} concentration will be decreased, resulting in vascular relaxation. These studies are consistent with the effect of PTH on the JG cells, and it is known that renin release is stimulated by a decrease in intracellular free Ca^{++} concentration. PTH, being able to block Ca^{++} channels in vascular smooth muscle, should therefore release renin from such modified vascular smooth muscle cells as the JG cells (Lindner et al., 1978).

It has been reported that PTH increased Ca^{++} content in many tissues (Michelalis, 1970; Wong & Cohn, 1975; Bogin et al., 1981) and this would seem to contradict our finding that PTH blocks Ca^{++} entry in vascular smooth muscle. This is not so. The effect of PTH on cellular Ca^{++} balance depends on the target organs involved. For example, while PTH relaxes many types of smooth muscle, it has positive chronotropic and inotropic effect on the heart (Tenner et al., 1983). Such a stimulatory effect would probably involve an increase in extracellular free Ca^{++} concentration. Electrophysiological studies showed that PTH probably opened calcium channel in cardiac smooth muscle cells (Kondo et al., 1985). These results indicate that the same hormone, PTH, in two different smooth muscles can produce opposite effects on cellular calcium balance. They are not mutually exclusive. More extensive studies on other smooth muscles and other target tissues are necessary. Also, it will be interesting to understand the difference in receptors or post-receptor mechanisms in the vascular and cardiac smooth muscles which respond to PTH in an opposite manner.

PRESENCE OF PTH OR PTH-LIKE SUBSTANCE IN NEURAL TISSUES

In addition to studying the effect of PTH on vascular smooth muscle, we investigated several other smooth muscle preparations in vitro. We observed that PTH relaxed uterine (Pang et al., 1981), gastrointestinal (Yang et al., 1985), tracheal (Yen et al., 1983) and vas deferens (Zhang et al., 1985) tissues. However, as stated earlier, PTH produced positive chronotropic and inotropic effect in cardiac preparations in vitro and in vivo (Kahot et al., 1981; Tenner et al., 1983). It is interesting that while PTH stimulates adenylate cyclase in both vascular and cardiac tissues, its effects on calcium channels, and hence net tissue responses, are opposite. When we compared the different effects of PTH on smooth muscles, it became obvious to us that the actions of PTH and isoproterenol, a beta-adrenergic agonist, are quite similar. In searching the literature, we found reports of PTH on hepatic (Neuman & Schneider, 1980) and adipose (Werner & Low, 1973) metabolism, and renin release. All these actions can also be elicited by beta-adrenergic stimulation. We do not believe that PTH produces these effects by stimulating beta-adrenergic receptors since propranolol, which blocked the action of isoproterenol in our smooth muscle assays, had no effect on the PTH actions. Nevertheless, these new actions of PTH do parallel those of beta-adrenergic stimulation (Pang et al., 1986b). What are the reasons for the similarities between beta-adrenergic stimulation and PTH actions? We hypothesized that PTH may exist as a neurotransmitter. If so, its co-release with NE would give meaning to the parallelism between the actions of these two chemical messengers. It is possible that NE is responsible for immediate but short effects and PTH for more sustained effects. This hypothesis also gives some physiological insight to these receptor-mediated actions by rather high PTH concentrations.

We began our search for PTH or a PTH-like substance in neural tissues by looking for PTH-like immunoreactivity in the plasma of fish, since this group is known to lack a parathyroid gland. Indeed, PTH immunoreactivity was demonstrated in the plasma of goldfish and trout. Of all the tissues analyzed, PTH immunoreactivity was found in boiled and dialyzed brain and pituitary glands of several species of fishes. The antisera used in these studies include two that recognized the C terminal sequence and one the N terminal sequence. In addition, these antisera did not cross-react with all the pituitary and hypothalamic peptides we have tested (Harvey et al., 1987). One of the antisera was also used to localize the PTH immunoreactivity in goldfish brain. A specific group of cells in the preoptic nucleus showed specific positive immunohistochemical staining which was absent when the antiserum was preabsorbed with extracted or synthetic PTH-(1-84). Furthermore, the fibres of these cells could be traced to terminate in the neurohypophysis (Kaneko & Pang, 1987). We then extended these exciting findings to other vertebrates. PTH immunoreactivity was detected in brain extracts of all vertebrate classes. In rat, mouse and guinea pig, the PTH concentrations were quite similar (Pang et al., 1987b). Immunocytochemical localization of the immunoreactivity in bullfrog and mouse showed the same anatomical distribution of these cells as in goldfish except that the fibres did not terminate in the neurohypophysis but rather in the hypophyseal portal system of the median eminence (Pang et al., 1987c). It is interesting that fishes lack the median eminence while all tetrapods have one. The important point is that all vertebrates have PTH or a PTH-like substance in the same group of cells in the brain. In guinea pig ileum neuroplex, PTH immunoreactivity was also detected by radioimmunoassay (RIA) (Fraser, Harvey & Pang, unpublished data). We conclude that PTH or a PTH-like substance is present in neural tissue either as a neurotransmitter or neurosecretory product. If it is a neurotransmitter, the local concentration will be sufficiently high to produce the reported effects of PTH. If it is present as a neurosecretory product to be released into blood, it is possible that this substance is not exactly PTH, but PTH-like. Such a molecule may be more effective than PTH itself and would explain why high concentrations of PTH are needed to mimic the effects of the PTH-like substance. These are speculations, and much more work is necessary to prove them. Our preliminary studies revealed that some of the immunoreactivity in salmon pituitary and rat hypothalamus extract appeared in the same fractions as that of synthetic hPTH-(1-84). This indicates substantial similarity between PTH and the neural immunoreactive PTH. Cytochemical demonstration of immunoreactive PTH in the neural tissue of the primitive hagfish and freshwater snails suggests that the neural IR-PTH is an old system (Kaneko & Pang, unpublished data; Wendelaar Bonga & Pang, unpublished data). If it is responsible for the "new" actions of PTH, this peptide and its actions may be rather "old" than "new".

CONCLUSION

PTH has many newly described actions, many of which parallel those of the beta-adrenergic system. If these actions are mediated by a PTH or PTH-like neurotransmitter or neurosecretory product, it would make the actions physiologically feasible. The presence of PTH or PTH-like immunoreactivity in vertebrate neural tissues certainly supports such an hypothesis. The purification and characterization of this peptide by biochemical or molecular genetic approaches will answer some of the questions raised above. It is possible that this PTH-like peptide is a PTH-gene-related peptide. Another interesting aspect of the study of these new actions of PTH is the elucidation of their cellular mechanism of action. Cyclic AMP and Ca^{++} are probably involved. What the temporal relationship is between these two intracellular messengers remains to be shown. The involvement of cellular calcium balance in the actions of PTH provides a new view of an old field. There have been many studies on the calcium dependence of hormonal action, but the investigation of how hormones affect cellular calcium balance is rather new. PTH, with paradoxical effects on two different smooth muscles, i.e. vascular and cardiac, provides a good example for investigation. The studies described so far should promote our understanding of these new or unusual actions of PTH. Such data are important in explaining some of the diverse clinical symptoms of parathyroid disorder. Some of these symptoms may be secondary to plasma Ca^{++} level abnormality, producing direct effects or indirect effects through neural and other hormonal regulations. However, some of these symptoms may be directly related to the "new" actions of PTH or a PTH-like substance.

REFERENCES

Bogin, E., Massry, S.G., and Harary, I., 1981, Effect of parathyroid hormone on rat heart cells, J. Clin. Invest., 67: 1215.

Berthelot, A. and Gairard, A., 1975, Effet de la parathormone sur la pression arterielle et la contraction de l'aorte isolee de rat, Experientia, 31: 457.

Brown, A.M., Kunze, D.L., and Yatani, A., 1984, The agonist effect of dihydropyridines on Ca channels, Nature, 311: 570.

Charbon, G.A., 1966, A diuretic and hypotensive action of a parathyroid extract, Acta Physiol. Pharmacol. Neerl., 14: 52.

Charbon, G.A. and Hulstaert, P.F., 1974, Augmentation of arterial hepatic and renal flow by extracted and synthetic parathyroid hormone, Endocrinology, 95: 621.

Chase, L.R. and Aurbach, G.D., 1968, Renal adenyl cyclase: anatomical separation of sites sensitive to parathyroid hormone and vasopressin, Science 159, 545.

Chase, L.R., Fiedark, S.A., and Aurbach, G.D., 1969, Activation of skeletal adenyl cyclase by parathyroid hormone in vitro, Endocrinology, 84: 761.

Collip, J.B. and Clark, E.P., 1925, Further studies on the physiological action of parathyroid hormone, J. Biol. Chem., 64: 133.

Crass, M.F., III and Pang, P.K.T., 1980, Parathyroid hormone: a coronary artery vasodilator, Science, 207: 1087.

Daugirdas, J.T., Al-Kudsi, R.R., Ing, T.S., Yang, M.C.M., Leehey, D.J., and Pang, P.K.T., 1986, Hemodynamic effects of bPTH-(1-34) and its analogue $Nle^{8,18}Tyr^{34}$ bPTH-(3-34) amide, Mineral Electrolyte Metab., 13: 33.

Dowe, J.P. and Joshua, I.G., 1987, In vivo arteriolar dilation in response to parathyroid hormone fragments, Peptides, 8: 443.

Handler, P. and Cohn, D.V., 1952, Effect of parathyroid extract on renal function, Am. J. Physiol., 169: 188.

Hardman, J.G., 1981, Cyclic nucleotides and smooth muscle contraction: some conceptual and experimental considerations, In: "Smooth Muscle: An Assessment of Current Knowledge" (E. Bulbring, A.F. Brading, A.W. Jones, and T. Tomita, eds.), University of Texas Press, Austin, p. 249.

Harvey, S., Zeng, Y.-Y., and Pang, P.K.T., 1987, Parathyroid hormone-
    like immunoreactivity in fish plasma and tissues, Gen. Comp.
    Endocrinol., in press.
Helwig, J.-J., Schleiffer, R., Judes, C., and Gairard, A., 1984, Distri-
    bution of parathyroid hormone-sensitive adenylate cyclase in iso-
    lated rabbit renal cortex microvessels and glomeruli, Life Sci.,
    35: 2649.
Helwig, J.-J., Yang, M.C.M., Bollack, C., Judes, C., and Pang, P.K.T.,
    1987, Structure activity relationship of parathyroid hormone:
    relative sensitivity of rabbit renal microvessel and tubule
    adenylate cyclases to oxidized PTH and PTH inhibitors, Eur. J.
    Pharmacol., in press.
Hester, R.K. and Weiss, G.B., 1981, Comparison of degree of dependence
    of canine arteries and veins on high and low affinity calcium for
    responses to norepinephrine and potassium, J. Pharmacol. Exp.
    Ther., 215: 239.
Hester, R.K., Weiss, G.B., and Fry, W.J., 1979, Differing actions of
    nitroprusside and D-600 on tension and ^{45}Ca fluxes in canine
    renal arteries, J. Pharmacol. Exp. Ther., 298: 155.
Hong, B.-S., Yang, M.C.M., Liang, J.N., and Pang, P.K.T., 1986,
    Correlation of structural changes in parathyroid hormone with its
    vascular action, Peptides, 7: 1131.
Huang, M. and Rorstad, O.P., 1984, Cerebral vascular adenylate cyclase:
    evidence for coupling to receptors for vasoactive intestinal
    peptide and parathyroid hormone, J. Neurochem., 43: 849.
Huang, M., Hanley, D.A., and Rorstad, O.P., 1983, Parathyroid hormone
    stimulates adenyl cyclase in rat cerebral microvessels, Life Sci.,
    32: 1009.
Kaneko, T. and Pang, P.K.T., 1987, Immunocytochemical detection of
    parathyroid hormone-like substance in the goldfish brain and
    pituitary gland, Gen. Comp. Endocrinol., in press.
Kahot, Y., Klein, K.L., Kaplan, R.A., Sanborn, W.G., and Kurokawa, K.,
    1981, Parathyroid hormone has a positive inotropic action in the
    rat, Endocrinology, 109: 2252.
Kondo, N., Shibata, S., Tenner, T.E., Jr., and Pang, P.K.T., 1985, The
    electrophysiological effects of PTH on cardiac tissues, Fed. Proc.,
    44: 1579 (Abstract).
Lindner, A., Tremann, J.A., Plantier, J., Chapman, W., Forrey, A.W.,
    Haines, G., and Palmeri, G.M., 1978, Effects of parathyroid hormone
    on the renal circulation and renin secretion in unanesthetized
    dogs, Mineral Electrolyte Metab., 1: 155.
Michelakis, A.M., 1970, Hormonal effects on cyclic-AMP in renal cell
    suspension system, Proc. Soc. Exp. Biol. Med., 135: 13.
Mitchell, R.D., Yang, M.C.M., and Pang, P.K.T., 1985, The role of extra-
    cellular Ca^{++} in vasoconstriction by arginine vasopressin, Fed.
    Proc., 44: 1111 (Abstract).
Narahashi, T., Tsunoo, A., and Yoshii, M., 1987, Characterization of two
    types of calcium channels in mouse neuroblastoma cells, J.
    Physiol., 383: 231.
Neuman, W.F. and Schneider, N., 1980, The parathyroid hormone-sensitive
    adenylate cyclase system in plasma membranes of rat liver, Endo-
    crinology, 107: 2082.
Nickols, G.A., 1985, Increased cyclic AMP in cultured vascular smooth
    muscle cells and relaxation of aortic strips by parathyroid
    hormone, Eur. J. Pharmacol., 116: 137.
Nickols, G.A., Metz, A.M., and Cline, W.H., Jr.,1986, Vasodilation of
    the rat mesenteric vasculature by parathyroid hormone, J.
    Pharmacol. Exp. Ther., 236: 419.

Pang, P.K.T., Harvey, S., Fraser, R., and Kaneko, T., 1987b, Para-thyroid hormone-like immunoreactivity in brains of tetrapod verte-brates, Am. J. Physiol., submitted for publication.

Pang, P.K.T., Hong, B.-S., Yen, L., and Yang, M.C.M., 1984, Parathyroid hormone: a specific potent vasodilator, In: "Contributions to Nephrology", Vol. 41 (G.M. Berlyne and S. Biovannetti, eds.), Karger, Basel, p. 137.

Pang, P.K.T., Kaneko, T., and Harvey, S., 1987c, Immunocytochemical dis-tribution of PTH-immunoreactivity in vertebrate brains, Am. J. Physiol., submitted for publication.

Pang, P.K.T., Shew, R.L., and Sawyer, W.H., 1981, Inhibition of uterine contraction by synthetic parathyroid hormone fragment, Life Sci., 28, 1317.

Pang, P.K.T., Yang, M.C.M., Keutmann, H.T., and Kenny, A.D., 1983, Structure-activity relationship of parathyroid hormone: separation of the hypotensive and hypercalcemic properties, Endocrinology, 112: 284.

Pang, P.K.T., Yang, M.C.M., and Sham, J.S.K., 1987a, Parathyroid hormone and calcium entry blockade in a vascular tissue, Life Sci., sub-mitted for publication.

Pang, P.K.T., Yang, M.C.M., Shew, R., and Tenner, T.E., Jr., 1985, The vasorelaxant action of parathyroid hormone fragments on isolated rat tail artery, Blood Vessels, 22: 57.

Pang, P.K.T., Yang, M.C.M., and Tenner, T.E., Jr., 1986b, Beta-adrenergic-like actions of parathyroid hormone, Trends Pharmacol. Sci., 7: 340.

Pang, P.K.T., Yang, M.C.M., Tenner, T.E., Jr., Kenny, A.D., and Cooper, C.W., 1986a, Cyclic AMP and the vascular action of parathyroid hormone, Can. J. Physiol. Pharmacol., 64: 1543.

Rambausek, M., Ritz, E., Rascher, W., Kreusser, W., Mann, J.F., Kreye, V.A., and Mehls, O., 1982, Vascular effects of parathyroid hormone (PTH), Adv. Exp. Med. Biol., 151: 619.

Schleiffer, R.A., Berthelot, A., and Gairard, A., 1979, Action of para-thyroid extract on arterial blood pressure and on contraction and ^{45}Ca exchange in isolated aorta of the rat, Eur. J. Pharmacol., 58: 163.

Spedding, M., 1987, Three types of Ca^{2+} channels explain discrepan-cies, Trends Pharmacol. Sci., 8: 115.

Stanton, R.C., Plant, S.B., and McCarron, D.A., 1985, cAMP response of vascular smooth muscle cells to bovine parathyroid hormone, Am. J. Physiol., 247, E822.

Tenner, T.E., Jr., Ramanadham, S., Yang, M.C.M., and Pang, P.K.T., 1983, Chronotropic actions of bPTH-(1-34) in the right atrium of the rat, Can. J. Physiol. Pharmacol., 61: 1162.

Weiss, G.B. (editor), 1981, "New Perspectives on Calcium Antagonists", Am. Physiol. Soc., Washington, D.C.

Werner, S., and Low, H., 1973, Stimulation of lipolysis and calcium accumulation by parathyroid hormone in rat adipose tissue *in vitro* after adrenalectomy and administration of high doses of cortisone acetate, Horm. Metab. Res., 5: 292.

Wong, G.L. and D.V. Cohn, 1975, Target cells in bone for parathormone and calcitonin are different: enrichment for each cell types by sequential digestion of mouse calveria and selective adhesion to polymeric surfaces, Proc. Natl. Acad. Sci. (U.S.A.), 72: 3167.

Yang, M.C.M., Kenny, A.D., and Pang, P.K.T., 1985, Effect of para-thyroid hormone on contraction of gastrointestinal tract in rat, In: "Current Trends in Comparative Endocrinology", Vol. 2 (B. Lofts and W.N. Holmes, eds.), Hong Kong University Press, Hong Kong, p. 1029.

Yang, M.C.M., Yen, L., and Pang, P.K.T., 1983, Mechanisms of hypotensive action of synthetic parathyroid hormone fragment [bPTH-(1-34)], Fed. Proc., 42: 848 (Abstract).

Yen, Y.C., Yang, M.C.M., Kenny, a.D., and Pang, P.K.T., 1983, Parathyroid hormone (PTH) fragments relax the guinea pig trachea *in vitro*, Can. J. Physiol. Pharmacol., 61: 1324.

Zhang, R.H., Yang, M.C.M., and Pang, P.K.T., 1985, The relaxing effect of parathyroid hormone on rat vas deferens, Fed. Proc., 44: 1579 (Abstract).

ROLE OF PARATHYROID HORMONE (PTH) IN THE BLOOD PRESSURE REGULATION

Kunitoshi Iseki

Second Department of Internal Medicine
Faculty of Medicine, Kyushu University
Fukuoka, Japan

INTRODUCTION

Since Handler et al (1) have reported that the parathyroid extract has the hypotensive effect, Pang and others (2,3,4) have confirmed and extended the findings. PTH has direct vasodilating action unrelated to alpha- or beta-adrenergic mechanisms (2). Also PTH has been shown to enhance calcium entry into and to increase calcium contents of many tissues (5). Clinically, it is well known that hypertension is common in subjects with primary hyperparathyroidism (6). Both acute and chronic renal failure are associated with secondary hyperparathyroidism (7).

Massry (1979) has hypothesized that excess PTH is a uremic toxin (8), and it may explain many uremic manifestations including a derangements in cardiovascular system. Campese et al (9) have reported that uremic patients display reduced pressor response to norepinephrine (NE), and this could be explained by excess PTH (10). Furthermore, uremic condition is accompanied with aggravated blood pressure response to acute hypercalcemia (11). To define the role of PTH in the regulation of blood pressure, we have observed the blood pressure response to norepinephrine (NE) and calcium infusion both in rats and human.

ROLE OF PTH IN REDUCED PRESSOR RESPONSE TO NE : ANIMAL STUDY

We have examined the effect of the intact 1-84 PTH and that of its amino-terminal 1-34 fragment on mean arterial pressure (MAP)(12). Bolus injections of 30 units of both 1-84 and 1-34 produced a significant decrease in MAP; however, the hypotensive response to 1-34 PTH was more marked than to 1-84 PTH (30 u/h). The infusion of 1-84 PTH (30 u/h) did not alter MAP, while the infusion of 1-34 PTH (30 u/h) led to a decrease in MAP from 124 tp 103 mmHg and to a rise in heart rate from 359 to 437 beats /min. The amino-terminal PTH may be a more potent vasodilator than 1-84 PTH. However, the physiological relevance of these short lived effect in the clinical setting is not clear. The pressure response to varying doses of NE was evaluated in several models using male Sprague-Dawley rats (10). To obtain uremic rats, 5/6 nephrectomy was performed and studies were done 14 days after the completion of the surgery. Parathyroidectomy (PTX) was performed by electrocautery with the success of the procedure ascertained by a decrease in plasma levels of calcium at least 2 mg/dl. To determine the pressure response to NE, the left carotid and one jugular vein were cannulated with PE-50 tubings. The tubings were led subcutaneously to

New Actions of Parathyroid Hormone
Edited by S. G. Massry and T. Fujita
Plenum Press, New York

emerge at the base of the neck and protected by wire springs. Experiments were performed 4 hours later, while the rats were awake, unrestrained and undisturbed. Blood pressure and heart rate were measured before and after a bolus injection of 10, 30, 100 and 300 ng of NE delivered in 0.1 ml of 0.9 % saline. Five minutes were allowed between the injection of the various doses. The increments in MAP in chronic renal failure (CRF) sham parathyroidectomized (PTX) rat were significantly less than in control and CRF-PTX rats. Treatment of CRF-sham PTX rats with indomethacin (3.3 mg/kg body weight, intraperitoneally, every 8 hours for 2 days) normalized the blood pressure response to NE. Treatment of control rats with indomethacin did not affect the response to NE. In the hind limb preparation, there was a significant shift to the right in the dose-response curve in CRF-sham PTX rats as compared to controls and CRF-PTX rats, indicating a decreased sensitivity to NE in CRF-sham PTX rats. There was no significant difference between the dose-response curve in the control and that in CRF-PTX rats.

Rascher et al proposed that the down-regulation of NE receptors is one other explanation for diminished NE responsiveness. They have denied the role of PTH, since in their 2 days hypocalcemic hypoparathyroid uremic rats did not show any difference in NE responsiveness with intact parathyroid uremic rats. The reason why it is different from our study is not clear. The difference in calcium balance may explain the difference in pressure response to NE, since we studied 7 days after PTX with water supplemented 8 % calcium gluconate to maintain normal serum calcium concentration. Indomethacin has several actions other than the inhibition of cyclooxygenase (14), so that our findings do not specifically prove that prostaglandins are responsible for vascular subsensitivity to NE. Although we have shown that PTH infusion caused the increase in urinary excretion of vasodilatory prostaglandin (12).

ROLE OF PTH IN REDUCED PRESSOR RESPONSE TO NE : HUMAN STUDY

Campese et al (9) reported that patients with uremia display reduced pressor response to NE and showed dialysis treatment have improved the responsiveness. Collins et al (15) found that treatment of CRF patients with indomethacin improved or normalized the pressor response to NE. They supported the notion that the reduced pressor response to NE in uremia is due to increased production of prostaglandins induced by excess PTH. We have observed the pressor response to NE in 5 hemodialysis patients who have performed subtotal parathyroidectomy (unpublished). After PTX, all patients showed improved pressor response to NE at a dose of NE 100 ng/kg/min. These clinical evidences are consistent with the notion that PTH is playing a role in reduced pressor response to NE in uremia. Since circulating NE is usually elevated in uremia (16,17), we could not exclude the possibility of the down-regulation of NE receptors. Campese (18) has suggested the possibility that PTH may directly and/or indirectly affect the activity of the sympatho-adrenal system.

ROLE OF PTH IN ACUTE HYPERCALCEMIC HYPERTENSION : ANIMAL STUDY

To study the blood pressure response to acute hypercalcemia, we have infused calcium (calcium chloride) in 5 % dextrose (19). The infusion of 5 % dextrose to normal rats produced no significant changes in the concentration of serum calcium or in MAP. The infusion of calcium at increasing doses of 50, 75, or 100 mg elemental calcium/kg body weight over 2 hours caused a rise in serum calcium, and there was a significant correlation between the amount of calcium infused and the increments in the concentration of serum calcium. The rise in serum calcium was associated with an increase in MAP, with the dose of 50 mg/kg causing a rise of 3.8 mmHg, 75 mg/kg producing a rise of 17 mmHg, and 100 mg/kg inducing a rise of 23 mmHg, the changes in MAP were directly and significantly related to the

changes in serum calcium. To determine the role of PTH, we have compared
the hypertensive effect of acute hypercalcemia between normal (sham PTX)
and PTX rats. Despite a similar increment in serum calcium (+7.4 vs +7.3
mg/dl), the rise in MAP was significantly higher in the sham PTX rats (+20
mmHg) than in the PTX rats (+7 mmHg). This difference could not be
attributed to the high calcium intake by the PTX rats, since sham PTX rats
receiving similar high calcium intake in their drinking water displayed a
rise in MAP of 19 mmHg with a rise of 7.4 mg/dl in serum calcium concentration. The simultaneous infusion of PTH 1-84 and calcium to PTX rats caused
a rise of 6.4 mg/dl in serum calcium concentration and an increment of 17
mmHg in MAP which was not different from that seen in the sham PTX rats
receiving calcium infusion and PTH and was significantly higher than in PTX
rats receiving calcium infusion only. The infusion of PTH alone to sham PTX
rats did not cause a significant change in serum calcium concentration.

Berl T et al (20) denied the contribution of PTH, since blood pressure
response in PTX rats receiving calcium was not significantly different from
control rats. With small increase in serum calcium concentration (less than
5 mg/dl), it would not be enough to produce the difference in blood pressure
response. Also the difference in the rate of increase in serum calcium
concentration (+3.7 mg/dl/30 min vs +7.5 mg/dl/120 min, Berl T et al vs ours)
and the difference in drinking water in PTX rats (calcium chloride 1 g/dl vs
calcium gluconate 8 g/dl, Berl T et al vs ours) may explain the discrepancy
in the results. Zawada et al (21) suggested the importance of serum magnesium
in acute hypercalcemic hypertension in dog study.

In uremic rats (5/6 nephrectomy), the infusion of 40 mg/kg body weight/2h
caused a significant rise in serum calcium levels (+6.1 mg/dl) and a significant rise in MAP (+23 mmHg). This change in MAP was significantly higher
than that observed in CRF-PTX rats (+9.2 mmHg), despite no significant
difference in the increment in serum calcium concentration. Similarly, the
infusion of 75 mg/kg/2h of calcium to CRF-sham PTX and CRF-PTX rats produced
comparable increments in serum calcium levels (+17.5 vs +15.2 mg/dl), but the
rise in MAP was significantly higher in the CRF-sham PTX rats (+38.6 mmHg)
than in CRF-PTX rats (+23.9 mmHg).

To evaluate the effects of similar changes in serum calcium concentration on MAP in the presence or absence of renal failure, regression analysis
of the data for various study groups were performed. For any rise in serum
calcium concentration, the increment in MAP in CRF-sham PTX rats was greater
than in normal, sham PTX and CRF-PTX rats, whereas the changes in MAP in the
latter two groups of animal were not different. Accordingly, the lack of a
significant difference between the slopes of the regression lines of the
normal and sham PTX rats combined and of the CRF-PTX rats may be due to
other consequences of CRF, other than PTH, that may also facilitate the
hypertensive action of hypercalcemia (22).

ROLE OF PTH IN ACUTE HYPERCALCEMIC HYPERTENSION : HUMAN STUDY

Weidmann et al (11) have reported that the propensity for an increase
in blood pressure was not related to pre-existing hypertension, but was
markedly influenced by the degree of renal insufficiency. They have suggested that uremia may increase the sensitivity of the cardiovascular and the
central nervous system to certain effects of calcium ion. Gennari et al
(22) found that following acute and comparable increments in the concentration of serum calcium produced by calcium infusion in 10 normal individuals
and in 5 subjects with postsurgical hypoparathyroidism, MAP increased significantly only in the normal subjects. They have confirmed our hypothesis
that the effect of calcium on arterial pressure is realized under intact
parathyroid function. Role of calcitonin was suspected, since calcium
infusion increased the levels of serum calcium paralelled with an increase
in circulating calcitonin. McCarron et al (24) have suggested that hypercalcemic hypertension is more dependent on the suppression of PTH than the
rise in serum calcium concentration in posttransplant hyperparathyroidism.

SUMMARY

Our animal and human studies and other human studies are consistent with the notion that PTH is playing a role in blood pressure regulation. However, several discrepances in animal study regarding blood pressure response to NE infusion and acute hypercalcemia do exist. In NE infusion, down-regulation of NE receptors could be the other explanation for the diminished responsiveness to NE. In acute hypercalcemia, acute depression of PTH and hypomagnesemia may modify the blood pressure response.

Although, the precise mechanisms of PTH action on blood are not clear, we have confirmed the clinical significance of excess PTH on the regulation of blood pressure. PTH action may be mediated through increased production of vasodilating prostaglandins and permissive role for calcium entry into cells.

REFERENCES

1. Handler P., Cohn D.V.: Effect of parathyroid extract on renal function. Am J Physiol 169: 188-193, 1952.
2. Pang P.K.T., Tenner T.E., Yee J.A., Yang M., Janssen H.F.: Hypotensive action of parathyroid hormone preparations on rats and dogs. Proc Natl Acad Sci USA 77: 675-678, 1980.
3. Hashimoto K., Nakagawa Y., Shibuya T., Satoh H., Ushijima T., Imai S.: Effects of parathyroid hormone and related polypeptides on the heart and coronary circulation of dogs. J Cardiovascular Pharm 3: 668-676, 1981.
4. Nakamura R., Watanabe T., Sokabe H.: Acute hypotensive action of para-thyroid hormone-(1-34) fragments in hypertensive rats (41253). Proceedings Soc Experimental Bio Med 168: 168-171, 1981.
5. Bogin E., Massry S.G., Haraly I.: Effects of parathyroid hormone on rat heart cells. J Clin Invest 67: 1215-1227, 1981.
6. Hellstrom J., Birks G., Edvall C.A.: Hypertension inhyperparathyroidism. Br J Urol 30: 13-24, 1958.
7. Massry S.G., Coburn J.W., Peacock M., Kleeman C.R.: Turnover of endo-genous parathyroid hormone in uremic patients and those undergoing hemo-dialysis. Trans Am Soc Artif Intern Organs 18: 416-422, 1972.
8. Massry S.G.: Is parathyroid Hormone a Uremic Toxin ? Nephron 19: 125-130, 1979.
9. Campese V.M., Romoff M.S., Levitan D., Lane K., Massry S.G.: Mechanisms of autonomic nervous system dysfunction in uremia. Kidney Int 20: 246-253, 1981.
10. Iseki K., Massry S.G., Campese V.M.: Evidence for a role of PTH in the reduced pressor response to norepinephrine in chronic renal failure. Kidney Int 28: 11-15, 1985.
11. Weidmann P., Massry S.G., Coburn J.W., Maxwell M.H., Atleson J., Kleeman C.R.: Blood pressure effects of acute hypercalcemia. Ann Intern Med 76: 741-745, 1972.
12. Saglikes Y., Massry S.G., Iseki K., Nadler J.L., Campese V.M.: Effect of PTH on blood pressure and response to vasoconstrictor agonists. Am J Physiol 248: F674-F681, 1985.
13. Rascher W., Schomig A., Kreye V.A., Ritz E.: Diminished vascular response to noradrenaline in experimental chronic uremia. Kidney Int 21: 20-27, 1982.
14. Rascher W., Dietz R., Schomig A., Burkart G., Gross F.: Reversal of corticosterone-induced supersensitivity of vascular smooth muscle to noradrenaline by arachidonic acid and prostacyclin. Eur J Pharmacol 68: 267-273, 1980.
15. Collins J., Massry S.G., Campese V.M.: Parathyroid Hormone and the Altered Vascular Response to Norepinephrine in Uremia. Am J Nephrol 5: 110-113, 1985.

16. Campese V.M., Iseki K., Massry S.G.: Plasma catecholamines and Vascular Reactivity in Uremia and Dialysis Patients. Contr Nephrol 41: 90-98, (Karger, Basel 1984).
17. Ksiazek A.: Beta dopamine hydroxylase activity and catecholamine levels in the plasma of patients with renal failure. Nephron 24: 170-174,1979.
18. Campese V.M.: Calcium, Parathyroid Hormone, and Sympatho-adrenal System. Am J Nephrol 6, suppl, 29-32, 1986.
19. Iseki K., Massry S.G., Campese V.M.: Effects of hypercalcemia and para-thyroid hormone on blood pressure in normal and renal failure rats. Am J Physiol 250: F924-F929, 1986.
20. Berl T., Levi M., Ellis M., Chaimovitz C.: Mechanism of Acute Hyper-calcemic Hypertension in the Conscious Rat. Hypertension 7:923-930, 1985.
21. Zawada E.T., TerWee J.A., McClung D.E.: Magnesium prevents acute hyper-calcemic hypertension. Nephron 47: 109-114, 1987.
22. Massry S.G., Iseki K., Campese V.M.: Serum Calcium, Parathyroid Hormone, and Blood Pressure. Am J Nephrol 6, suppl, 19-28, 1986.
23. Gennari C., Nami R., Bianchini C., Aversa A.M.: Blood pressure effects of acute hypercalcemia in normal subjects and thyroparathyroidectomized patients. Mineral Electrolyte Metab 11: 369-373, 1985.
24. McCarron D.A., Muther R.S., Plant S.B., Krutzik S.: Parathyroid Hormone : A Determinant of Posttransplant Blood Pressure Regulation. Am J Kid Dis 1: 38-44, 1981.

CALCIUM AND CALCIUM REGULATING HORMONES IN HUMAN HYPERTENSION

Lawrence M. Resnick

Cardiovascular Center, The New York Hospital-Cornell
Medical Center
525 East 68th Street, Starr-4, New York, 10021

INTRODUCTION

Although the importance of calcium in cardiovascular physiology is historically well established, its relevance to the regulation of blood pressure has only recently become a topic of clinical significance. More than one hundred years ago, Sidney Ringer first demonstrated the involvement of calcium in cardiac muscle contraction (1). As part of a final common pathway by which neural as well as hormonal inputs alter muscle contraction, calcium has also become central in our attempts to better understand the regulation of peripheral vasoconstrictor tone and thus of blood pressure homeostasis. Developing in a parallel fashion, calcium has also been shown to be involved in the mechanism of stimulus-secretion coupling, and is thus critical for endocrine secretion. It is not surprising therefore, that hypertensive disease, characterized as it is by increased peripheral vasoconstrictor tone and a variety of other cardiovascular, endocrine, and neural abnormalities, is witnessing intense, calcium-directed research seeking to define how calcium at molecular and biochemical levels may contribute to the hypertensive process.

At the other end of the spectrum, Addison described the ability of oral calcium supplementation to lower blood pressure in patients with essential hypertension as early as 1924 (2). However, the relevance of clinical aspects of calcium metabolism to blood pressure phenomena, including the dietary intake, absorption, distribution, and excretion of calcium, have not been adequately investigated, and only within the last decade has a significant literature begun to appear. These studies suggest that alterations of calcium metabolism exist in a variety of hypertensive syndromes. Attempts have been made to explain clinical effects of altered calcium intake directly at the cellular level by considering molecular and biochemical details of calcium's involvement in membrane ion pump mechanisms, transducing enzyme systems such as phospholipases and protein kinases, and in muscle calcium-protein interactions leading directly to vasoconstriction.

We have attempted to investigate human hypertension clinically, and have also demonstrated a variety of alterations in calcium metabolism in this syndrome (3). Our approach has focussed on the clinical as well as biochemical heterogeneity of human hypertension and has emphasized a shift

New Actions of Parathyroid Hormone
Edited by S. G. Massry and T. Fujita
Plenum Press, New York

of calcium metabolism in both directions away from average normotensive values among different hypertensive populations. These alterations may have both diagnostic and therapeutic relevance in identifying specific hypertensive subgroups, e.g., those whose blood pressure is sensitive to the effects of dietary salt loading, as being those most likely to benefit from increased dietary calcium supplementation. Lastly, we have hypothesized a role for the calcium regulating hormones parathyroid hormone (PTH), calcitonin (CT), and 1,25 dihydroxyvitamin D (1,25D), coordinately with the renin-aldosterone system, in the normal regulation of blood pressure and volume homeostasis.

Calcium Metabolism is Altered in Human Hypertension

A wide range of alterations in calcium metabolism have been reported in hypertension. Early epidemiologic evidence suggested that circulating calcium and blood pressure were directly related - the higher the serum total calcium, the higher the blood pressure (4). More recently, a similar, strikingly positive relationship was demonstrated between intracellular cytosolic free calcium in platelets and blood pressure (5). Once again, the higher the cytosolic free calcium, the greater the blood pressure. The hypercalcemia of primary hyperparathyroidism is routinely associated with increases in blood pressure (6), as is iatrogenic hypercalcemia, whether as acute intravenous loads or chronically as in vitamin D intoxication (7). Conversely, hypocalcemia may be associated with hypotension (8). These data collectively suggest that alterations in calcium metabolism may exist in blood pressure disorders, and that a calcium surfeit contributes to its underlying pathophysiology. However, equally suggestive are data indicating exactly the opposite, that a calcium deficit characterizes the hypertensive state. Epidemiologic surveys of diverse ethnically and geographically defined groups indicate a rather consistent pattern - an inverse relationship between assessed dietary calcium intake and concurrent blood pressure. The higher the measured blood pressure, the lower the ingested calcium (9,10). At the same time relative to renal sodium excretion, calcium excretion is excessive among hypertensive subjects, a greater loss of calcium resulting at any given level of sodium intake (11). Lower serum ionized calcium levels have also been measured in some hypertensives (12). Lastly, dietary calcium supplementation in various rat models of hypertension, and in human hypertensives as well, may in at least some circumstances lower blood pressure (13-15). Hence, a deficit of calcium has also been claimed as central to the pathogenesis of hypertension. These apparently paradoxical data have made the contribution of calcium metabolism to hypertension still undefined and controversial.

We believe that analyzing hypertension as if it were of uniform underlying pathophysiology, considering all hypertensives as one homogeneous group is mistaken and contributes to ongoing artificial controversies, obscuring the central role calcium plays in the pathophysiology of hypertension. We began investigating calcium metabolism in hypertension by measuring circulating levels of ionized calcium and of the calcium regulating hormones, parathyroid hormone (PTH), calcitonin (CT) and 1,25 dihydroxy vitamin D (1,25D) in subjects with primary, essential hypertension (16,17). Distinct pathophysiologic subgroups were identified by means of renin-sodium profiling. The renal pressor hormone, renin, released by the juxtaglomerular apparatus in response to a variety of ionic, neural, humoral and direct pressure-stretch stimuli, both reflects and contributes to pressure and volume homeostasis. Of interest, renin, like parathyroid hormone, is unusual among hormones, increasing intracellular calcium levels associated with suppression of cellular hormone secretion. Approximately one-third of hypertensive individuals have renin levels inappropriately suppressed compared to normotensive subjects at the same average level of urinary sodium excretion. These subjects are more commonly found in black and elderly hypertensive populations in whom sodium-volume factors may predominate. On the other hand, inappropriately high levels of renin usually signify angiotension II dependent hypertension, in which sodium-volume mechanisms appear to be less clinically relevant. Thus, renin-sodium profiling may allow for a more pathophysiologically oriented way of categorizing hypertensive subjects, and has allowed us to more logically fashion appropriate antihypertensive treatment regimens (18).

When patients were categorized in this manner, serum ionized calcium levels in hypertensives were within the normal range, but were distinguishably different among different renin subgroups (16) (Figure 1a). Low renin hypertensives had lower average serum ionized calcium values while high renin subjects had values higher than other hypertensive or normotensive control subjects. With considerable overlap observed between individual subjects within renin subgroups, we sought to establish the pathophysiologic rather than just the statistical significance of the small ionized calcium changes within the normal range by measuring the calcium regulating hormones PTH, CT, and 1,25D. What we found was that each of the calcium regulating hormonal species measured was likewise shifted (17). Like serum ionized calcium values themselves however, each

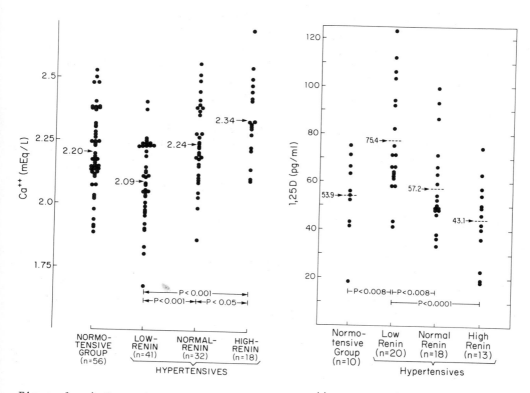

Figure 1. a) Serum ionized calcium levels (Ca^{++}) in normotensive and in renin subgroups of essential hypertensive subjects; b) Serum 1,25 dihydroxyvitamin D (1,25D) levels in normotensive and renin subgroups of essential hypertensive subjects (16,17).

145

Table 1. Calcium Regulating Hormones in Essential Hypertension

Group	PTH		CT	1,25D
N1-BP (n=10)	244 ± 21	(254) (±42)	68.0 ± 6.5	53.9 ± 5.3
Lo-RH (n=20)	433** ± 38	(398)** (±31)	56.4 ± 1.8	75.4*** ± 5.5
N1-RH (n=18)	318* ± 22	(307)† (±33)	66.2# ± 4.0	57.2†† ± 4.3
Hi-RH (n=13)	292 ± 37	(311) (±39)	84.3***,†††† ± 3.9	43.1††† ± 4.6

*p<0.05
**p<0.01   vs. N1-BP
***p<0.008

†p<0.05
††p<0.008   vs. LoRH   #p<0.005 vs. HiRH
†††p<0.0001
††††p<0.00001

*and t for values in parentheses are mean adjusted for covariance of
urinary sodium excretion.

p-values for CT an 1,25 D are for pooled variance-T statistics
(Bonferroni)

hormone was deviated in opposite directions away from average normotensive
values, appropriate for and thus presumably secondary to the altered circulating concentrations of calcium (Table 1). Thus, PTH values were
consistently elevated in low renin subjects, appropriate for the lower
ionized calcium values found in these patients. Similarly, 1,25D values
were elevated in these subjects while calcitonin levels were lower, again
exactly what one would expect if calcium levels were physiologially sensed
as being significantly lower in these individuals (Figure 1b). Conversely,
high renin subjects had elevated CT levels and suppressed values for both
PTH and 1,25D compared to the other hypertensive subjects, again
consistent with the higher average circulating ionized calcium levels
observed in these subjects. Low renin essential hypertensive subjects are
thus acting as if they have a "calcium deficit" while high renin
hypertensive subjects, as a group, act as if a calcium surfeit was
present. It may be that apparently paradoxical calcium-related
abnormalities of hypertensive subjects previously reported may at least
partly reflect different hypertensive populations, with calcium metabolism
shifted in each in different directions away from average normotensive
values.

The Relevance of Altered Calcium Metabolism in Clinical Hypertension

Dietary Salt Sensitivity in Hypertension: When salt provokes altered calcium
metabolism, it exacerbates hypertension.

What might be the potential clinical significance, if any, of these
subtle shifts in calcium metabolism among different renin-defined subgroups o:
essential hypertension? We reasoned that if these calcium metabolic shifts
contributed to the pathogenesis of the hypertension, then maneuvers which wer

known to exacerbate hypertension ought to necessarily provoke and/or exacerbate those same alterations in calcium metabolism. We therefore studied the short- and longer-term effects of dietary salt loading on blood pressure and calcium metabolism. Essential hypertensive subjects were randomly allocated to metabolic balance diets containing 10 and 200 mEq of sodium chloride for five days each. Longer-term studies among essential hypertensives provided for low sodium chloride (<50 mEq/day) and high sodium chloride (>200 mEq/day) diets for one month each under outpatient supervision (19,20).

In each group of studies, consistent relationships were observed between the ability of salt to raise blood pressure and its ability to alter calcium metabolism. Salt raised pressure significantly in approximately one-half of the hypertensive subjects in both short- and long-term studies, while pressure actually declined in some patients with salt loading. Regardless of the magnitude of the blood pressure change, continuous relationships were observed between the change in diastolic pressure on high vs. low dietary salt, and salt-induced changes in both serum ionized calcium (r=-0.72, p<0.001, short-term; r=-0.78, p<0.001 - long-term) and 1,25D (r=0.82, p<0.001, short-term; r=0.71, p<0.001, long-term) (Figure 2). Salt raised pressure the most in those individuals in whom it most lowered ionized calcium levels and most elevated levels of 1,25D - provoking exactly those calcium metabolic changes characteristic of and originally observed in low renin hypertension . It thus appears that the originally observed "calcium deficient" ionic and hormonal pattern observed in low renin patients is of pathophysiologic significance for hypertension, contributing to and/or reflective of dietary salt sensitivity. Interestingly, preliminary studies by others also suggested that salt loading in normotensive subjects may elevate PTH and 1,25D levels, although pressure measurements were not reported in that study (21). Conversely, when extremes of dietary salt intake did not result in significant changes in blood pressure, significant changes in serum ionized calcium were also not observed (22).

Oral Calcium Supplementation in Hypertension: When calcium reverses altered calcium metabolic indices, calcium reverses hypertension.

Although the above results indicated to us that the ability of salt to raise blood pressure was associated with its ability to alter calcium

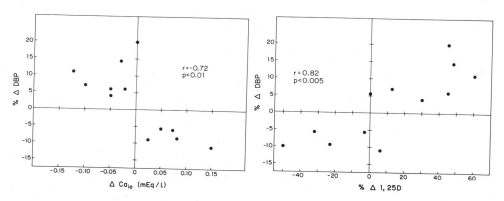

Figure 2. Dependence of salt-induced blood pressure effects on salt-induced changes in calcium metabolism. ΔCa_{io} -salt-induced change in serum ionized calcium, %Δ 1,25D - percent change in 1,25 dihydroxyvitamin D (19).

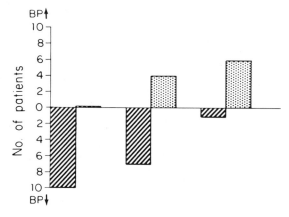

Figure 3. The effect of short-term calcium supplementation on blood
pressure in relation to initial plasma renin activity (24).

metabolism, the two phenomenon need not have been causally linked, the
salt-induced blood pressure rise perhaps not dependent on the salt-induced
calcium metabolic shifts. We thus proceeded to supplement hypertensive
patients with 2 grams per day of calcium carbonate in four divided doses
under a variety of conditions, a) in short-term studies of hypertensive
patients on metabolic balance diets; b) in longer-term outpatient studies;
and c) on high vs. low dietary salt intakes. In each instance, calcium
supplementation lowered blood pressure preferentially among those subjects
with lower plasma renin activity (23) (Figure 3), lower initial serum
ionized calcium levels (24) (Figure 4), and among those who were salt-
sensitive (25) (Figure 5). Of note, while dietary calcium supplementation
did not elevate circulating ionized calcium levels themselves, it always

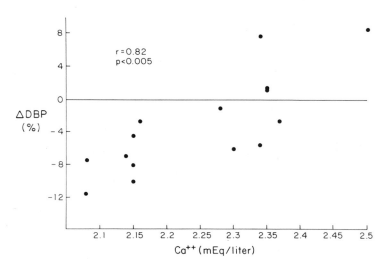

Figure 4. The effect of long-term (6 mos.) oral calcium supplementation on
blood pressure in relation to pre-treatment serum ionized calcium
(24).

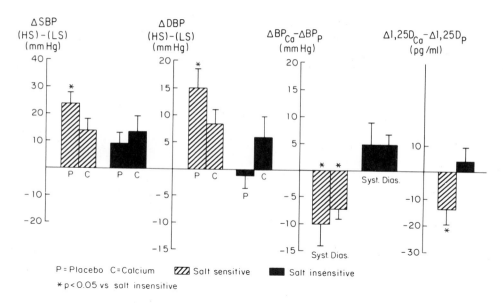

Figure 5. Calcium supplementation lowers pressure best in salt-sensitive
         hypertension (25).

reversed the elevated PTH and 1,25D levels characteristic of the low-
renin, salt sensitive patient. Indeed, it was only among salt sensitive
subjects that calcium supplementation significantly lowered 1,25D levels,
and only among salt sensitive patients did calcium supplementation blunt
salt induced elevations in blood pressure. Interestingly also were
pressor responses to oral calcium supplementation observed in subjects
with high renin and higher initial ionized calcium levels, and among those
who were salt insensitive. Once again, these results reflect the different and often opposite clinical responses to the same dietary maneuver.
These data thus emphasize the heterogeneity of hypertensive mechanisms
among different hypertensive subjects, and suggest the relevance of
calcium metabolic indices in identifying and perhaps underlying this
heterogeneity.

Hence, the subtle shifts in calcium metabolism initially observed
among different renin subgroups of essential hypertensives and induced by
dietary salt loading in salt sensitive individuals, are indeed of clinical
relevance to hypertension. Specifically, sodium-volume dependent
hypertension is a "calcium-dependent" hypertension in which salt induces
the "calcium metabolic deficit" characteristic of the low renin state:
lower serum ionized calcium and elevated 1,25D levels. It is especially
in this form of hypertension, that calcium supplementation reverses and/or
blunts both the blood pressure and these same calcium variables that
sodium loading exacerbates.

The Relationship of Calcium Regulating Hormones to the Renin-Aldosterone
System in Hypertension: Why Does Calcium Supplementation Lower Blood
Pressure? Role of 1,25D vs. PTH.

We wondered whether the observed "see-saw like" opposing effects of
dietary salt vis-a-vis dietary calcium on blood pressure were due to opposite
salt and calcium-induced effects on circulating calcium ion levels per se, or
to induced alterations in calcium regulating hormones, or both. We reasoned
that adding 1,25D therapy to oral calcium supplementation would, by enhancing
calcium absorption, provide a more positive calcium balance than calcium
supplementation alone. If total body calcium balance and/or circulating

Table 2. Metabolic Effects of Calcium with and Without 1,25
Dihydroxyvitamin D

Rx	Δ Ca^{++} (%)	Δ PTH (%)	Δ1,25 D (%)	Δ PRA (%)
Ca^{++}	3.2 ±3.0	-35.7 ±11.6	-53 ±15	38 ±8.3
Ca^{++} + 1,25 D	2.3 ±1.1	-20 ± 7.7	63* ±21	-31* ±9.5

*$p < 0.001$ vs. Ca^{++} alone

calcium levels were themselves critical to the observed dietary mineral-
induced blood pressure effects, then the addition of 1,25D to calcium
itself would potentiate calcium effects on blood pressure. Interestingly,
exactly the opposite was observed (26,27).

Essential hypertensive patients on metabolic balance diets, already
receiving 2 grams per day of supplemental calcium, were then given 1,25D,
0.25 mcg per day for three additional days. While calcium supplementation
lowered blood pressure preferentially among low renin hypertensives, who
had lower initial levels of serum ionized calcium (Figures 3,4) the
addition of 1,25D to calcium reversed the calcium effects and elevated
pressure in these same patients (Figure 6). Conversely, blood pressure
was ameliorated by calcium plus 1,25D in those high renin, higher initial
ionized calcium patients in whom calcium alone exerted a pressor effect.
Comparing the effects of these two calcium maneuvers on circulating
hormone levels was also revealing (Table 2). Calcium supplementation
alone suppressed endogenous PTH and 1,25D levels, and elevated plasma
renin activity without significantly elevating serum ionized calcium
levels. Calcium given with additional exogenous 1,25D also suppressed PTH

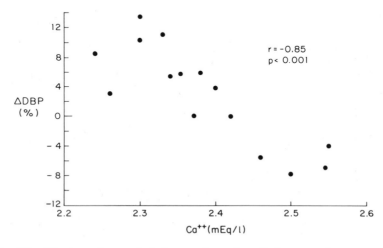

Figure 6. BP effects of co-administered oral calcium supplementation with
1,25 dihydroxyvitamin D. Blood pressure changes were compared on
the basis of initial serum ionized calcium levels (Ca$^{++}_{io}$) (27).

levels while not significantly elevating serum ionized calcium. However, circulating 1,25D levels rose significantly, compared to calcium supplementation alone, and plasma renin activity was suppressed. These opposite hormonal effects parallel their opposite blood pressure effects. It thus appears that 1) PTH is probably of little significance in mediating the blood pressure effects of oral calcium supplementation, since it was suppressed by both calcium-related maneuvers, each having opposite blood pressure consequences; 2) at least part of the mechanism by which increased oral calcium intake influences blood pressure is by virtue of its ability to suppress circulating 1,25D levels; 3) the inverse relation of plasma renin activity to 1,25D observed in steady-state screening of hypertensive populations is also consistently observed dynamically. Calcium supplementation in suppressing endogenous 1,25D, elevates plasma renin activity. This further strengthens the linkage between the renin-aldosterone system and calcium regulating hormones; and lastly 4) the fact that calcium supplementation lowers blood pressure best among those subjects in whom it reverses those various renin and calcium hormonal deviations initially observed in low renin and salt-sensitive hypertensive subjects, emphasizes the clinical relevance of these hormonal deviations in the pathogenesis of the hypertensive process.

Primary Aldosteronism Alters the Relation of PTH to 1,25D: A Role for Mineralocorticoids in Regulating Renal 1,25D?

In essential hypertension, although alterations in calcium regulating hormones may be relevant to the expression of the elevated blood pressure, they don't seem to be primary defects. Indeed, the hyperparathyroidism and the associated elevations of circulating 1,25D observed in low renin and salt-sensitive forms of hypertension were appropriate for and thus presumably secondary to the lower serum ionized calcium levels measured in those hypertensive states. Conversely, the calcium hormonal patterns observed in high renin, salt-insensitive hypertensives, suggestive of a calcium surfeit, are exactly what one would expect for the higher than average normotensive values for circulating ionized calcium measured in these subjects. These altered extracellular distributions of serum ionized calcium are themselves as yet unexplained, and we have hypothesized how they may reflect primary underlying abnormalities of cellular calcium handling (3). Nevertheless, these calcium hormonal changes appear to be necessary for the expression of the elevated blood pressure and are linked to the activity of the renin-aldosterone system as described above.

Unlike essential hypertension, however, in primary aldosteronism, relationships between calcium hormones and circulating calcium levels are abnormal and suggest primary effects of mineralocorticoid excess on the renal production of 1,25D, independently of standard calcium signals. Although it has been appreciated that mineralocorticoid excess causes renal calcium wasting and negative calcium balance (28,29), only recently has it been clinically recognized that the syndrome of primary aldosteronism is routinely associated with secondary hyperparathyroidism (30). Serum ionized calcium levels in primary aldosteronism, a syndrome with the greatest degree of renin suppression, are even lower than in low renin essential hypertensive subjects. Appropriately, PTH levels are even higher than in low renin essential hypertension. At the same time, however, serum 1,25D levels are paradoxically suppressed in primary aldosteronism compared with low renin essential hypertension. This has also been found in DOC-saline hypertensive rats compared with sodium chloride-loaded control rats - lower calcium levels with concurrent paradoxically lower 1,25D levels (Figure 7). Furthermore, the normal, direct, positive relationship between PTH and 1,25D is reversed in this syndrome. The higher the 1,25D, the lower the PTH, implying perhaps an intact feedback relationship between 1,25D and PTH, but at the same time implying that neither calcium itself nor PTH are primary influences on circulating 1,25D levels in primary aldosteronism. We hypothesize that mineralocorticoid hormones, here in opposition to physiologically "appropriate" calcium-related inputs, participate in the control of 1,25D synthesis (31).

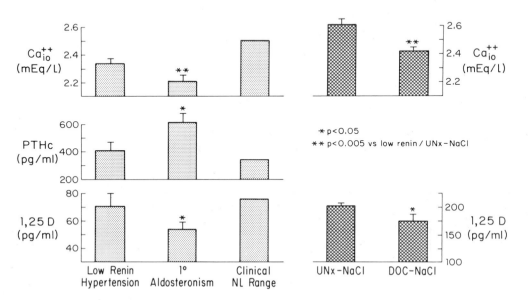

Figure 7. Calcium metabolic indices in primary aldosteronism and experimental mineralocorticoid excess. Ca_{io}^{++}-serum ionized calcium, PTH_c - C-terminal PTH levels, 1,25D -1,25 dihydroxyvitamin D (31).

Summary and Overall Hypothesis

What emerges from this data is an appreciation of a critical role for calcium regulating hormones coordinately with renin-aldosterone system, linking the humoral control of monovalent and divalent cation metabolism, in transducing dietary mineral signals at the cellular level. The resultant steady-state alterations in the distribution of calcium and magnesium intracellularly and between intracellular and extracellular compartments in a variety of different tissues directly influences 1) cardiac hemodynamic function, 2) central nervous and peripheral vasoactive hormone release, 3) peripheral smooth muscle vasoconstrictor tone, and hence the resultant blood pressure. This pattern of relationships is illustrated in Figure 8. This scheme, in which the ability of an altered dietary mineral balance to affect blood pressure is necessarily mediated by and in turn affects mono- and divalent cation regulating hormones, provides a perspective for better understanding both the biochemical and clinical heterogeneity of hypertension.

Specifically, this may help to resolve the bothersome observations 1) that a variety of genetically inherited ion transport defects found in hypertension are also found in normotensive family relatives and hence cannot by themselves explain elevated blood pressure, and 2) that chronic dietary sodium excess and/or calcium deficiency also do not usually result in clinical hypertension. Therefore, in neither case can these factors be considered "causes" of hypertension although they may each represent necessary but not sufficient condition. In essential hypertension for instance, different primary genetically inherited or acquired alterations in cellular ion transport systems may result in the heterogeneous distribution of serum ionized calcium we have observed. These in turn, create the metabolic setpoints of these two hormone systems - i.e., the renin-aldosterone system and calcium regulating hormones, which would lead to hypertension only when access to dietary minerals such as sodium chloride, potassium, calcium, and magnesium, is also shifted significantly each mineral either enhancing or suppressing these pathophysiologic hormone shifts. A high dietary salt intake in the setting of high endogenous 1,25D and secondary hyperparathyroidism would result in accelerated calcium transport intracellularly and thus the vasoconstriction, enhanced cardiovascular function, and increased central neural hormonal release often observed in salt-sensitive hypertension. In the absence of this skewed metabolic profile, dietary salt loading would result in no elevation in blood pressure. Furthermore, by helping to offset the calcium metabolic profile characterizing the low renin and salt-sensitive state, dietary calcium supplementation blunts the pressor effects of salt and in already salt loaded people, is significantly antihypertensive. These considerations also appear to help explain the heterogeneous blood pressure responses to a variety of different pharmacologic agents, including newer drug classes as calcium channel antagonists and converting enzyme inhibitors (18,32).

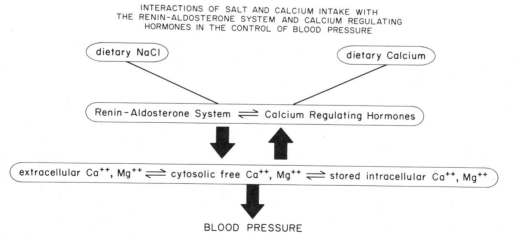

INTERACTIONS OF SALT AND CALCIUM INTAKE WITH
THE RENIN-ALDOSTERONE SYSTEM AND CALCIUM REGULATING
HORMONES IN THE CONTROL OF BLOOD PRESSURE

Figure 8. Hypothetical scheme in which the renin-aldosterone system and calcium regulating hormones coordinately transduce environmental dietary-mineral signals at the cellular level, thereby mediating the contributions of dietary minerals to blood pressure (17).

Knowing how these hormonal systems operate to preside coordinately over blood pressure homeostasis will not only afford additional meaningful insights into the pathophysiology of hypertension, but will allow us diagnostically to identify subgroups of hypertensives for whom more physiologic, individualized therapy can be constructed. Ultimately, long-term prophylactic strategies to prevent the onset of hypertensive disease might be developed.

REFERENCES

1. S. Ringer, A third contribution regarding the infusion of the inorganic constituents of the blood on the ventricular contraction, J. Physiology (Lond.), 4, 222-225 (1883).
2. W.L.T. Addison, The use of calcium chloride in arterial hypertension, Canad. Med. Assoc. J., 14, 1059-1061 (1924).
3. L.M. Resnick, Uniformity and diversity of calcium metabolism in hypertension: A conceptual framework, Am. J. Med, 82 (Suppl 1B), 16-26 (1987).
4. H. Kesteloot and J. Geboers, Calcium and blood pressure, Lancet, 1:813-315 (1982).
5. P. Erne, P. Bolli, E. Burgissen, and F.R. Buhler, Correlation of platele calcium with blood pressure: Effect of antihypertensive therapy, N. Engl. J. Med., 319:1084-1088 (1984).
6. G.S. Brinton, W. Jubiz, and L.D. Lagerquist, Hypertension in primary hyperparathyroidism: The role of the renin-angiotensin system, J. Clin. Endocrinol. Metab., 41:1025-1029 (1975).
7. P. Weidmann, S.G. Massry, J.W. Coburn, M.H. Maxwell, J. Atleson, C.R. Kleeman, Blood pressure effects of acute hypercalcemia: Studies in patients with chronic renal failure, Ann. Intern. Med., 76:741-745 (1972).
8. G.H.A. Clowes, Jr., and F.A. Simeone, Acute hypocalcemia in surgical patients, Ann. Surg., 145:530-540 (1957).
9. D. McCarron, C.D. Morris, J.H. Henry, and J.L. Standon, Blood pressure and nutrient intake in the United States, Science, 224:1392-1398 (1984).
10. S. Achley, E. Connor-Barrett, and L. Suary, Dairy products, calcium and blood pressure, Am. J. Clin. Nutr., 38:457-461 (1983).
11. P. Strazzullo, V. Nunziata, M. Cirillo, et al, Abnormalities of calcium metabolism in essential hypetension. Clin. Sci., 65:137-141 (1983).
12. D.A. McCarron, Low serum concentrations of ionized calcium in patients with hypertension, N. Engl. J. Med., 307:226-228 (1982).
13. S. Ayachi, Increased dietary calcium lowers blood pressure in the spontaneous hypertensive rat, Metabolism, 28:1234-1238 (1979).
14. J.M. Belizan, J. Villar, O. Pineda, A.E. Gonzalez, E. Soing, G. Garrera, R. Sibrian, Reduction of blood pressure with calcium supplementation in young adults, JAMA, 249:1161-1165 (1983).
15. D.A. McCarron, and C.D. Morris, Blood pressure response to oral calcium in persons with mild to moderate hypertension. Ann. Intern. Med., 103:825-831 (1985).
16. L.M. Resnick, J.H. Laragh, J.E. Sealey, and M.H. Alderman, Divalent cations in essential hypertension: Relations between serum ionized calcium, magnesium and plasma renin activity. N. Engl. J. Med., 309:888-891 (1983).
17. L.M. Resnick, F.B. Müller, and J.H. Laragh, Calcium regulating hormones in essential hypertension: Relation to plasma renin activity and sodium metabolism, Ann. Intern. Med., 105:649-654 (1986).
18. L.M. Resnick, and J.H. Laragh, Renin, calcium metabolism and the pathophysiologic basis of antihypertensive therapy, Am. J. Cardiol., 56:68H-74H (1985).

19. L.M. Resnick, J.P. Nicholson, and J.H. Laragh, Alterations in calcium metabolism mediate dietary salt sensitivity in essential hypertension, Trans. Assoc. Amer. Physicians, 98:313-321 (1985).

20. L.M. Resnick, J.P. Nicholson, and J.H. Laragh, Sodium sensitivity and calcium regulating hormones in essential hypertension, J. Am. Coll Cardiol., 5:436 (1985).

21. N.A. Breslau, J.L. McCurie, J.E. Zerwith, C.Y.C. Pak, The role of dietary sodium on renal excretion and intestinal absoprtion of calcium and on vitamin D metabolism, J. Clin. Endocrin. Metab., 55:369-372 (1982).

22. D.A. McCarron, L.I. Rankin, M.L.U. Bennett, S. Krutzik, M.R. McClung, F.C. Luft, Urinary calcium excretion at extremes of sodium intake in normal man, Am. J. Nephrol., 1:84 (1981).

23. L.M. Resnick, J.E. Sealey, and J.H. Laragh, Short and long-term oral calcium alters blood pressure (BP) in essential hypertension, Fed. Proc., 42(3):300 (1983).

24. L.M. Resnick, J.P. Nicholson, and J.H. Laragh, Calcium metabolism and essential hypertension - relationship to altered renin system activity, Fed. Proc., 45:2739-2745 (1986).

25. L.M. Resnick, B. Di Fabio, R.M. Marion, G.D. James, and J.H. Laragh, Dietary calcium modifies the pressor effects of dietary salt intake in essential hypertension, J. Hypertension, 4(Suppl 6):S679-S681 (1986)

26. L.M. Resnick, and J.H. Laragh, Does dihydroxyvitamin D (1,25 D) cause low renin hypertension?, Hypertension, 6:792 (1984).

27. L.M. Resnick, Calcium and vitamin D metabolism in the pathophysiology of human hypertension, In: Am. Inst. Nutr. Proceedings - Nutrition '87, 110-115 (1987).

28. R. Luft, and B. Sjogren, Some aspects of the metabolic effect of deoxycorticosterone acetate, Metabolism, 2:313-321 (1953).

29. S. Massry, J.W. Coburn, L.W. Chapman, C.R. Kleeman, The effect of long-term deoxycorticosterone acetate administration on the renal excretion of calcium and magnesium, J. Lab. Clin. Med., 71:212-219 (1968).

30. L.M. Resnick, and J.H. Laragh, Calcium metabolism and parathyroid function in primary aldosteronism, Am. J. Med., 78:385-390 (1985).

31. L.M. Resnick, J.M. Gertner, and J.H. Laragh, Abnormal vitamin D metabolism in primary aldosteronism and experimental mineralcorticoid excess, J. Hypertension, 5 (1987), in press.

32. L.M. Resnick, J.P. Nicholson, and J.H. Laragh, Calcium, the renin-angiotensin system, and the hypertensive response to nifedipine, Hypertension, 10:254-258 (1987).

VENTRICULAR ARRHYTHMIAS IN HEMODIALYSIS PATIENTS:

A STUDY OF INCIDENCE AND CONTRIBUTORY FACTORS

Ken-ichi Kimura*, Kaoru Tabei**, Toshio Nakayama*,
Yasushi Asano**, and Saichi Hosoda*

Departments of *Cardiology and **Nephrology
Jichi Medical School
Minamikawachi, Tochigi, Japan

ABSTRACT

One hundred patients undergoing maintenance hemodialysis for chronic renal failure were evaluated by Holter ECG monitoring for a 72-hour period from the day of hemodialysis therapy. Eighteen patients (the frequent group) who had more than 700 premature ventricular contractions (PVCs) per day were found among these 100 patients. In those eighteen, the PVCs were recorded frequently during and for 4 hours after hemodialysis. The values of the serum calcium concentration times those of phosphorus, which are thought to be an index of parathyroid function, were significantly higher in the frequent group than in patients without PVCs (the no arrhythmia group) or in those with fewer PVCs (less than 700 beats per day; sporadic group). Also, in the frequent group, the percent fractional shortening of the left ventricle, as measured by 2-dimensional echocardiography, was significantly lower than those in the no arrhythmia and sporadic groups. From these results, we conclude that the pathogenesis of the PVCs in chronic renal failure resulted partially from impaired cardiac performance and accelerated parathyroid function.

INTRODUCTION

Owing to advances in hemodialysis techniques and their application, the number of long-term hemodialysis patients has been increasing markedly in Japan. As a result, cases of secondary hyperparathyroidism have also increased in frequency. It has been recognized that hyperparathyroidism secondary to chronic renal disease may be exacerbated by lon-term hemodialysis. Parathyroid hormone (PTH) is thought to be one of the uremic toxins[1] that causes anemia, uremic osteitis fibrosa, and/or peripheral neuropathy. Recently, PTH has been shown to cause deterioration of cardiac function[2], inhibition of the vascular response to norepinephrine[3], and so-called uremic cardiomyopathy[4]. On the other hand, it is now well documented that cardiac arrhythmia has been encountered frequently in uremic patients who have undergone regular hemodialysis[1,5,6]. There remains controversial, however, regarding the factors that contribute to cardiac arrhythmias. Several likely factors have been suggested, including rapid fall of serum potassium during hemodialysis[6], abnormal plasma catecholamine levels[7], uremic cardiomyopathy[4], and the use of digitalis[8], the mechanisms of these arrhythmias

New Actions of Parathyroid Hormone
Edited by S. G. Massry and T. Fujita
Plenum Press, New York

has not been defined with any certainty. We have recently encountered a
very interesting case whose ventricular arrhythmia was markedly diminished
after parathyroidectomy, suggesting that PTH may have caused the
ventricular arrhythmia. The experience of this case led us to study the
correlations between maintenance hemodialysis and the prevalence of
ventricular arrhythmias. We also evaluated factors that may contribute
to the development of such arrhythmia.

CASE REPORT

A 43 year old man had been receiving regular hemodialysis therapy
for 12 years. He had experienced pulse deficit during hemodialysis
therapy for 2 years, and had suffered from ankle and knee joint pain over
the same period. Clinical findings such as a Rugger jersey appearance
and a salt-and-pepper appearance on bone X-ray films, a high plasma
concentration of c-terminal parathyroid hormone (c-PTH; 25.6 ng/ml), and
enlarged parathyroid glands led us to diagnose secondary hyperparathyroidism. After the admission, 72 hours of continuous Holter
monitoring was performed and the ECG showed frequent mono-morphic PVCs
(711 beats per day). However, 72-hour Holter monitoring revealed only 1
PVC a day on the 7th day after parathyroidectomy (Fig. 1).

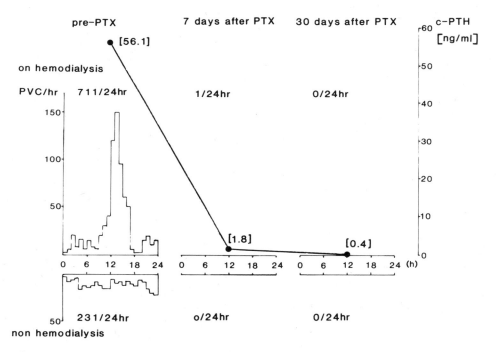

Fig. 1.   A 43 year old man with secondary to hyperparathyroidism. The
upper part of the left column shows the amount of PVC on
hemodialysis day, and the lower part, the amount of PVC on
non-hemodialysis day. The number of PVCs increased during
and for 4 hours after hemodialysis. 72 hours of Holter
monitoring showed only 1 PVC a day on the 7th day after
parathyroidectomy, as shown in the middle column. The
concentration of the c-PTH was also significantly diminished
after parathyroidectomy.

PATIENTS AND METHODS

One hundred patients with chronic renal failure (59 males, 41 females; mean age, 50.6 years) undergoing regular maintenance hemodialysis were the subjects of this investigation. The mean duration of hemodialysis was 40.8 months (range: 1 month to 15 years). The causes of chronic renal failure were chronic glomerulonephritis in 37 cases, diabetic nephropathy in 20, and nephrosclerosis in 9; and in the remaining 34 cases the causes varied but included gout and systemic lupus erythematosus. Hemodialysis was performed by the standard technique with hollow fiber type dialyzers for a mean of 4.0 hours (range 3 to 5 hours) 2 or 3 times per week. The dialysate contained (mEq/L) Na 135, K 2.5, Cl 107, Ca 3.0, Mg 1.5, bicarbonate 27.5, and acetate 7.5 (AK-solita C, Shimizu Co., Japan). Holter monitoring was carried out for a continuous 72-hour period, which included the day on which hemodialysis was performed. Two-dimensional echocardiogram were obtained in all cases prior to hemodialysis (Toshiba SSA-40A, Toshiba Electric Co., Japan). Laboratory tests were performed prior to treatment on the day of hemodialysis. The patients were classified into three groups according to the number of recorded PVCs. Patients in the no arrhythmia group had no PVCs during the 72 hours of monitoring; those in the sporadic group had fewer than 700 arrhythmic beats/day; and those in the frequent group had more than 700/day. The data were statistically analyzed by Student's nonpaired tests, the nonparametric test, and nonparametric rank correlation. P values less than 5 % were considered to be significant.

RESULTS

Incidence of PVCs

Of the 100 patients, 77 had ventricular arrhythmias. Eighteen of these were classified in the frequent group, and 59 of these were classified in the sporadic group. The grade of ventricular arrhythmias, according to the classification of Lown's[9], 11 patients in frequent group (61 %) and 16 in sporadic group (27 %) were classified into more than grade 3, i.e. multi-morphic PVCs, non-sustained and sustained ventricular tachycardia. In the frequent group, the grades of Lown's were getting worse in 13 patients (72 %) during and after hemodialysis. On the other hand, in sporadic group, the grades were getting worse in 40 patients (68 %) during and after hemodialysis. Thus, the grades of Lown's were deteriorated by hemodialysis therapy in both of sporadic and frequent groups. Moreover, in sporadic group, 7 patients showed sustained ventricular tachycardia only during hemodialysis (Fig. 2). The frequency of PVCs was significantly higher in older patients.

Factors affecting PVCs

Eight of the 18 patients with frequent PVCs had cardiac disorders, including aortic or mitral valve disease (4 cases) and myocardial infarction (2 cases) (Table 1).
The products of serum calcium times serum phosphorus were significantly higher in the frequent group than those in the no arrhythmia group (54.7 ± 3.5 vs 43.8 ± 3.2; $p < 0.005$). The estimated free calcium concentration, calculated from the total calcium concentration minus the albumin concentration (assuming that 1 mg/dl calcium binds to 1 g/dl albumin), was significantly higher in the frequent group than in the no arrhythmia group (5.56 ± 0.23 vs 5.13 ± 0.29; $p < 0.05$). Plasma free fatty acid was also high in the frequent group compared to those in the sporadic and no arrhythmia groups. There were no other significant

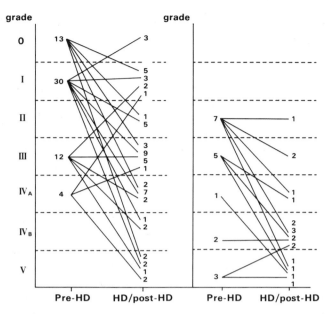

Fig. 2. The grade of ventricular arrhythmias, according to the classification of Lown, deteriorated during and after hemodialysis in the 59 patients with sporadic PVCs and in the 18 with frequent PVCs.

intergroup differences in hematological and biochemical data. The ECG findings revealed that the corrected QT interval was significantly prolonged in the frequent group in comparison with the no arrhythmia group (0.52 ± 0.02 vs 0.44 ± 0.01 sec; p<0.001). The left ventricular end-diastolic dimension as measured by 2-dimensional echocardiography tended to be large in the frequent group, but this finding was not statistically significant. The percent fractional shortening of the left ventricle was significantly diminished in the frequent group as compared to that in the no arrhythmia group (40.7 ± 1.9 vs 30.7 ± 1.8 %; p<0.005).

DISCUSSION

In this study, it was apparent that ventricular arrhythmias occurred frequently in patients on chronic maintenance hemodialysis. Despite the considerable improvements in dialysis techniques, patients with end-stage renal disease who are on chronic hemodialysis have a yearly mortality of 10 %. Cardiovascular disease such as congestive heart failure, cardiac arrhythmias, and acute myocardial infarction[10,11] are responsible for 30 to 50 % of this mortality[18,19]. This high susceptibility to cardio-vascular mortality is not restricted to elderly patients but accounts for 50 % of deaths in children on hemodialysis as well[12]. The precise contribution of cardiac arrhythmias to increased cardiovascular mortality in stable end-stage renal disease patients on chronic hemodialysis has not been determined. There is epidemiologic evidence, however, that the occurrence of significant ventricular arrhythmias, particularly in the

Table 1. Correlation between heart disease and PVCs.

	(+)	(−)	
PVC (−)	2	21	23
PVC (+)	15	44	59
PVC (++)	8	10	18
Total	25	75	100

p<0.05

Table 2. Underlying cardiac disorders.

	AS	AR	MR	angina	OMI	other
PVC (+)				1		1
PVC (−)		3	5	2	2	3
PVC (++)	2	1	1		2	2

AS: aortic stenosis, AR: aortic regurgitation,
MR: mitral regurgitation, OMI: old myocardial infarction.

presence of underlying heart disease, may increase these patients' susceptibility to fatal arrhythmias[13,14]. In fact, we observed 5 deaths from ventricular tachycardia/fibrillation in patients on maintenanace hemodialysis[15]. In 4 of these 5 cases, serious arrhythmias were documented from 1 to 2 weeks before death, and nonsustained ventricular tachycardia was noted in all 5 for 18 to 48 hours after hemodialysis. When we studied these phenomena in 100 hemodialysis patients, we found the indicence of PVCs to be significantly higher during and for 4 hours after hemodialysis than before hemodialysis (p<0.05). Complex PVCs and nonsustained ventricular tachycardia frequently appeared during hemodialysis. We used the index of calcium times phosphorus to estimate parathyroid function[16], and found that this index was significantly higher in the frequent PVC group than that in no arrhythmia group. As mentioned before, in a 43 year old male patient who underwent parathyroidectomy for secondary hyperparathyroidism associated with long-term hemodialysis, the significant postoperative decrease in the serum c-PTH concentration (25.6 to 1.8 ng/ml), was paralleled by a dramatic fall in the number of PVCs recorded during 24-hour Holter monitoring, from 711 beats to 1 beat per day. These findings suggest that parathyroid hormone may play a role in the genesis of PVCs in uremic individuals.

Ramires et.al.[5] reported that the c-PTH concentration was significantly higher in patients with cardiac arrhythmias than in those without arrhythmias, and suggested that PTH might be an arrhythmogenic agent in uremic patients. Calcium ions have received attention recently for their possible roles in the amelioration of the adverse effects of myocardial ischemia and in the genesis of arrhythmias[17].

We concluded that depressed cardiac performance and accelerated parathyroid function are major contributors to the pathogenesis of PVCs uremic patients.

ACKNOWLEDGEMENT

This work was supported by a Research Grant for Cardiovascular Disease (59C-5) from the Ministry of Health and Welfare of Japan.

REFERENCES

1. S.G. Massry, D.A. Goldstein: The search for uremic toxin(s)'X''X'= PTH. Clin. Nephrol. 11: 181-189 (1979).

2. U. Gafter, A. Battler, M. Eldar, D. Zevin, H.N. Neufeld, J. Levi: Effect of hyperparathyroidism on cardiac function in patients with end-stage renal disease. Nephron 41: 30-33 (1985).

3. J. Collins, S.G. Massry, V.M. Camperse: Parathyroid hormone and the altered vascular response to norepinephrine in uremia. Am. J. Nephrol. 5: 110-113 (1985).

4. R.J.S. McGonigle, M.B. Fowler, A.B. Timmis, M.J. Weston, V. Parsons: Uremic cardiomyopathy: Potential role of vitamin D and parathyroid hormone. Nephron 36: 94-100 (1984).

5. G. Ramirez, C.D. Brueggemeyer, I.L. Newton: Cardiac arrhythmias on hemodialysis in chronic renal failure patients. Nephron 36: 212-218 (1984).

6. G. Morrison, E.L. Michelson, S. Brown, J. Morganroth: Mechanism and prevention of cardiac arrhythmias in chronic hemodialysis patients. Kidney Int. 17: 811-819 (1980).

7. G.N. Corder, J. Sharma, R.H. McDonald: Variable levels of plasma catecholamines and dopamine beta-hydroxylase in hemodialysis patients. Nephron 25: 267-272 (1980).

8. V. Wizemann, W. Kramer, T. Funke, G. Schutterle: Dialysis-induced cardiac arrhythmias: Fact or fiction? Nephron 39: 356-360 (1985).

9. B. Lown, M. Wolf: Approaches to sudden death from coronary heart disease. Circulation 44: 130 (1971).

10. B.T. Burton, K.K. Krueger, F.A. Bryan, Jr.: National registry of long-term dialysis patients. J.A.M.A. 218: 718-722 (1971).

11. A. Lindner, B. Charra, D.J. Sherrard, B.H. Scribner: Accelerated atherosclerosis in prolonged maintenanace hemodialysis. New Engl. J. Med. 290: 697-701 (1974).

12. K. Scharar, F.P. Brunner, H. von Dehn, H.J. Gurland, H. Harlen, F.M. Parsons: Combined report on regular dialysis and transplantation of children in Europe. 1971. Proc. Eur. Dial. Transplant Ass. 10: 58 (1973).

13. M. Rodstein, L. Wolloch, R. Gubner: Mortality study of the significance of extrasystoles in an insured population. Circulation 44: 617-625 (1971).

14. B.N. Chiang, L.V. Perlman, L.D. Ostrander, Jr., F.H. Epstein: Relationship of premature systoles to coronary heart disease and sudden death in the Tecumseh epidemiologic study. Ann. Intern. Med. 70: 1159-1166 (1979).

15. K. Kimura, K. Tabei, S. Hosoda: Selection of the treatment and tachyarrhythmia in various myocardial disorders--with regard to the myocardial damage in uremic patients. Nagoya, Japan, 1986 (Suppl.)

16. S.G. Massry, J.W. Coburn, M.M. Popovtzer, et.al.: Secondary hyperparathyroidism in chronic renal failure. The clinical spectrum in uremia, during hemodialysis and after renal transplantation. Arch. Intern. Med. 124: 431-441 (1969).

17. W.T. Clusin, M.R. Bristow, H.S. Karagueuzian, B.G. Katzung, J.S. Schroeder: Do calcium dependent ionic currents mediate ischemic ventricular fibrillation? Am. J. Cardiol. 49: 606-612 (1982).

PARATHYROID HORMONE AND MUSCLE

PARATHYROID HORMONE IN MUSCULAR DYSTROPHY

Genaro M.A. Palmieri, Tulio E. Bertorini,
David F. Nutting, and Abbie B. Hinton

Departments of Medicine, Neurology, and Physiology
and Biophysics. University of Tennessee-Memphis
Memphis, TN 38163

Fifty years ago, Houssay showed that pituitary ablation ameliorates the hyperglycemia of pancreatectomized dogs.[1] This approach was later applied to human diseases, such as diabetes mellitus and cancer. A conclusion of those studies is that under certain circumstances, hormones secreted in normal amounts may be deleterious in human disease. In this presentation we will discuss the role that normally functioning parathyroid glands may have in muscular dystrophy.

Muscle Ca in Muscular Dystrophy

Muscular dystrophy is a genetic condition in which structural and functional alterations of plasma membranes have been demonstrated in skeletal muscle[2,3] and erythrocytes[4]. These leaky membranes are probably responsible for many aspects of the pathogenesis of this disease. Pathologists were the first to observe that in skeletal muscle of patients with Duchenne muscular dystrophy (DMD), specific stains for Ca were highly positive[5,6]. We decided, therefore, to determine the Ca content in skeletal muscle of patients with DMD and other neuromuscular diseases, using well established techniques for mineral analysis of tissues[7]. Muscle Ca content was three times higher than normal in DMD (Table 1). This elevation was significantly greater than that seen in other neuromuscular diseases.

Since soft tissue calcification is the final result of a series of events resulting in cell death and tissue necrosis, it was important to determine if the accumulation of Ca was a pre-or post-necrotic phenomenon. In collaboration with Dr. F. Cornelio and co-workers from Milano, Italy, we were able to study the skeletal muscle of fetuses at risk for DMD and in a premature infant who later developed typical clinical and laboratory signs of DMD. In these subjects, no muscle necrosis was found in detailed histochemical examination, yet muscle Ca still was elevated, about three-fold[8]. These observations clearly show that the excessive Ca accumulation in muscular dystrophy proceeded the development of necrosis and support the hypothesis that the increased intracellular Ca accumulation may play a role in the progression of the dystrophic process[5, 9-13].

Table 1. Muscle Ca in Duchenne Muscular Dystrophy (Extracted from Bertorini et al[7], with permission).

Group (n)	Calcium*
A. Normal subjects (22)	8.49 ± 0.36
B. Duchenne muscular dystrophy (27)	24.63 ± 0.84
C. Denervating diseases# (14)	16.12 ± 1.07
D. Polymyositis-dermatomyositis (11)	15.77 ± 1.74
E. Other neuromuscular diseases** (11)	15.61 ± 1.82

* mEq/kg fat-free dry tissue, mean $\pm$ SEM
\# Peripheral neuropathies and spinal muscular atrophy
** Congenital myopathies, limb girdle muscular dystrophy and fascioscapulohumeral muscular dystrophy
A vs B, C, D, E: $p < 0.0001$; B vs C, D, E: $p < 0.0001$

The concentration of Ca in the cytosol is approximately $10^{-7}M$, but $10^{-3}M$ in the extracellular fluid, resulting in a 10,000-fold gradient from the extracellular and to the intracellular compartments. This provides a strong chemical driving force for Ca to enter cells, especially when cell membranes are leaky. Although minute elevations of cytosolic Ca play a role in cell activation under physiological circumstances[14], excessive cytosolic Ca impairs cellular function by reducing ATP synthesis[15, 16], and by stimulating Ca dependent neutral proteases[17-20] and phospholipases[21,22]. The fall in ATP alters Ca extrusion mechanisms, allowing more extracellular Ca to accumulate in the cell, causing more damage and eventually cell death. The cell, however, has safeguards and is able to sequester the excessive Ca in mitochondria and in the endoplasmic reticulum. When these reservoirs are overloaded, the tissue suffers the consequences of the excessive Ca accumulation. In fact, Wrogemann and co-workers[12,13] found increased Ca and altered physiology in mitochondria from dystrophic muscle.

Parathyroid Hormone and Cell Ca

It has been known for almost 20 years that parathyroid hormone (PTH) increases the flux of Ca into target cells[23,24]. Under physiological conditions, the transient elevation of cytosolic Ca plays the role of second messenger of hormonal action, but excessive PTH secretion, such as in hyperparathyroidism, causes intracellular accumulation of Ca[25] and leads to nephrocalcinosis and renal failure. Hyperparathyroidism, affects not just organs with high affinity receptors, such as bone and kidney; elevated Ca has been found in brain[26] and skeletal muscle[27]. Since these observations were also demonstrated in secondary hyperparathyroidism with normal or low serum Ca[26,27], it appears that excessive PTH, and not hypercalcemia, is the cause of the exaggerated Ca accumulation in soft tissues. Excessive PTH may also increase Ca flux into cardiac muscle, since adding PTH to heart cells in vitro stimulated their beating rate[28], a reflection of cytosolic Ca concentration. Moreover, the excess PTH eventually killed the heart cells.

Parathyroid Hormone and Muscular Dystrophy

Since we found a normal serum concentration of PTH in DMD (66.4 ± 2.3 pMol/L in 17 DMD boys and 65.4 ± 7.4 in 5 age-matched normal boys), the elevated muscle Ca in DMD could not be attributed to excessive secretion of PTH. We tested the hypothesis that "normal" circulating PTH could contribute to the excessive muscle Ca accumulation in muscular dystrophy. Dystrophic hamsters (BIO 14.6) and non-dystrophic hybrid hamsters (BIO F1B) were submitted to thyroparathyroidectomy (TPTX) at age 35d and maintained on a routine laboratory diet and freshly prepared L-thyroxine, 0.6 µg/100g body weight per day, injected subcutaneously. Control animals were injected with the same volume of vehicle. Fifty-five days after TPTX (age 90d) samples of heart ventricles, diaphragm, rectus femoris, and blood were obtained for chemical determinations. A detailed description of the methods appears elsewhere[29]. To assess the completeness of the TPTX, a careful examination of the trachea and adjacent area was performed under a dissecting microscope, and in addition serial sections of trachea and adjacent tissues were evaluated histologically. No remaining parathyroid tissue was observed. Histochemical examination of muscles and chemical analysis of tissues were carried out using a blind protocol. Table 2 shows the muscle Ca content. A marked elevation in Ca was observed in dystrophic hamsters. TPTX caused significant reduction in dystrophic, but not in normal animals.

No difference in magnesium content was observed comparing normal and dystrophic, intact and TPTX, hamsters.

Table 2. Effect of Parathyroid Ablation on Ca Content[*] of Heart (Ventricles), Diaphragm and Rectus Femoris of Normal and Dystrophic Hamsters. (Extracted from Palmieri et al[29], with permission).

Group(n)	Heart	Diaphragm	Rectus Femoris
A. Normal (6)	19.9 ± 0.1	11.3 ± 0.2	14.8 ± 0.3
B. Normal + TPTX (5)	19.6 ± 0.5	11.5 ± 0.2	15.1 ± 0.9
C. Dystrophic (10)	414 ± 37	80.6 ± 6.6	50.6 ± 9.5
D. Dystrophic + TPTX (9)	200 ± 17	60.6 ± 2.7	28.8 ± 2.9

*mEq/kg/fat-free dry tissue, mean ± SE.
 For all muscle types : A vs B: NS; A vs C: p<0.001; C vs D: p<0.05 (ANOVA).

Histological evaluation was done using an arbitary scale of 0-4 for each parameter examined; 0 represented absence of lesions and 4 severe involvement. Table 3 summarizes the results of ventricles and rectus femoris from TPTX and intact dystrophic hamsters.

In order to determine whether the TPTX-induced changes observed in muscle Ca content and histology in dystrophic hamsters represented improvement of the muscle, or arrest or retardation of the dystrophic process, we performed identical studies in 35d old dystrophic hamsters, the age in which TPTX has carried out. At this age, heart,

Table 3. Histological Findings, Effect of TPTX in Dystrophic
Hamsters (DH). (Extracted from Palmieri et al[29],
with permission).

| Lesion | Heart (n) | | Rectus femoris (n) | |
	DH (10)	DH + TPTX (9)	DH (10)	DH + TPTX (9)
Necrosis	1.6 + 0.2	1.2 + 0.1	1.6 + 0.2	1.6 + 0.3
Phagocytosis	2.3 + 0.3	2.0 + 0.2	2.7 + 0.2	2.3 + 0.4
Ca	2.3 + 0.2	1.8 + 0.3	0.5 + 0.2	1.3 + 0.2
Fibrosis	2.7 + 0.2	1.8 + 0.1*	0.5 + 0.2	0.6 + 0.3
Atrophy	------	-----	2.3 + 0.1	1.4 + 0.3*

Mean + SE of values obtained using a 0 ⟶ 4 scale; 0 represents
absence of lesions and 4 represents severe involvement. All
intact and TPTX normal hamsters were 0. Note the lack of difference in observed Ca deposits in spite of a 40-50% reduction in
chemical analysis of Ca in TPTX dystrophic hamsters (Table 1).
*p<0.02.

Although in general the lesions were less intense in TPTX dystrophic
hamsters, only fibrosis of the heart and atrophy in the rectus femoris
showed significant improvement.

diaphragm and rectus femoris Ca was already 2-5 fold higher in
dystrophic than in normal hamsters, but 2-4 fold lower than in 90d
old, TPTX dystrophic hamsters[29], suggesting that TPTX did not arrest,
but did retard the dystrophic process.

Plasma creatine kinase was elevated as expected in dystrophic
hamsters and was reduced by 65% following TPTX (Table 4). Plasma Ca
did not change 55d after TPTX (Table 3) on a diet containing 1.2% Ca.

Table 4. Hamster Plasma Creatine Kinase and Ca (Extracted from
Palmieri et al[29], with permission).

Group (n)	Ca mg/dl	CK U/ml
A. Normal (6)	10.8 + 0.2	28 + 5
B. Normal + TPTX (5)	11.4 + 0.3	45 + 9
C. Dystrophic (10)	10.9 + 0.2	1293 + 416
D. Dystrophic + TPTX (9)	10.6 + 0.4	424 + 61

CK comparison of A vs B: NS; A vs C: P<0.002; C vs D: P<0.02.
All Ca comparisons were non-significant.

Although no parathyroid tissue was detected in TPTX animals, the
normal levels of plasma Ca 55 d after TPTX prompted us to determine
the effect of acute TPTX in hamsters on plasma Ca. Six hours after
TPTX the plasma Ca was 5.8 + 0.58 mg/dl and 10.1 + 0.7 in sham-operated controls. This shows that acute, but not chronic, TPTX causes
hypocalcemia in hamsters on standard rodent laboratory diet.

This study clearly demonstrates that in dystrophic hamsters, TPTX causes a marked reduction in muscle Ca, plasma CK, and some amelioration of the histological lesions. These changes were independent of the levels of plasma Ca and were not observed in normal hamsters. Thus, PTH aggravates the dystrophic process, probably by enhancing the already increased Ca flux into muscle caused by a defective sarcolemma.

Diltiazem in Muscular Dystrophy

Since the elimination of a Ca-agonist, PTH, was beneficial in muscular dystrophy, we then studied the effects of the Ca-antagonist diltiazem in dystrophic hamsters, using a similar experimental design. Fifty-five days of treatment with diltiazem, 25mg/kg/d orally, resulted in beneficial effects almost identical to those observed in TPTX[30]. Thus, our studies suggest that the elimination of a Ca-agonist, PTH, or the administration of a Ca-antagonist, diltiazem, retarded the dystrophic process.

On the basis of our studies in dystrophic hamsters, a double blind clinical trial in DMD, was recently completed in our institution. We observed a beneficial trend and no side effects with the administration of diltiazem, 8mg/kg/d, to DMD boys for two years[31].

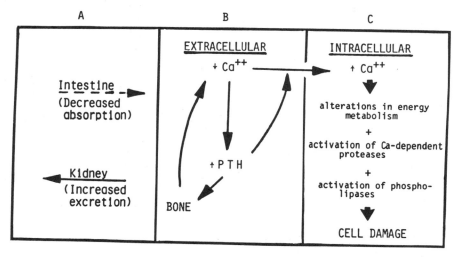

Figure 1. Hypothetical role of Ca balance in cellular Ca content. (A) Reduced absorption or increased excretion of Ca (unmatched by increased intestinal absorption) results in (B) hypocalcemia, that stimulates PTH secretion. PTH mobilizes Ca from bone (and increases renal Ca reabsorption), thus normalizing the extracellular Ca concentration. The elevated PTH also (C) stimulates Ca translocation into cells, particularly in the presence of congenital or acquired defective Ca exchange functions of plasma membranes. The excessive intracellular Ca could cause permanent or reversible cell damage. Thus, suppression of PTH secretion by exogenous Ca might prevent cell damage in certain diseases. (Reproduced from Palmieri et al[35], with permission).

On the basis of these findings, we may extend our hypothesis to other diseases in which cell Ca homeostasis may be altered. In muscular dystrophy the defective plasma membrane has a genetic cause. There are other conditions in which acquired alteration of plasma membranes occur, such as in acute pancreatitis[32]. In experimental acute pancreatitis in dogs we observed a 100% increment in skeletal muscle Ca after 24-48 hours[33]. A review on altered cell Ca metabolism in human diseases has been published elsewhere[34]. It is premature to implicate PTH in the pathogenesis of these disorders, but our studies on muscular dystrophy suggest that PTH, albeit in normal concentrations, may have a deleterious effect in conditions associated with altered plasma membranes. In these conditions it may be worthwhile to reduce PTH secretion to a minimum, and this could be accomplished by maintaining an adequate balance of Ca. The hypothetical role of Ca balance in cellular Ca content, via PTH has been discussed previously[35] and is illustrated in Figure 1. This hypothesis may explain the observed beneficial effect of Ca supplementation in arterial hypertension[36] and in the prevention of colonic cancer[37].

ACKNOWLEDGMENTS

This work was supported, in part by grant RR002211 from the U.S. Public Health Service and a grant from the Muscular Dystrophy Association.

The authors wish to thank the skillful editorial assistance of Ms. Donna Stallings.

REFERENCES

1. B.A. Houssay, The hypophysis and metabolism. Carbohydrate metabolism, N Eng J Med 214: 971 (1936).
2. B. Mokri and A.G. Engel, Duchenne dystrophy: electron microscope findings pointing to a basic or early abnormality in the plasma membrane of the muscle fiber, Neurology 25: 1111 (1975).
3. A.D. Roses, M.H. Herbstreith, and S.H. Appel. Membrane protein kinase alteration in Duchenne muscular dystrophy, Nature (Lond) 254: 350 (1975).
4. S. Araki, and S. Mawatari, Ouabain and erythrocyte-ghost adenosine triphosphatase, Arch Neurol 24: 187 (1974).
5. M.A. Oberc, and W.K. Engel, Ultrastructural localization of calcium in normal and abnormal skeletal muscle, Lab Invest 36: 566 (1977).
6. J.B. Bodensteiner, and A.G. Engel, Intracellular calcium accumulation in Duchenne dystrophy and other myopathies: a study of 567,000 muscle fibers in 114 biopsies, Neurology 28: 439 (1978).
7. T.E. Bertorini, S.K. Bhattacharya, G.M.A. Palmieri, C.M. Chesney, D. Pifer, and B. Baker, Muscle calcium and magnesium content in Duchenne muscular dystrophy, Neurology 32: 1088 (1982).
8. T.E. Bertorini, F. Cornelio, S.K. Bhattacharya, G.M.A. Palmieri, I. Dones, F. Dworzak, and B. Brambati, Calcium and magnesium content in fetuses at risk and pre-nectrotic Duchenne muscular dystrophy, Neurology 34: 1436 (1984).
9. K.O. Godwin, J. Edwardly, and C.N. Fuss, "Retention of 45Ca in rats and lambs associated with the onset of nutritional dystropy, Aust J Biol Sci 28: 457 (1975).
10. S. Ebashi, and H. Sugita, The role of calcium in physiological

and pathological processes of skeletal muscle, in: "Current Topics in Nerve and Muscle Research". A.J. Aguayo, G. Karpati (eds). ICS No. 455, p. 73. Excerpta Medica, Amsterdam (1979).

11. K. Lossnitzer, J. Janke, B. Hein, M. Stauch, and A. Fleckenstein, Disturbed myocardial calcium metabolism: a possible pathogenetic factor in the hereditary cardiomyopathy of the Syrian hamster", in: " Recent Advances in Studies on Cardiac Structure and Metabolism". No. 6. A. Fleckenstein and G. Rona (eds), p. 207. University Park Press, Baltimore (1975).

12. K. Wrogemann, B.E. Jacobson, and M.C. Blanchaer, On the mechanism of a calcium-associated defect of oxidative phosphorylation in progressive muscular dystrophy, Arch Biochem Biophys 159: 267 (1973).

13. K. Wrogemann, and S.D. Pena, Mitochondrial calcium overload: A general mechanism for cell-necrosis in muscle diseases, Lancet 1: 672 (1976).

14. H. Rasmussen, Pathways of amplitude and sensitivity modulation in the calcium messenger system, in: "Calcium and cell function", W.Y. Cheung (ed). Vol. IV p. 1. Academic Press, New York (1983).

15. A. Fleckenstein, Myokardstoffwechsel und Nekrose, in: VI Symposium der Deutsch. Ges. fur Fortschritte auf dem Gebiet der Inneren Medizin uber 'Herzinfarkt und Schock'. L. Heilmeyer and H.J. Holtmeier (eds), p. 94. Georg Thieme Verlag, Stuttgart (1968).

16. A. Fleckenstein, J. Janke, H.J. Doring, and O. Leder, Myocardial fiber necrosis due to intracellular calcium overload; a new principle in cardiac pathophysiology, in: "Myocardial Biology. Recent Advances in Studies on Cardiac Structure and Metabolism". No. 4, N.S. Dhalla (ed), p. 563, University Park Press, Baltimore (1974).

17. W.R. Dayton, D.E. Goll, M.G. Zeece, R.M. Robson, and W.J. Reville, A Ca^{++}-activated protease possibly involved in myofibrillar protein turnover. Purification from porcine muscle, Biochemistry 15: 2150 (1976).

18. N.C. Kar, and C.M. Pearson, A calcium-activated neutral protease in normal and dystrophic human muscle, Clin Chim Acta 73: 293 (1976).

19. C.J. Duncan, Role of intracellular calcium in promoting muscle damage: a strategy for controlling the dystrophic condition, Experientia 34: 1531 (1978).

20. J.S. Neerunjun, and V. Dubowitz, Increased calcium-activated neutral protease activity in muscles of dystrophic hamsters and mice, J Neurol Sci 40: 105 (1979).

21. S. Mittnacht, Jr., C.S. Sherman, and J.L. Farber, Reversal of ischemic mitochondrial dysfunction, J Biol Chem 254: 9871 (1979).

22. D.E. Epps, J.W. Palmer, H.H. Schmid, and D.R. Pfeiffer, Inhibition of permeability-dependent Ca^{2+} release mitochondria by N-acylethanolamines, a class of lipids synthesized in ischemic heart tissues, J Biol Chem 257: 1383 (1982).

23. A.B. Borle, Calcium transport in cell culture and the effects of parathyroid hormone, in: "Parathyroid Hormone and Thyrocalcitonin (Calcitonin)". R.V. Talmage and L.F. Belanger (eds). ICS No. 159, p. 258 Excerpta Medica, Amsterdam (1968).

24. A.B. Borle, Control, modulation and regulation of cell calcium, Rev Physiol Biochem Pharmacol 90: 13 (1981).

25. A.B. Borle, and I. Clark, Effects of phosphate-induced hyperparathyroidism and parathyroidectomy on rat kidney calcium in vivo, Am J Physiol 241: E136 (1981).

26. A.I. Arieff, and S.G. Massry, Calcium metabolism of brain in acute renal failure: effects of uremia, hemodialysis and parathyroid hormone, J Clin Invest 53: 387 (1974).

27. R. Guisado, A.I. Arieff, and S. Massry, Muscle water and electrolytes in uremia and the effects of hemodialysis, J Lab Clin Med 89: 322 (1977).

28. E. Bogin, S.G. Massry, and I. Harary, Effect of parathyroid hormone on rat heart cells, J Clin Invest 67: 1215 (1981).

29. G.M. Palmieri, D.F. Nutting, S.K. Bhattacharya, T.E. Bertorini, and J.C. Williams, Parathryoid ablation in dystrophic hamsters: effects on calcium content and histology of heart, diaphragm and rectus femoris, J Clin Invest 68: 646 (1981).

30. S.K. Bhattacharya, G.M.A. Palmieri, T.E Bertorini, and D.F Nutting, Effect of the calcium antagonist diltiazem in dystrophic hamsters, Muscle Nerve 5: 73 (1982).

31. T.E. Bertorini, G.M.A. Palmieri, J.W. Griffin, M. Igarashi, J. McGee, R. Brown, D.F. Nutting, A.B. Hinton, and J.G. Karas, Effect of chronic treatment with the calcium antagonist diltiazem in Duchenne muscular dystrophy, Neurology, in press.

32. D.E. Bockman, W.R. Schiller, C. Suriyapa, J.H. Mutchler, and M.C. Anderson, Fine structure of early experimental acute pancreatitis in dogs, Lab Invest 28: 584 (1973).

33. S.K. Bhattacharya, R.W. Luther, J.W. Pate, A.J. Crawford, O.F. Moore, J.A. Pitcock, G.M.A. Palmieri, and L.G. Britt, Soft tissue calcium and magnesium content in acute pancreatitis in the dog: Calcium accumulation, a mechanism for hypocalcemia in acute pancreatitis, J Lab Clin Med 105: 422 (1985).

34. H. Rasmussen, and G.M.A. Palmieri, Altered cell calcium metabolism and human diseases, in: "Calcium in biological systems", R.P. Rubin, G.B. Weiss, and J.W. Putney (eds). p. 551 Plenum Publishing Corp. New York (1985).

35. G.M. Palmieri, A.B. Hinton, T.E. Bertorini, S.K. Bhattacharya, and D.F. Nutting, Muscle calcium accumulation in muscular dystrophy, in: "Intracellular calcium regulation". H. Boder, K. Gietzen, J. Rosenthal, R. Rudel, and H.V. Wolf (eds). p. 335. Manchester University Press, Manchester (1986).

36. D.A. McCarron, and C.D. Morris, Blood pressure response to oral calcium in persons with mild to moderate hypertension, Ann Int Med 103: 825 (1985).

37. M. Lipkin, and H. Newmark, Effect of added dietary Ca on colonic epithelial cell proliferation in subjects at high risk for familial colonic cancer, N Engl J Med 313: 1381 (1985).

HISTOLOGIC STUDIES IN MUSCLE OF HYPERPARATHYROIDISM

Tulio E. Bertorini

University of Tennessee, Memphis
Memphis Neuroscience Center
Memphis, Tennessee

INTRODUCTION

Patients with hyperparathyroidism may develop persistent proximal muscle weakness with the clinical characteristics of a myopathy [1-8]. This condition is distinct from the clinical constellation of weakness, lassitude, nausea, and vomiting that is associated with hypercalcemia [9,10]. The so-called hyperparathyroid myopathy has a more chronic course, often with muscular wasting, whereas hypercalcemia-induced symptoms are temporary and rapidly reversible.

In parathyroid myopathy, the trunk and limbs are predominantly affected, although weakness may also be seen in the neck flexors. Patients may have a waddling gait, and muscular wasting with pain are common findings [11]. The severity of weakness varies, and appears to be related to the duration of the hyperparathyroidism before diagnosis and treatment. Serum levels of calcium [3,4] and parathyroid hormone (PTH) [11] are not correlated with severity.

Important clinical findings include the presence of normal or hyperactive deep tendon reflexes, an unusual tongue tremor, minor sensory deficits (particularly vibratory sense) and, occasionally, an encephalopathy [11].

There seems to be a relationship between hyperparathyroidism and amyotrophic lateral sclerosis (ALS) [11,12]. However, most patients with hyperparathyroid myopathy show no evidence of corticospinal tract involvement or typical ALS.

Myopathy has been reported in both primary and secondary hyperparathyroidism [12,13]. Incidences of 70% and 80% have been reported in two series [12,14], but other investigators have found lower incidences [15-17]. With earlier recognition and treatment of hyperparathyroidism, before muscle weakness develops [18], the condition will probably be seen less frequently.

New Actions of Parathyroid Hormone
Edited by S. G. Massry and T. Fujita
Plenum Press, New York

Nerve conduction velocities are often normal in primary hyperparathyroidism, although mildly decreased values are seen in some cases [19]. In the secondary form, abnormal velocities may result from the neuropathy of kidney disease.

Electromyographic studies in patients with parathyroid myopathy classically show the presence of brief polyphasic motor units, as seen in other myopathies [11,16,20], despite the presence in pathologic studies of atrophic angular fibers [11] -- a finding that is characteristic of denervating diseases such as neuropathies. Denervation potentials, however, are usually absent [21]. Abnormalities in neuromuscular transmission have also been reported [22], but Ljunghall et al. [19] found little evidence of a neuromuscular transmission defect in a study using single fiber electromyography. The latter result could be explained at least in part by the fact that mild cases were studied.

There seem to be two types of hyperparathyroid myopathy. An extremely rare form is characterized by a necrotizing muscle disease that may be accompanied by skin ulcerations and elevation of serum enzymes [5,23]. The second more frequent form has a more indolent course, shows no evidence of muscle necrosis, and is usually associated with normal serum enzymes. Generally, muscle histochemistry reveals evidence of fiber atrophy, mainly of type II fibers as seen in disuse and other endocrine "myopathies" [24], some of the atrophic fibers are similar to what is found in neuropathies [11]. However, others have reported normal histology [3] or some degree of myofiber degeneration and regeneration [4].

The necrotizing form of hyperparathyroid myopathy seems clearly correlated with the presence of severe intramuscular arteriolar calcification, which may play a pathogenic role [23]. The pathogenesis of the non-necrotizing form is unclear, but its relationship to increased levels of parathyroid hormone is supported by the observation of PTH-induced muscle weakness experimentally, in humans [25]. In addition, muscle weakness improves following successful surgery in patients with hyperparathyroidism [26,27]. The pathologic findings suggest disuse atrophy, and the presence of angular fibers also indicates a neurogenic component, which has been postulated to result from damage to terminal nerve branches or the nerve cell [11].

Parathyroid hormone is known to increase the influx of calcium into the cytosol [28-30], and increased calcium has been demonstrated in muscle [31], brain [32], and soft tissues [33] in hyperparathyroidism. This calcium accumulation could activate neutral proteases [34,35] and overload mitochondria, thus impairing oxidation and triggering muscle necrosis [36,37], and may be the cause of muscle cell damage in the rare necrotizing myopathy of hyperparathyroidism. Because necrosis is unusual in hyperparathyroidism, these mechanisms cannot totally explain the muscle weakness seen in many of these patients, although it is conceivable that increased calcium could affect muscle function without causing necrosis.

To address issues related to the causes of parathyroid myopathy and to delineate its histopathology, we performed detailed histochemical and morphometric analyses of muscle biopsies in patients with primary and secondary hyperparathyroidism and various degrees of muscle weakness.

Specifically, we studied muscle fiber size and distribution, histologic evidence of necrosis, calcium accumulation in cells and vessels, and signs for denervation and reinnervation.

MATERIAL AND METHODS

Seven patients with primary and three with secondary hyperparathyoidism were studied (see Table I). All patients had parathyroid hyperplasia or adenoma; muscle weakness ranged from mild to moderate in nine patients, one patient who had not developed weakness was also studied.

Muscle biopsies were obtained at the time of parathyroidectomy; specimens were taken from the sternocleidomastoid muscles in seven patients and from a limb in three patients. The muscle was quickly frozen and preparations were made using a complete battery of histochemical stains, including ATPase, an oxidase stain (NADH-TR), nonspecific esterase, alkaline and acid phosphatases, Alizarin Red S, modified trichrome, and hematoxylin and eosin [24,38]. Quantitative analyses were done to assess the number of internalized nuclei, necrotic fibers, and angular atrophic esterase-positive fibers. Electron microscopic studies were made using standard techniques [24,38].

The two major muscle fiber types were analyzed histographically using the ATPase stain at pH 9.4. Mean fiber diameter [39] was calculated randomly in 200 fibers, excluding those that appeared clearly atrophic and angulated. (These measurements could not be done in one patient because the specimen was inadequate.) Atrophic and hypertrophic factors were calculated [40]. Percentages of fibers of both types was also determined.

Nonrandom distribution of fibers, which would indicate reinnervation and grouping, was assessed by calculating the co-dispersion index using techniques previously reported [41]. Results were compared with seven normal controls and from the literature.

TABLE I
PATIENTS STUDIED

AGE/SEX	DIAGNOSIS	SYMPTOMS
45/F	Primary hyperparathyroidism	Mild weakness, osteopenia, back pain
57/M	Primary hyperparathyroidism	Moderate weakness, decreased endurance, back pain
69/F	Primary hyperparathyroidism	Mild weakness
59/F	Primary hyperparathyroidism	Mild weakness, bone pains
72/F	Primary hyperparathyroidism	Very mild weakness, decreased muscle mass
71/F	Primary hyperparathyroidism	Mild weakness
53/F	Primary hyperparathyroidism	No weakness, bone pains
48/F	Secondary hyperparathyroidism	Mild weakness
43/M	Secondary hyperparathyroidism	Moderate weakness, neuropathy
48/M	Secondary hyperparathyroidism	Moderate weakness

RESULTS

Analysis of the biopsies revealed no evidence of fiber necrosis or other findings typically associated with myopathies, such as split fibers or increased endomysial connective tissue and fat. Increased numbers of internalized nuclei were seen in only two cases, both with secondary hyperparathyroidism. Electron microscopy showed only very rare fibers with slight disruption of the myofilaments. Calcium accumulation was not seen in muscle fibers, contrary to findings in other types of myopathies [42]. Calcium deposits were present in intramuscular arterioles in all patients (see Figure 1). However, this finding is not unique to this patient group; we have observed such deposits occasionally in other unrelated disorders and rarely in normal biopsies, particularly from elderly individuals. Some of the arterioles appeared thickened on electron microscopy, which also showed thickened basal lamina in some capillaries. Acid phosphatase activity, which is associated with activation of lysosomes and might indicate a prenecrotic stage, was only slightly increased in granular form in one patient. Increased alkaline phosphatase activity in muscle fiber, which occurs with cell regeneration [43], was not observed.

Results of the histometric analyses are summarized in Table II. Type I fibers were normal in all of the biopsies studied except one, and in two cases, type II fibers showed a mildly increased diameter when compared with our controls. However, these diameters were within the accepted normal ranges in the literature [24]. (Figure 2 shows as an example histograms made from calculations of fiber diameter in two cases compared with a normal control.) Standard deviations of type I fiber diameters greater than 0.25 of the mean were seen in three of eight biopsies, indicating an increased variation of fiber size. Increased variation of type II fiber size was seen in five cases. This mildly increased variation in fiber size, which is sometimes viewed as indicating myopathy, could also be secondary to various degrees of fiber atrophy and is seen in neurogenic diseases.

The atrophic factor was increased in type I fibers in one case and in type II fibers in another. The hypertrophic factor was increased in type I fibers in three biopsies and type II fibers in one. The number of atrophic angular esterase-positive fibers was calculated and graded + if there were 5 to 10 per lower power field and ++ if there were 10 to 15. They were increased in five (of seven) patients with primary hyperparathyroidism and two (of three) with secondary hyperparathyroidism (see Figure 1). Small, round, esterase-positive fibers were seen in eight biopsies.

The co-dispersion index, as indicator of the loss of random distribution of fibers [41], is considered normal when values are below 0.30 based on our normal controls. This index was slightly increased in three of our cases, which might indicate mildly increased fiber segregation. Fiber type grouping was not observed in any biopsy. A slight increase in the predominance of type II fibers was seen in three biopsies when compared with normal subjects. However, this was within normal limits in the literature. Also, because these findings sometimes correspond to the depth of the section, they are probably not significant. The biopsy of the patient with no weakness had atrophic angular fibers and arteriolar calcification, the co-dispersion index was slightly increased but the specimen was too small and inappropriate for adequate histometric determinations.

DISCUSSION

Our studies in hyperparathyroid patients with mild to moderate weakness confirmed the findings of others [11]. The main pathologic abnor-

TABLE II

RESULTS OF HISTOMETRIC ANALYSES OF MUSCLE BIOPSIES

	Fiber Diameter (μm)		Atrophic Angular/Round		Percentage of Fiber Types*		Co-dispersion Index	Atrophic Factor I / II		Hypertrophic Factor I / II	
	I	II	-	-	% I	% II	0-030	<150	<250	<300	<400
NL	54 ± 6.5	46 ± 7.4									
P	43 ± 7	47 ± 11	+	+	31	69	0.325	48	30	0	15
P	79 ± 15	94 ± 28	2+	+	33	67	0.109	30	37	1800	2400
P	55 ± 12	48 ± 12	+	0	25	75	0.124	61	60	143	216
P	50 ± 12	50 ± 10	0	+	32	68	0.229	30	0	72	76
P	41 ± 9	40 ± 8	0	+	49	51	0.340	69	113	0	0
P	54 ± 14	45 ± 16	2+	+	29	71	0.290	16	177	213	109
P	--	--	+	0	--	--	0.370	--	--	--	--
S	68 ± 20	56 ± 17	0	+	45	55	0	11	92	989	340
S	56 ± 14	69 ± 18	2+	+	28	72	0.039	160	146	66	60
S	69 ± 18	49 ± 24	1+	+	47	53	0.081	74	755	479	255

* Normal percentage of type I fibers from 30-60; Normal percentage of type II fibers from 50-70

P = Primary hyperparathyroidism; S = Secondary hyperparathyroidism

Specimen for patient #7 was not adequate for all measurements.

mality was muscle atrophy, characterized by the presence of small angular
fibers that are frequently associated with neurogenic atrophy. We also
found small, round fibers, some of which were esterase-positive and may
have been in the process of denervation. There was no evidence of cell
necrosis or histologic accumulation of calcium, indicating that necrosis
does not play a significant role in muscle weakness in most patients with
hyperparathyroidism. In contrast to the findings of others, type II muscle
fiber atrophy was not a prominent finding, and mean fiber diameters were
not significantly abnormal.

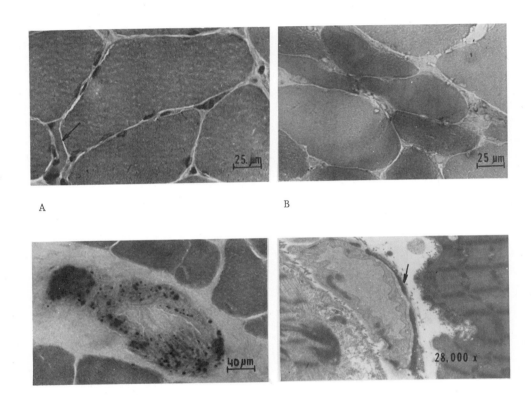

Figure 1. (A) Modified trichrome stain of muscle biopsy from patient 2
(Table II), showing atrophic angular fiber (arrow); (B) Nonspecific
esterase stain, showing esterase-positive atrophic fibers; (C) Alizarin
Red S stain, showing calcium deposits in walls of small intramuscular
vessel; (D) Electron micrograph showing calcium deposits in walls of
small intramuscular vessel.

Arteriolar calcification was the most frequent pathologic abnormality
and might explain, at least in part, the increased calcium content that has
been reported in muscle extracts. We do not have any evidence that this
played a role in muscle weakness, as it appears to do in the unusual
necrotizing form of hyperparathyroid myopathy. We cannot rule out,
however, the possibility that soluble calcium was increased in muscle
fibers affecting their function, and yet was not detected by our histologic
techniques.

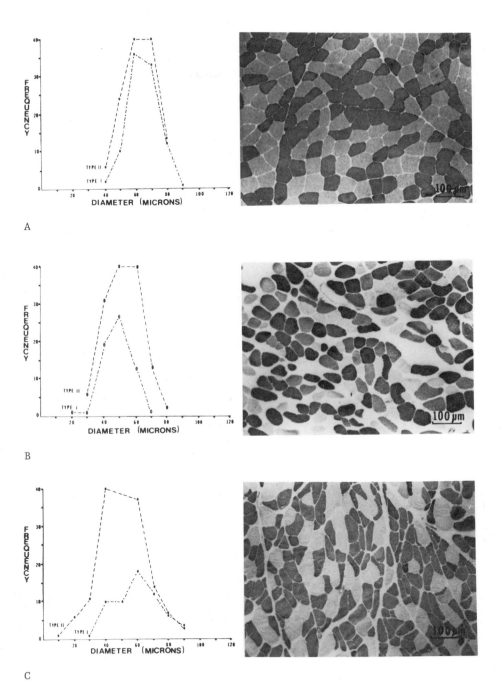

Figure 2. Histograms and ATPase (pH 9.4) stains of a normal (A) and two hyperparathyroid patients. Case #1 (B) and #6 (C), notice round atrophic fibers in B, and in C the angular atrophic fibers appear dark on this stain but also many appear dark on NADH-TR and nonspecific esterase (as in denervation).

The cause of the "neurogenic" atrophy seen in most of these patients remains unexplained. We did not find evidence of peripheral neuropathy by examination or by standard electrophysiologic techniques. It could be that the disease affects the motor neuron itself, and in some patients this condition does resemble a motor neuron disorder [11,12].

Another explanation is that a factor like parathyroid hormone, calcium, or some unknown substance might cause damage to the terminal nerve branches, producing isolated atrophy [11]. But this seems unlikely in view of the absence of significant denervation potentials on electromyography. Also against this hypothesis is the absence of the significant sprouting and fiber type grouping that is seen in other neurogenic conditions. It is conceivable that we did not detect grouping because the myopathy in our patients was very mild, although, others [11] have not observed this feature in more severe cases. A dysfunction of few terminal axonal branches and lack of sprouting could explain the brief motor units seen on electromyography.

It is also possible that weakness is caused by a disorder of neuromuscular transmission, such as that in myasthenia gravis [11], producing a "functional denervation" of muscle fibers. Indeed, in myasthenia, one can find atrophic angular fibers, type II fiber atrophy without histologic grouping and brief motor units without denervation potentials on EMG, as in hyperparathyroidism. Others have demonstrated abnormalities in neuromuscular transmission in hyperparathyroid patients with myopathy [22], this was not confirmed by single fiber electromyography [19]. Finally, it is conceivable that the condition affects muscle cells in a form that resembles, but is not caused by, nerve damage.

In conclusion, although the weakness in hyperparathyroidism resembles a myopathy, and PTH have effects in muscle that might trigger necrosis, the results of our pathologic studies indicate that the condition is not necessarily a myopathy. The most consistent finding is that of arteriolar calcification which is accompanied by fiber atrophy as in "neurogenic" diseases, but without nerve sprouting which is seen in these conditions.

Acknowledgements

I would like to thank Dr. Genaro Palmieri for allowing us to study his patients. Helen Ham and Christy Wright for invaluable secretarial and editorial assistance and for excellent technical assistance, Jean Elmendorf, Frank Maretta, Lou Grubbs and Linda Horner.

REFERENCES

1. A. Bischoff, and L. Esslen, Myopathy with primary hyperparathyroidism, Neurology (MN) 15:64, (1965).
2. B. Frame, E.G. Heinze, Jr., M.A. Block, and G.A. Manson, Myopathy in primary hyperparathyroidism. Observation in three patients, Ann Intern Med 68:1022, (1968).
3. R. Smith, and G. Stern, Muscular weakness in osteomalacia and hyperparathyroidism, J Neurol Sci 8:511, (1969).
4. E.J. Cholod, M.D. Haust, A.J. Hudson, and F.N. Lewis, Myopathy in primary familial hyperparathyroidism. Clinical and morphologic studies, Am J Med 48:700, (1970).
5. W.W. Goodhue, J.N. Davis, and R.S. Porro, Ischemic myopathy in uremic hyperparathyroidism, JAMA 221:911, (1972).

6. C. Richet, M. Sourdel, and A. Pergola, Syndromes parathyroidomusculaires; myopathies sclèreuses lièes à des troubles parathyroidiens, J Méd Franc 26:377, (1937).

7. T.R. Murphy, W.H. ReMine, and M.K. Burbank, Hyperparathyroidism: Report of a case in which parathyroid adenoma presented primarily with profound muscular weakness, Staff Meetings of the Mayo Clinic 35:629, (1960).

8. R. Smith, and G. Stern, Myopathy in osteomalacia and hyperparathyroidism, Brain 90:593, (1967).

9. F. Albright, The parathyroid - Physiology and therapeutics, JAMA 117:527, (1941).

10. E.H. Norris, Collective review. The parathyroid adenoma: A study of 322 cases, International Abstr Surg 84:1, (1947).

11. B.M. Patten, J.P. Bilezikian, L.E. Mallette, A. Prince, W.K. Engel, and G.D. Aurbach, Neuromuscular disease in primary hyperparathyroidism, Ann Intern Med 80:182, (1974).

12. C.T. Vicale, The diagnostic features of a muscular syndrome resulting from hyperparathyroidism, osteomalacia owing to renal tubular acidosis and perhaps to related disorders of calcium metabolism, Trans Am Neurol Assn 74:143, (1949).

13. L.E. Mallette, B.M. Patten, and W.K. Engel, Neuromuscular disease in secondary hyperparathyroidism, Ann Intern Med 82:474, (1975).

14. J. Lemann, and A.A. Donatelli, Calcium intoxication due to primary hyperparathyroidism. A medical and surgical emergency, Ann Intern Med 60:447, (1964).

15. G. Karpati, and B. Frame, Neuropsychiatric disorders in primary hyperparathyroidism clinical analysis with review of the literature, Arch Neurol 10:387, (1964).

16. G.D. Aurbach, L. Mallette, B. Patten, D. Heath, J. Doppman, and J. Bilezikian, Hyperparathyroidism: Recent studies, Ann Intern Med 79:566, (1973).

17. A.B. Gutman, P.L. Swenson, and W.B. Parsons, The differential diagnosis of hyperparathyroidism, JAMA 103:87, (1934).

18. G. Åkerström, R. Bergström, L. Grimelius, H. Johansson, S. Ljunghall, B. Lundström, M. Palmér, J. Rastad, and C. Rudberg, Relation between changes in clinical and histopathological features of primary hyperparathyroidism, World J Surg 10:696, (1986).

19. S. Ljunghall, G. Åkerström, G. Johansson, Y. Olsson, and G. Stålberg, Neuromuscular involvement in primary hyperparathyroidism, J Neurol 231:263, (1984).

20. J.W. Prineas, A.S. Mason, R.A. Henson, Myopathy in metabolic bone disease, Brit Med J 1:1034, (1965).

21. R.A. Henson, The neurologic aspects of hypercalcemia; with special reference to primary hyperparathyroidism, J Roy Coll Phys 1:41, (1966).

22. P.E. Kaplan, J.R. Hines, J.E. Leestma, and H.J. Ruder, Neuromuscular junction transmission defect in a patient with primary hyperparathyroidism, Electromyograph Clin Neurophysiol 20:259, (1980).

23. J.A. Richardson, G. Herron, R. Reitz, and R. Layzer, Ischemic ulcerations of the skin and necrosis of muscle in azotemic hyperparathyroidism, Ann Intern Med 71:129, (1969).

24. V. Dubowitz, ed., Muscle Biopsy. A Practical Approach (2nd ed.), Bailliere Tindall, London, (1985).

25. J.L. Johnson, R.M. Wilder, Experimental chronic hyperparathyroidism: Metabolism studies in man, Am J Med Sci 182:800, (1931).

26. E. Wersäll-Robertson, B. Hamberger, H. Ehrén, E. Eriksson, and P. Granberg, Increase in muscular strength following surgery for primary hyperparathyroidism, Acta Med Scand 220:233, (1986).

27. I. Hedman, G. Grimby, and L. Tisell, Improvement of muscle strength after treatment for hyperparathyroidism, Acta Chir Scand 150:521, (1984).

28. A.B. Borle, Calcium transport in cell culture and the effects of parathyroid hormone, in, Parathyroid Hormone and Throcalcitonin (Calcitonin), R.V. Talmage and L.F. Belanger, eds., Excerpta Medica, Amsterdam, 258, (1968).

29. H. Rasmussen, and P. Bordier, eds., The Physiological and Cellular Basis of Metabolic Bone Disease, The Williams and Wilkins Co., Baltimore, MD, 124, (1974).

30. E. Bogin, S.G. Massry, and I. Harary, Effect of parathyroid hormone in rat heart cells, J Clin Invest 67:1215, (1981).

31. R. Guisado, A.T. Arieff, and S. Massry, Muscle water and electrolytes in uremia and the effects of hemodialysis, J Lab Clin Med 89:322, (1977).

32. A.T. Arieff, and S.G. Massry, Calcium metabolism of brain in acute renal failure: Effects of uremia, hemodialysis, and parathyroid hormone, J Clin Invest 53:387, (1974).

33. J.W. Berkow, B.S. Fine, and L.E. Zimmerman, Unusual ocular calcification in hyperparathyroidism, Am J Ophthalmol 66:812, (1968).

34. W.R. Dayton, D.E. Goll, M.G. Zeece, R.M. Robson, and W.J. Reville, A Ca^{++}-activated protease possibly involved in myofibrillar protein turnover. Purification from porcine muscle, Biochemistry 15:2150, (1976).

35. W.R. Dayton, W.J. Reville, D.E. Goll, and M.H. Stromer, A Ca^{++}-activated protease possibly involved in myofibrillar protein turnover. Partial characterization of the purified enzyme, Biochemistry 15:2159, (1976).

36. K. Wrogemann, and S.D.J. Pena, Mitochondrial calcium overload: A general mechanism for cell-necrosis in muscle diseases, Lancet 1:672, (1976).

37. S. Ebashi, and H. Sugita, The role of calcium in physiological and pathological processes of skeletal muscle. in Topics in Nerve and Muscle Research, A.J. Aguayo and G. Karpati, eds., Excerpta Medica, Amsterdam, 75, (1979).

38. T.E. Bertorini, Y. Yeh, C. Trevison, E. Stadlan, S. Sabesin, and S. DiMauro, Carnitine palmityl transferase deficiency: Myoglobinuria and respiratory failure, Neurology 30:263, (1980).

39. M.H. Brooke, and W.K. Engel, The histographic analysis of human muscle biopsies with regard to fiber types. 1. Adult male and female, Neurology 19:221, (1969).

40. M.H. Brooke, and W.K. Engel, The histographic analysis of human muscle biopsies with regard to fiber types. Diseases of the upper and lower motor neuron, Neurology 19:378, (1969).

41. J.M. Lester, D.I. Silber, M.H. Cohen, R.P. Hirsch, W.G. Bradley, and J.F. Brenner, The co-dispersion index for the measurement of fiber type distribution patterns, Muscle & Nerve 6:581, (1983).

42. T.E. Bertorini, S.K. Bhattacharya, G.M.A. Palmieri, C. Chesney, D. Pifer, and B. Baker, Muscle calcium and magnesium content in Duchenne muscular dystrophy, Neurology 32:1088, (1982).

43. T.E. Bertorini, Histopathology of the inflammatory myopathies, in, Polymyositis and Dermatomyositis, M.C. Dalakas, ed., Butterworth Publishers, Woburn, MA, (1987).

PARATHYROID HORMONE AND GASTROINTESTINAL SMOOTH MUSCLE

Lester L.S. Mok, May C.M. Yang, Peter K.T. Pang,
James C. Thompson and Cary W. Cooper

Depts. of Pharmacology and Toxicology and Surgery, Univ. of
Texas Med. Branch, Galveston, TX, USA and Dept. of Physiology
Univ. of Alberta, Edmonton, Alberta, Canada

INTRODUCTION

Bone and kidney are well-recognized, classical target tissues for parathyroid hormone (PTH). However, considerable recent work has shown clearly that PTH also is a potent and effective agent in causing relaxation of vascular smooth muscle (1-3). Such work has confirmed and greatly extended earlier observations that PTH was hypotensive by virtue of its ability to relax certain vascular beds (4).

PTH has been shown to affect smooth muscle contractility in tissues other than blood vessels, e.g. in the trachea, uterus and vas deferens (5-7). An early preliminary report also indicated that PTH caused relaxation of gastrointestinal smooth muscle (8). The studies described here were designed to examine further the effect of PTH on GI smooth muscle. In particular, we wished to explore the nature and specificity of the effect and to determine which regions of the GI tract were responsive. Ultimately our goal is to understand the mechanism of action and to elucidate the physiologic relevance of the effect.

METHODS

Sprague-Dawley rats were fasted overnight and anesthetized with ether. The GI tract was exposed, and portions of it were removed for study. Tissue was mounted in a 3 ml tissue chamber so that tension could be developed along the longitudinal axis. Fundic and colonic longitudinal strips were cut for use. Duodenal and ileal segments were left as cylindrical sections in order to maintain appropriate tension. These procedures have been described previously in detail (9).

One gram resting tension was applied to each tissue, and the change in tissue tension was monitored using a strain gauge transducer and polygraph. Tissue was perfused at $37^\circ C$ in a non-recirculating fashion with oxygenated Medium 199 or with Earle's salt solution; either medium proved satisfactory. Test agents were added directly to the tissue bath to give the concentrations desired. Changes in tension before and after treatment were compared for each strip (e.g., see Fig. 1), and a paired t-test was used to assess whether changes were significant ($p < .05$). Values are shown, however, as mean $\pm SE$ (N=4-8 rats/group).

In some experiments effects of PTH on resting tension were examined. In others, the ability of PTH to inhibit agonist-induced contraction was studied. Classical adrenergic or cholinergic blocking agents, as well as PTH analogs, were used to examine specificity and to identify potential transmitter systems which might mediate an indirect action of PTH.

RESULTS

Figure 1 shows a representative tracing. With colonic strips, as shown here, the tissue maintained a suitable resting tension and effects of PTH on resting tension could be evaluated. PTH effectively lowered resting tension; no prior contraction of tissue was required. Other preparations of the GI tract, however, sometimes did not maintain a stable resting tension, and in this case we examined the ability of PTH to counteract agonist-induced contraction.

Nature of PTH Effect

As shown in Figure 1, PTH produced relaxation of GI smooth muscle within minutes of exposure of the tissue to the peptide. The relaxation persisted as long as the peptide was administered, and it disappeared when peptide was washed out.

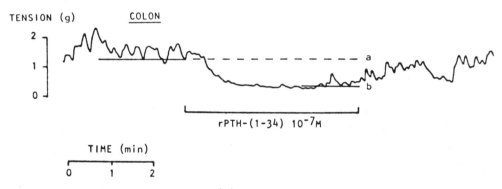

Fig. 1. Ability of 100 nM rat (r) PTH 1-34 to cause relaxation of rat colonic smooth muscle. In subsequent figures, the change (Δ) in tension before and after treatment was calculated as b-a.

GI Responsiveness and Dose-Effect Relationships

Figure 2 shows cumulative dose-response curves for rPTH 1-34 or bovine (b) PTH 1-34 using various regions of the GI tract. The results illustrate that the ability of PTH to cause relaxation was dose-dependent and that the peptide produced relaxation of smooth muscle throughout the length of the GI tract from the stomach to the colon. Table 1 also illustrates that all GI regions were responsive to PTH and further shows that the effect of PTH was apparent regardless of the agonist used to

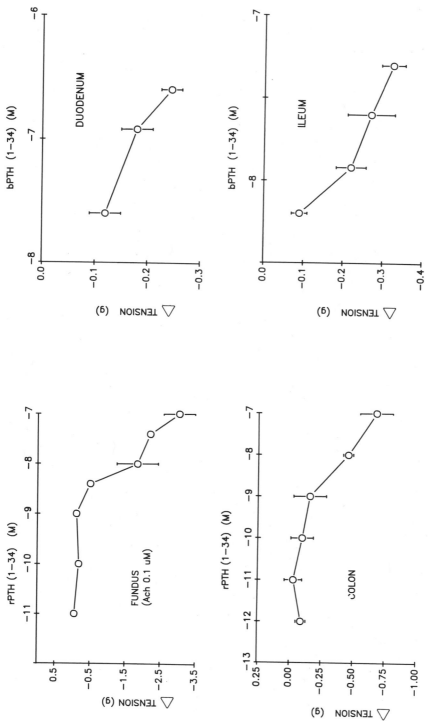

Figure 2. Log dose-effect curves showing ability of rPTH 1-34 or bPTH 1-34 to cause relaxation of GI smooth muscle in various regions of the GI tract (ACh = acetylcholine). Doses were given over 5 min periods without intervening washout.

Table 1. Ability of PTH (10 nM) to inhibit agonist-induced contraction.

Tissue	Agonist	Inhibition by PTH
Fundus	Acetylcholine (1 uM)	+
	Carbachol (0.5 uM)	+
	Bombesin (10 nM)	+
	PGE_2 (5.7 uM)	+
	KCl (15 mM)	+
Duodenum	Carbachol (1 uM)	+
Ileum	Carbachol (0.5 uM)	+
Colon	Acetylcholine (1 uM)	+

induce contraction. Our most extensive studies have been done in the colon, where the ED_{50} for rPTH was found to be 5.2 nM and in the stomach (fundus) where the IC_{50} for relaxation of acetylcholine-induced contraction was 5.8 nM (9).

Specificity

The effect of PTH to cause relaxation of GI smooth muscle is specific. Figures 3 and 4 illustrate that non-PTH peptides or proteins, e.g. albumin, salmon calcitonin, and rat calcitonin gene-related peptide (CGRP) were ineffective in causing relaxation even at high doses. Figures 4-6 further illustrate the specificity of the PTH effect by showing that the N-terminally truncated synthetic PTH analogs, bPTH 7-34 and bPTH 3-34, unlike bPTH 1-34, were ineffective in causing relaxation. However, as Figures 5 and 6 show, these PTH analogs could counteract the relaxant effect of PTH 1-34 when they were present together with PTH 1-34 in equimolar amounts (Fig. 5) or in a molar excess (Fig. 6).

It is well recognized that the N-terminal portion of the PTH 1-84 molecule is the region responsible for classical biological actions. Likewise, it is well known that oxidation of the methionine residues at positions 8 and 18 can destroy activity and that loss of activity due to oxidation is avoided by substitution of norleucine for methionine in synthetic PTH analogs. Figure 7 shows that oxidation of bPTH 1-34 with H_2O_2 destroyed the ability of the peptide to cause GI smooth muscle relaxation. Conversely, such treatment of the $(Nle^{8,18}, Tyr^{34})$ bPTH 1-34 analog in no way affected its ability to cause relaxation (Fig. 7).

Mechanism of Action

Results shown in Table 2 reveal that the ability of PTH to relax GI smooth muscle was unaffected by the presence of classical blockers of neurotransmission. The doses of blockers employed were high and, for most of them, we showed in related studies that they were effective in blocking the appropriate cholinergic or adrenergic transmitter effects in our GI smooth muscle preparations. Therefore the relaxant effect of PTH is not mediated indirectly by an effect on classical neurotransmitters.

The ability of PTH to cause relaxation of GI smooth muscle likely involves initially an interaction of the peptide with specific PTH receptors on the smooth muscle cell membrane. However, this interaction has not yet been demonstrated directly. We currently are trying to do this using radioiodinated PTH.

186

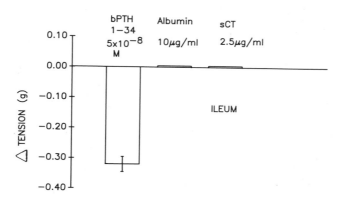

Fig. 3. Relaxation of ileal smooth muscle by bPTH 1-34 but not by bovine
serum albumin or salmon calcitonin (sCT).

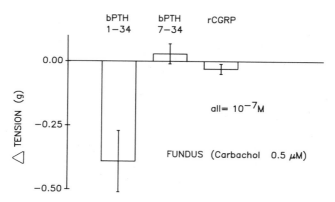

Fig. 4. Ability of PTH 1-34, but not PTH 7-34 or rat CGRP to cause
relaxation of GI smooth muscle.

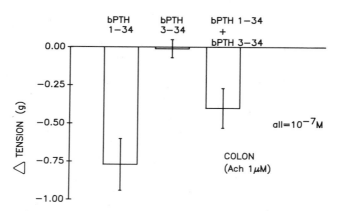

Fig. 5. Ability of PTH 3-34 to counteract relaxant effect of PTH 1-34 on colonic strips but not to cause relaxation itself (PTH 1-34 + PTH 3-34 vs PTH 1-34 = p < .05).

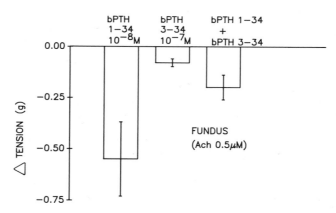

Fig. 6. Ability of PTH 3-34 to counteract relaxant effect of PTH 1-34 on fundic strips but not to cause relaxation itself (PTH 1-34 + PTH 3-34 vs PTH 1-34 = p < .05).

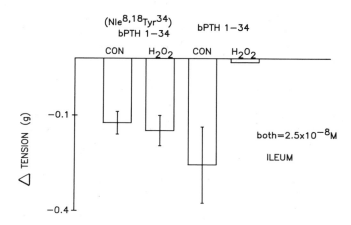

Fig. 7. Prior treatment with H_2O_2 abolishes ability of bPTH 1-34 to cause relaxation but does not affect action of Nle substituted PTH analogs (CON = Control).

Table 2. Ability of drugs to inhibit PTH-induced (10 nM) relaxation in the rat colon.

Drugs	Inhibition
$^{8,18}Nle, ^{34}Tyr$ -bPTH-(3-34) (0.1 uM)	+
Propranolol (1 uM)	−
Phentolamine (10 uM)	−
Atropine (1 uM)	−
Hexamethonium (5 mM)	−
Tetrodotoxin (1 uM)	−

In vascular smooth muscle the relaxant effect of PTH has been linked to the classical intracellular messenger, cAMP (3,10,11). Presumably receptor operated Ca channels and calmodulin-dependent cellular events are influenced by PTH-receptor interactions. In GI smooth muscle the cellular mediators of PTH are, as yet, unidentified. It is true that cAMP can, in theory, mediate relaxation. Our own studies (Figure 8) illustrate that cAMP analogs, like PTH, can produce relaxation of GI smooth muscle. However, in studies not shown we have been unable to demonstrate an unequivocal cAMP or cGMP increase in smooth muscle tissue in response to PTH. In these same studies we have been able to show, in GI smooth muscle, a clear-cut tissue cAMP response to isoproterenol and a striking cGMP response to nitrate. Therefore, we remain skeptical that cyclic nucleotides will prove to be the key intracellular mediators of PTH action in GI smooth muscle. Ca^{++} undoubtedly is a key factor, and we have some evidence using Ca-free medium that contraction involving both mobilization of intracellular Ca^{++} and influx of extracellular Ca^{++} are influenced by PTH. However, much additional work is required and, future studies surely should address the potential roles of inositolphosphates, diacylglycerol and protein kinase C as potential mechanisms mediating PTH action in the gut (12).

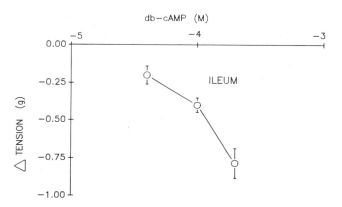

Fig. 8. Dose-response curve showing ability of dibutyryl cAMP to cause relaxation of GI smooth muscle.

SUMMARY

We have shown that PTH is a potent GI smooth muscle relaxant. The effect occurs with segments of the GI tract from stomach to colon. The action of PTH dose-dependent, specific, and not mediated by cholinergic or adrenergic transmitters. Most likely, the effect of PTH involves GI smooth muscle cell PTH receptors, but the mechanism of action and physiologic relevance of the relaxant effect remain to be elucidated.

ACKNOWLEDGMENT

This work was supported by USPHS Program Project Grant AM35608 and by USPHS Biomedical Research Support Grants RR05427 and RR07205.

REFERENCES

1. P.K.T. Pang, T.E. Tenner, Jr., J.A. Yee, M. Yang, and H.F. Janssen. Hypotensive actions of parathyroid hormone preparations on rats and dogs. Proc. Nat. Acad. Sci. USA 77: 675 (1980).

2. P.K.T. Pang, M.C.M. Yang, R. Shew, and T.E. Tenner, Jr. The vasorelaxant action of parathyroid hormone fragments on isolated rat tail artery. Blood Vessels 22: 57 (1985).

3. G.A. Nickols. Increased cAMP in cultured vascular smooth muscle cells and relaxation of aortic strips by parathyroid hormone. Eur. J. Pharmacol. 116: 137 (1985).

4. G.A. Charbon. A diuretic and hypotensive action of parathyroid extract. Acta. Physiol. Pharmacol. Neerl. 14: 52 (1966).

5. Y.C. Yen, M.C.M. Yang, A.D. Kenny, and P.K.T. Pang. Parathyroid hormone (PTH) fragments relax the guinea pig trachea in vitro. Canad. J. Physiol. Pharmacol. 61: 1324 (1983).

6. R.L. Shew and P.K.T. Pang. Effects of bPTH fragments (1-34), (3-34), and (7-34) on uterine contraction. Peptides 5: 485 (1984).

7. R.H. Zhang, M.C.M. Yang and P.K.T. Pang. The relaxing effect of parathyroid hormone on rat vas deferens. Fed. Proc. 44: 1650, 1985.

8. M.C.M. Yang, A.D. Kenny, and P.K.T. Pang. Effect of parathyroid hormone on rat gastrointestinal contraction in vitro. In: "Current Trends in Comparative Endocrinology", B. Lofts and W.N. Holmes, ed., Hong Kong Univ. Press, Hong Kong, p. 1029 (1985)

9. L.L.S. Mok, C.W. Cooper, and J.C. Thompson. Relaxation of rat gastrointestinal smooth muscle by parathyroid hormone. J. Bone Min. Res. 2: 329 (1987).

10. G.A. Nickols, M.A Metz, and W.H. Cline, Jr. Endothelium-independent linkage of parathyroid hormone receptors of rat vascular tissue with increased adenosine 3',5'-monophosphate and relaxation of vascular smooth muscle. Endocrinology 119: 349 (1986).

11. P.K.T. Pang, M.C. Yang, T.E. Tenner, Jr., A.D Kenny, and C.W. Cooper. Cyclic AMP and the vascular action of parathyroid hormone. Can. J. Physiol. & Pharmacol. 64: 1543 (1987).

12. H. Rasmussen, Y. Takuwa, and S. Park. Protein kinase C in the regulation of smooth muscle contraction. FASEB J. 1: 177 (1987).

EFFECT OF INFECTION ON CARDIAC AND SKELETAL MUSCLE CALCIUM CONTENT

IN THE RAT ENDOCARDITIS MODEL

L.M. Baddour, M.M. Hill, A.B. Hinton and G.M.A. Palmieri

Department of Medicine, University of Tennessee-Memphis

Memphis, TN 38163

There is a 10,000 fold gradient of Ca across the plasma membrane of every cell. The Ca concentration in the extracellular compartment is 10^{-3}M and only 10^{-7}M in the cytosol. Under normal circumstances, this gradient is tightly maintained by the very low permeability of plasma membranes for Ca. In some diseases, however, there is a loosening of this control and Ca intrudes into the cell causing reversible or irreversible cell damage. Elevation of cytosolic calcium, reduces ATP synthesis depriving the cell of the energy needed for maintaining its normal functions (1,2). Thus the efficiency of the Ca pumping mechanisms decreases, resulting in additional cellular Ca accumulation, causing more cell damage. High cytosolic Ca also causes cell injury and eventual cell death by stimulation of Ca-activated neutral proteases (3,4) and phospholipases (5,6).

Alterations of cellular Ca homeostasis plays a role in the pathogenesis of a variety of human disorders. In some, such as Duchenne muscular dystrophy, there is a genetic structural defect of plasma membranes that allows an exaggerated influx of Ca into muscle cells. In other diseases, such as acute pancreatitis, the defect is acquired. This subject was recently reviewed by Rasmussen and Palmieri (7).

Hypocalcemia may occur in severe infections, particularly in septic shock (8). Zaloga and Chernow (9) found reduced blood Ca^{2+} in 12 of 60 patients with septic shock. Although, some alterations in calciotropic hormones were observed in those patients, there is no definitive explanation for the acute hypocalcemia in sepsis. The possibility that excessive translocation of calcium into the cellular compartment may occur in infection has not been explored. We therefore tested this hypothesis in the rat model of experimental endocarditis.

Methods: The procedure used to produce endocarditis in rats has been previously described in detail (10). Briefly, an intracardiac catheter is placed in the left ventricle, via the right common carotid artery, of 150-200g Sprague-Dawley rats. Two days later, 10^7 colony-forming units of <u>Staphylococcus epidermidis</u> suspended in 1ml of 0.15M Nace solution is injected through the tongue vein of animals. Ninety six hours after bacterial challenge, samples of the right ventricle and rectus femoris were obtained for chemical analysis. The aorta and left ventricle were opened and vegetations were excised, weighed and homogenized. The vegetations and catheters were cultured in broth. In addition, quantitative cultures of the vegetation suspensions were performed. No gross abnormalities were observed in the right ventricle which was not catheterized in these experiments. Control rats were subjected to identical procedures, but sterile saline solution instead of bacterial inocula was injected. Calcium was measured in acid extracts of dry, defatted samples of right ventricle and rectus femoris as previously reported (11,12).

Results: There was similar tolerance to the procedures in infected and control rats. A significant increase (p=0.01) in Ca content in the right ventricle of infected animals (Table 1) was observed. The Ca content of the rectus femoris of infected rats was elevated in several animals, but as a group it did not show statistical significance.

Table 1. Muscle Ca* in Endocarditis Content in Infected and Noninfected Rats.

Right Ventricle (n)		Rectus Femoris (n)	
Control (4)	32.49 $\pm$ 6.39	(6) 23.71 $\pm$ 2.37	
Infected (12)	72.51 $\pm$ 12.58	(12) 51.90 $\pm$ 16.04	
p=0.01		NS	

*mEq/kg/fat free dry tissue, mean $\pm$ SE.

Discussion: This preliminary observation clearly demonstrates that rats which develop experimental endocarditis due to <u>S. epidermidis</u> have a marked increase in the Ca content of the right ventricle. The skeletal muscle also showed some increment in calcium accumulation. In choosing the present experimental model, we avoided the technically simpler intraperitoneal bacterial inoculation model. The intraperitoneal infection could have caused peritonitis and pancreatitis, and prior studies of noninfectious acute pancreatitis have demonstrated elevated skeletal muscle Ca by 100% in dogs (13).

Since the relatively mild infection in the present study caused a 120% increment in the myocardium of the right ventricle, it is conceivable that the hypocalcemia of septic shock could be explained, in part, by an excessive translocation of Ca from the extracellular to the intracellular compartment. Parathyroid hormone (PTH) could accentuate the cellular damage caused by excessive intracellular Ca during infection by stimulating Ca entry into cells (14). Although this hypothesis needs to be explored, it is tempting to speculate that suppression of PTH secretion by maintaining an adequate intake of Ca could be beneficial during infection, since Wood (15) reported more than 150 years ago that administration of Ca had a positive effect in the treatment of tuberculosis. Moreover, vitamin D promotes antituberculosis resistance (16), and calcitriol stimulates macrophages-induced inhibition of tubercle bacilli replication, _in vitro_ (17). Thus, Ca, PTH and vitamin D may play an important role in infection.

REFERENCES

1. A. Fleckenstein, Myokardstoffwechsel und Nekrose, _in_: VI Symposium der Deutsch. Ges. fur Fortschritte auf dem Gebiet der Inneren Medizin uber 'Herzinfarkt und Schock'. L. Heilmeyer and H.J. Holtmeier (eds), p. 94. Georg Thieme Verlag, Stuttgart (1968).
2. A. Fleckenstein, J. Janke, H.J. Doring, and O. Leder, Myocardial fiber necrosis due to intracellular calcium overload; a new principle in cardiac pathophysiology, _in_: "Myocardial Biology. Recent Advances in Studies on Cardiac Structure and Metabolism". No. 4, N.S. Dhalla (ed), p. 563, University Park Press, Baltimore (1974).
3. W.R. Dayton, D.E. Goll, M.G. Zeece, R.M. Robson, and W.J. Reville, A Ca++-activated protease possibly involved in myofibrillar protein turnover. Purification from porcine muscle, _Biochemistry_ 15: 2150 (1976).
4. N.C. Kar, and C.M. Pearson, A calcium-activated neutral protease in normal and dystrophic human muscle, _Clin Chim Acta_ 73: 293 (1976).
5. S. Mittnacht, Jr., C.S. Sherman, and J.L. Farber, Reversal of ischemic mitochondrial dysfunction, _J Biol Chem_ 254: 9871 (1979).
6. D.E. Epps, J.W. Palmer, H.H. Schmid, and D.R. Pfeiffer, Inhibition of permeability-dependent Ca^{2+} release mitochondria by N-acylethanolamines, a class of lipids synthesized in ischemic heart tissues, _J Biol Chem_ 257: 1383 (1982).
7. H. Rasmussen, and G.M.A. Palmieri, Altered cell calcium metabolism and human diseases, _in_: "Calcium in biological systems", R.P. Rubin, G.B. Weiss, and J.W. Putney (eds). p. 551 Plenum Publishing Corp. New York (1985).
8. B. Taylor, W.J. Sibbald, M.W. Edmonds, R.L. Holliday, and C. Williams, Ionized hypocalcemia in critically ill patients with sepsis, _Can J Surg_ 21: 429 (1978).
9. G.P. Zaloga, and B. Chernow, The multifactorial basis for hypocalcemia during sepsis. Studies of the parathyroid hormone-vitamin D axis, _Ann Int Med_ 107: 36 (1987).
10. L.M. Baddour, G.D. Christensen, M.G. Hester, and A.L. Bisno, Production of experimental endocarditis by coagulase-negative staphylococci: variability in species virulence, _J Infect Dis_ 150: 721 (1984).
11. S.K. Bhattacharya, J.C. Williams, and G.M.A. Palmieri, Determination of calcium and magnesium in cardiac and skeletal muscle by atomic absorption spectroscopy using stoichiometric nitrous oxide-acetylene flame, _Anal Lett_ 12: 1451 (1979).
12. G.M. Palmieri, D.F. Nutting, S.K. Bhattacharya, T.E. Bertorini, and J.C. Williams, Parathyroid ablation in dystrophic hamsters: effects on calcium content and histology of heart, diaphragm and rectus femoris, _J Clin Invest_ 68: 646 (1981).
13. S.K. Bhattacharya, R.W. Luther, J.W. Pate, A.J. Crawford, O.F. Moore, J.A. Pitcock, G.M.A. Palmieri, and L.G. Britt, Soft tissue calcium and magnesium content in acute pancreatitis in the dog: Calcium accumulation, a mechanism for hypocalcemia in acute pancreatitis, _J Lab Clin Med_ 105: 422 (1985).

METABOLIC EFFECTS OF PARATHYROID HORMONE

PARATHYROID HORMONE AND LIPID METABOLISM

T. Drüeke, J.-B. Roullet and B. Lacour
INSERM U 90, Département de Néphrologie
and Service de Biochimie, Hôpital Necker
Paris, France

KNOWN EFFECTS OF PARATHYROID HORMONE ON LIPID METABOLISM : CONTROVERSIAL REPORTS IN THE LITERATURE

In addition to its well known actions on classic target organs, it has become apparent in recent years that parathyroid hormone (PTH) exerts effects in many other tissues. Thus, PTH has also well-defined effects on lipid metabolism. The hormone stimulates adipose tissue lipolysis in vitro in the experimental animal (1) as well as in the man (2-4). The administration of parathyroid extract into dogs and into human beings induces an increase in serum free fatty acids (3,5).

In primary hyperparathyroidism (I° HPTH), contradictory findings have been reported. Thus, two reports have indicated a decrease in serum cholesterol concentrations (6,7) and one study a decrease in serum triglyceride (TG) concentration (7). The latter was normalized after parathyroidectomy (PTx). However, other authors found an increase in the incidence of type IV hyperlipidemia in I° HPTH (8) and an improvement after PTx. Still others did not find any change of serum lipids in the presence of longstanding hyperparathyroidism (9).

In the experimental animal with normal renal function, PTx was associated with a decrease in serum total cholesterol and TG (10). However, other authors did not observe an effect of PTx on the catabolism of Intralipid^R, a TG-rich emulsion (11).

In uremic patients with II° HPTH, the authors of two studies reported that PTx was not associated with an improvement of lipid disturbances (6,12). Others were unable to correlate serum PTH and TG concentration (13). An inverse relation between both parameters has even been reported by one group (14).

In uremic animals, a significant decrease in serum total cholesterol, phospholipids and/or TG following PTx has been reported by several groups of authors (15-17).

PERSONAL STUDIES

Studies in the experimental animal

We performed several experiments in rats with normal function in order to obtain further insight into the possible role of PTH in lipid metabolism (18). Two experimental models of HPTH were used : an endogenous, nutritional type, and an exogenous type. The endogenous state of HPTH was induced using a calcium-poor (0.02%) diet during 4 weeks, and the exogenous state by thrice daily injections of parathyroid extract (PTE, 5 USP/100 g body weight) during 8 days. Control animals received sham injections of vehicle solution only. In addition, an experimental model of hypoparathyroidism was also created using total PTx by electro-coagulation. The latter group as well as a sham-operated group of rats were studied 2 weeks after surgery.

All lipid studies were done at 9:00 am, after an overnight fast of 16 hr. Blood for analysis of lipid parameters was obtained by jugular vein puncture under light ethyl ether anesthesia. Plasma post-heparin lipolytic activity (PHLA), an intravenous fat tolerance test (IVFTT) using Intralipid^R, intestinal absorption of TG using [^{3}H]-triolein, and hepatic TG secretion rate (TGSR) were performed as described (18).

The results of the experimental study in rats indicated the following :

1) The endogenous type of HPTH was associated with a significant increase in serum total cholesterol and TG concentrations. It was also associated with a significant decrease in the serum clearance rate of intravenously infused Intralipid^R.

2) Endogenous HPTH induced a significant increase in hepatic TG content, as compared to values of control rats. Intestinal absorption of [^{3}H]-triolein was comparable in both groups of rats. Furthermore, the hepatic TGSR of the hyperparathyroid rats was lower than that of control animals.

3) The exogenous type of HPTH was also accompanied by a slight increase in serum cholesterol and TG concentrations as well as a decrease in plasma PHLA but the changes did not reach the level of statistical significance.

4) In the hypoparathyroid state, a significant decrease in serum cholesterol and TG levels and a significant rise in plasma PHLA were observed when compared to control rats.

We concluded from these studies that the hyperparathyroid state induces an increase in serum cholesterol and TG concentrations, the latter being due not to increased hepatic production or intestinal lipid absorption, but to decreased peripheral removal. The hypoparathyroid state is associated with changes opposite in direction. The reason why the changes observed were more prominent with the endogenous type than with the exogenous type of HPTH is unclear. It is possible that the exogenous HPTH was too short in duration and/or too mild to allow marked changes to occur.

Studies in patients with I° HPTH and II° HPTH

In an attempt to better understand the various and apparently inconsistent lipid disturbances of I° and II° HPTH in man, we undertook studies of lipoprotein metabolism in such patients before and after surgical PTx (19).

Patients with I° HPTH. Eighty-six patients (mean age±SEM, 48.5±1.37 yr) were compared to 22 healthy control subjects who were matched for age and sex. Mean serum TG levels of the patients were significantly higher than that of the healthy volunteers : 1.51±0.09 (SEM) vs. 1.01±0.09 mM (p<0.001). Serum HDL-TG, total cholesterol, HDL-cholesterol, LDL-cholesterol, and apolipoproteins (apo) A and B, however, were comparable between both groups.

Serum lipid parameters could be evaluated in 60 patients before and 5-7 days after PTx (short-term follow-up), and in 13 patients also more than 1 year after surgery (long-term follow-up). Whereas all the above lipoprotein values decreased significantly during the short-term observation period, only serum total TG and HDL-TG remained diminished in the long term. In contrast, serum total cholesterol, HDL-cholesterol, and LDL-cholesterol were found increased at that time.

Patients with II° HPTH. Thirty-four chronic hemodialysis patients with severe II° HPTH were studied before and after PTx. Their mean age was 49.7±2.07 yr. They were being treated by dialysis for a mean duration of 73.8±5.73 mo. (range, 1-137 mo.). At the time of study, their dialysis time was 3x4 hr/week in most instances. Their serum HDL cholesterol and serum HDL-phospholipids were decreased as compared to the healthy subjects : 0.93±0.06 vs 1.22±0.08 mM, p<0.01, and1.18±0.06 vs 1.53±0.07 mM, p<0.001, respectively. Their serum total TG were increased : 2.17±0.19 vs 1.01±0.09 mM.

The short term effects of PTx after 7-14 days were the following : Total serum cholesterol, TG, phospholipids, and LDL-cholesterol decreased significantly. Serum total apo-B decreased slightly, but not significantly. No change occurred for cholesterol, TG, or apo-A content of HDL.

Twelve to 18 months after PTx, 11 hemodialysis patients, who were in a comparable nutritional and clinical status, were studied again. Serum TG remained significantly decreased. However, the other lipid parameters had returned to values observed before surgery.

Taken together, the present data obtained in patients with I° and II° HPTH before and after PTx show that PTH appears to exert deleterious effects on the metabolism of TG-rich lipoproteins in man. These effects can be corrected by PTx in patients with I° HPTH since the patients' serum and lipoprotein TG concentrations returned towards normal after PTx. After a prolonged time interval following surgical correction of HPTH, serum TG levels remained in the normal range. In uremic patients with II° HPTH, an excessive PTH secretion appears to be only one of the factors contributing to their well-known lipid disturbances. Many of the perturbations of lipoprotein metabolism during chronic renal failure appear not to depend directly on PTH excess. However, PTx was capable of reducing the elevated serum TG levels of these patients in the long-term, without correcting them totally.

Collectively, the data of our experimental and human studies as well as at least some reports of the literature point to an association of HPTH with perturbations of TG metabolism. Such changes may be more or less pronounced, depending probably on the severity of the hyperparathyroid state and possibly also on environmental factors such as dietary habits and physical activity. It is still not known whether the disturbances of the metabolism of TG-rich lipoproteins are mainly due to increased hepatic production or rather to decreased peripheral removal. It is conceivable that both mechanisms be involved but to a varying extent from one particular situation to another.

REFERENCES

1. Werner, S.; Löw, H. Stimulation of lipolysis and calcium accumulation by parathyroid hormone in rat adipose tissue after adrenalectomy and administration of high doses of cortisone acetate. Horm. Metab. Res. 5: 292-296 (1973)

2. Gozariu, L.; Forster, K.; Faulhaber, J.D. et al. Parathyroid hormone and calcitonin : Influences on lipolysis of human adipose tissue. Horm. Metab. Res. 6: 243-245 (1974)

3. Sinha, T.K.; Thajchayapon, G.P.; Queener, S.F. et al. On the lipolytic action of parathyroid hormone in man. Metabolism 25: 251-260 (1976)

4. Ziegler, R.; Jobst, W.; Minne, H. et al. Calciotropic hormones and lipolysis of human adipose tissue : Role of extracellular calcium as conditioning but not regulating factor. Endokrinologie 75: 577-588 (1980)

5. Hallberg, D.; Werner, S. Circulatory and lipolytic effects of parathyroid hormone.Horm. Metab. Res. 9: 424-428 (1977)

6. De Moor, P.; Creyttens, G.; Bouillon, R. et al. Results obtained in 75 patients operated upon for hyperparathyroidism. Ann. Endocrinol. (Paris) 34: 616-620 (1973)

7. Christensson, T.; Einarsson, K. Serum lipids before and after parathyroidectomy in patients with primary hyperparathyroidism. Clin. Chim. Acta 78: 411-415 (1977)

8. Ljunghall, S.; Lithell, H.; Vessby, B. et al. Glucose and lipoprotein metabolism in primary hyperparathyroidism. Effects of parathyroidectomy. Acta Endocrinol (Copenh) 89: 508-589 (1978)

9. Vaziri, N.D.; Wellikson, L.; Gwinup, G. et al. Lipid fractions in primary hyperparathyroidism before and after surgical cure. Acta Endocrinol (Copenh) 102: 539-542 (1983)

10. Paloyan, E.; Kolar, J.; Castles, J. et al. The role of parathyroid hormone in lipid metabolism. Fed. Proc. 22: 676 (1963)

11. Heuck, C.C.; Ritz, E. Does parathyroid hormone play a role in lipid metabolism? Contrib. Nephrol. 20: 118-128 (1980)

12. Lazarus, J.M.; Lowrie, E.G.; Hampers, C.L. et al. Cardiovascular disease in uremic patients on hemodialysis. Kidney Int. (suppl.) 7: 167-175 (1975)

13. Schaefer, K.; Offermann, G.; von Herrath, D. et al. Failure to show a correlation between serum parathyroid hormone, nerve conduction velocity and serum lipids in hemodialysis patients. Clin. Nephrol. 14: 81-88 (1980)

14. Brunzell, J.D.; Goldberg, A.P. Hormonal regulation of human adipose tissue lipoprotein lipase, in: Schettler, G. et al., editors: Atherosclerosis IV. Berlin, Springer publ., 1977, p. 336

15. Cantin, M. Kidney, parathyroid, and lipemia. Lab. Invest. 14: 1691-1698 (1965)

16. Alfrey, A.C.; Tomford, R.C; Karlinsky, M.L. Effect of parathyroidectomy on nephrotic serum nephritis (abstract). Kidney Int. 18: 530 (1980)

17. Ritz, E.; Heuck, C.C.; Boland, R. Phosphate, calcium, and lipid metabolism. Adv. Exp. Med. Biol. 128: 197-208 (1980)

18. Lacour, B.; Basile, C.; Drüeke, T.; Funck-Brentano, J.-L. Parathyroid function and lipid metabolism in the rat. Miner. Electrolyte Metab. 7: 157-165 (1982)

19. Lacour, B.; Roullet, J.B.; Liagre, A.M. et al. Serum lipoprotein disturbances in primary and secondary hyperparathyroidism and effects of parathyroidectomy. Am. J. Kidney Dis. 8: 422-429 (1986)

IS PTH ASSOCIATED WITH LIPID METABOLISM?

Yoshiki Nishizawa, Hitoshi Tanishita, Hitoshi Goto,*
Satoshi Hagiwara, Takami Miki, Shuzo Otani,*
and Hirotoshi Morii

Second Department of Internal Medicine, and*Department of Biochemistry, Osaka City University Medical
School
1-5-7, Asahi-machi, Abeno-ku, Osaka 545, Japan

INTRODUCTION

There is evidence that parathyroid hormone (PTH) acts on
tissues other than the skeletal system and renal cortex: it
seems to affect muscles, the nervous system, and adipose
tissue, in particular. PTH influences both protein (1) and
glucose metabolism (2). In lipid metabolism, PTH stimulates
lipolysis of adipose tissues in vitro (3, 4, 5) and in vivo
(6). However, reports about the effect of parathyroidectomy
(PTX) on the serum lipid level in patients with primary hyperparathyroidism are contradictory, and there are only a few
studies about the action of PTH on lipoprotein lipase (LPL).

In this study, we investigated the direct action of PTH
on lipid metabolism other than lipolysis, and evaluated the
mechanisms by which PTH accelerates hyperlipidemia.

SUBJECTS AND METHODS

Clinical study: Thirty patients with chronic renal
failure who had been treated by hemodialysis for five years or
more and who had never been given any vitamin D analogues or
calcitonin preparations were selected for a retrospective
study of patients with secondary hyperparathyroidism. The
mean period of hemodialysis was 5 years and 2 months, and the
mean age at the first hemodialysis treatment was 45.3 ± 12.4
years. Twenty-three of the patients were men and seven
women.

Serum lipids were assayed before and after PTX in the hemodialysed patients with secondary hyperparathyroidism and in
other patients with primary hyperparathyroidism. Five
patients with chronic renal failure (three men and two women)
with a mean age of 41.4 ± 5.2 years and a mean duration of
hemodialysis of 7 years and 11 months underwent PTX because of
severe hyperparathyroidism. Ten patients with primary hyperparathyroidism (7 men and 3 women) with a mean age of $56.1 \pm
15.5$ years were also subjects for this study of PTX.

New Actions of Parathyroid Hormone
Edited by S. G. Massry and T. Fujita
Plenum Press, New York

Study of uremic rats: Male Wistar rats were divided into four groups; a non-uremic group with sham-PTX, a non-uremic group with PTX, a uremic group with sham-PTX, and a uremic group with PTX. Chronic uremia was induced surgically in two stages by a modification of the method of Bagdade and co-workers (7). First, 2/3-nephrectomy was performed, and then the contralateral kidney was removed 1 week later. PTX was done 12 weeks after the second nephrectomy. The rats were starved overnight after PTX and killed the next day. Blood urea nitrogen (BUN) was 48.9 ± 20.4 mg/dl for the sham-PTX groups and 40.4 ± 11.7 mg/dl for the PTX groups.

Culture conditions for cells: SaOS2 cells (ATCC, HTB 85) are human osteogenic sarcoma cells, that may have the PTH receptor (8). Cells were cultured in McCoy 5A medium containing 10% FCS in a suspension of 1.5×10^5 cells/ml for 7 to 9 days under 5% CO_2 and 95% air at $37\,^\circ$C.

Adipocytes were prepared from epididymal and retroperitoneal fat from male SD rats 5 weeks old that had food freshly available. The preparation procedure was as described by Gliemann and co-workers (9). The incubation medium was Krebs-Ringer bicarbonate buffer containing 4% albumin, 0.55 mM glucose, 25 mM Hepes, and 0.3% collagenase.

Hepatocytes were isolated from SD rats 6 weeks old by perfusion of the liver with Ca^{++}-free Hanks-Hepes solution and then Hanks-Hepes solution containing 0.05% collagenase. The cells were cultured as monolayers in William medium E containing 10% FCS, 10^{-6} M dexamethasone, 2×10^{-6} M insulin, and antibiotics in a humidified chamber at $37\,^\circ$C under 5% CO_2 and 95% air.

Assay of post-heparin lipolytic activity (PHLA): In the experiment with uremic rats, heparin (250 U/kg body weight) was injected intravenously and post-heparin plasma was prepared from blood sampled 15 min later. PHLA, the sum of the total activities of LPL and hepatic triglyceride lipase (HTGL), was measured by the method of Nilsson-Ehle and Schotz (10). After the mixture of artificial lipid particles with 1.4 umol of [14 C]triolein and stock serum as activator were incubated for 2 min at $37\,^\circ$C, 20 ul of sample plasma was added into the mixture in the presence of 0.045 mmol for PHLA assays or of 0.3 mmol for HTGL activity assays. The mixture was incubated for 10 min at $37\,^\circ$C, and the reaction was stopped by addition of Belfrage's solution and 0.5 N NaOH. The radioactivity of the supernatant was counted.

Assay of HTGL in the hepatocytes: Isolated rat hepatocytes were cultured for 24 hours with or without 10^{-8} M PTH 1-84, and the cells were washed 3 times with PBS. Cells were cultured in Hanks-Hepes solution containing artificial lipid particles of 0.75 uCi/ml [14 C]triolein with or without PTH or heparin. Then the cells were washed five times with PBS and dissolved in 0.5 N NaOH. The activity of HTGL was expressed as the incorporation of [14 C]triolein into the cells [activity = (cpm in cells after incubation/mg protein) - (cpm in cells at time 0/mg protein)].

Measurements of lipogenesis: In hepatocytes and SaOS2 cells, lipogenesis was measured in a modification of the method by Nakamura and coworkers (11). Cells incubated in Hanks-Hepes solution containing 1 uCi/ml [14 C]acetic acid and PTH for 2 hours at $37\,^\circ$C under 5% CO_2 and 95% air. The resulting supernatant was extracted with diethyl ether after the harvest of the cells. The extract was evaporated under N_2, dissolved in 100 ul of diethyl ether, and used in thin layer chromatography (Silica gel 60, Merk; hexane:diethyl ether:acetate = 70:20:1, w/w). After the scratching off of spots of each lipid fraction, their radioactivity was measured.

Lipogenesis in the adipocytes was measured by a modification of the method by Moody et al. (12) One milliliter of the cell suspension was incubated in a 20-ml scintillation vial with KRB buffer containing 4% albumin, 0.55 mM glucose, 25 mM Hepes, [3 H]glucose (1 uCi/ml), and PTH or not with shaking at 37 °C. Incubation was stopped by the addition of 200 ul of 8 N H_2SO_4, and the cell solution was mixed and extracted with 15 ml of toluene scintillator.

The results are expressed as means + S.D. and the significance of differences was evaluated by Student's t-test.

RESULTS

Levels of cholesterol and triglycerides (TG) in 170 hemodialysed patients: One year after the start of hemodialysis, level of serum cholesterol was 156 + 34 mg/dl in men and 160 + 35 mg/dl in women, and of TG was 159 + 79 mg/dl in men and 130 + 45 mg/dl in women (Fig. 1). Hypertriglyceridemia was seen in 45% of the patients, and hypercholesterolemia in only 5%. These findings mean that type IV hyperlipidemia is the most frequently seen type in the uremic patients.

Retrospective study: Changes in alkaline phosphatase (AP), cholesterol, and TG in the 30 patients who had never

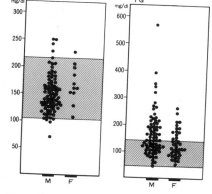

Fig. 1 Levels of cholesterol and TG in patients treated by HD one year after start of HD treatment. Shaded bands show normal limits.

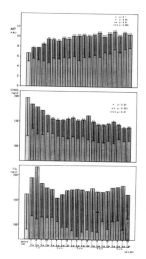

Fig. 2 Serum levels of AP and lipids for 5 years from the start of HD in patients with end-stage renal disease.

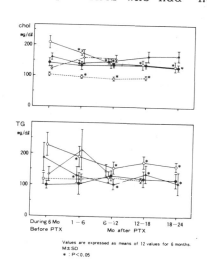

Values are expressed as means of 12 values for 6 months.
M±SD
* : P<0.05

Fig. 3 Levels of serum lipids after PTX in patients treated HD.

been treated with vitamin D analogues or calcitonin preparations are shown in Fig. 2. AP increased during treatment, which suggested that secondary hyperparathyroidism develops even in hemodialysed patients. The levels of cholesterol decreased significantly after treatment started. However, TG stayed at the same high level despite hemodialysis, perhaps because of the progress of the secondary hyperparathyroidism. The correlation of laboratory data from these 30 patients obtained at the same time after treatment started is shown in Table 1, where significance is shown by the shading. AP was correlated with TG, beta-lipoprotein, and phospholipids. PTH was not correlated with these lipids, perhaps because the c-PTH level was variable among these hemodialysed patients. Therefore, serum levels of TG may be influenced by secondary hyperparathyroidism.

Table 1 Relationship between lipids and other factors in patients treated by HD.

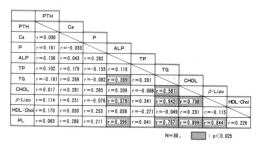

	PTH	Ca	P	ALP	TP	TG	CHOL	β-Lipo	HDL-Chol
PTH									
Ca	r=0.030								
P	r=0.161	r=−0.033							
ALP	r=0.136	r=0.043	r=0.282						
TP	r=0.102	r=0.179	r=−0.155	r=0.119					
TG	r=−0.161	r=0.269	r=−0.082	r=0.389	r=0.201				
CHOL	r=0.017	r=0.281	r=0.285	r=0.209	r=−0.008	r=0.581			
β-Lipo	r=0.114	r=0.251	r=−0.076	r=0.376	r=0.241	r=0.942	r=0.708		
HDL-Chol	r=0.170	r=0.030	r=0.253	r=0.038	r=−0.271	r=−0.049	r=0.231	r=−0.115	
PL	r=0.063	r=0.288	r=0.211	r=0.396	r=0.041	r=0.767	r=0.899	r=0.844	r=0.226

N=30,　▨ : p<0.025

Effect of PTX on serum lipids in hemodialysed patients: The mean values of serum cholesterol and TG for the five parathyroidectomized patients during the six months before and after the operation are shown in Fig. 3. One patient had a low level of cholesterol before surgery and the others had normal levels. Two of the five patients had high levels of TG at this time. The serum level of cholesterol decreased after PTX in the patient whose mean cholesterol before surgery was the highest of the five patients. In the two patients with hypertriglyceridemia, the serum TG decreased into the normal range, and remained normal in the following 30 months.

Effect of PTX on serum lipids in primary hyperparathyroidism: The mean cholesterol was 202.5 ± 51.7 mg/dl before and 193.8 ± 31.7 mg/dl after PTX and the mean TG was 128.6 ±

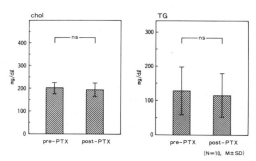

Fig. 4 Levels of serum lipids before and after PTX in patients with primary hyperparathyroidism.

Table 2 Levels of apoproteins before and after PTX in patients with primary hyperparathyroidism.

	pre-PTX	post-PTX	p
A 1	130.2 ± 16.8	120.6 ± 13.2	ns
A 2	29.0 ± 4.3	27.4 ± 3.7	ns
B	110.2 ± 29.7	97.4 ± 29.0	ns
C 2	5.6 ± 1.7	4.5 ± 1.9	ns
C 3	9.4 ± 2.5	8.2 ± 2.6	ns
E	4.5 ± 0.5	4.8 ± 0.9	ns

(N=10, M±SD)

69.9 mg/dl before and 115.5 ± 65.3 mg/dl after PTX in ten parathyroidectomized patients with primary hyperparathyroidism. There was no significant difference before and after PTX (Fig. 4). The levels of apoprotein in the serum before and after PTX were not significantly different (Table 2); they were already in the normal range before the operation.

Effect of PTX on serum lipids in uremic rats: The TG level decreased significantly and cholesterol tended to decrease after PTX (Fig.5), as earlier reports (13, 14) has already shown.

Effect of PTX on PHLA in uremic rats: PHLA decreased in uremia even after PTX. HTGL activity was suppressed in the uremic rats, and decreased still more after PTX. LPL activity, however, was at the same level in the uremic rats as in the controls, and increased after PTX (Fig. 6).

Effect of PTH on HTGL activity in vitro: The HTGL activity of the cells decreased with the addition of 10^{-8} M PTH 1-84 for 24 hours before the assay (12056 ± 318 cpm/mg protein/2 hr in PTH group and 15564 ± 504 cpm/mg protein/2 hr in control group; p < 0.0003). Therefore, PTH directly decreased HTGL activity.

Effect of PTH on lipogenesis in vitro: Cholesterol and TG production increased in SaOS2 cells when the concentration of PTH 1-34 was 10^{-8} M (Table 3). In rat adipocytes, PTH 1-34 stimulated lipid production (Fig. 7). Also, PTH 1-84 increased lipogenesis in SaOS2 cells and adipocytes (data not shown). PTH 1-34 did not affect the production of cholesterol or TG by rat hepatocytes at any concentration from 10^{-9} to 10^{-7} M, but PTH 1-84 increased lipid synthesis in those cells at the concentrations of 10^{-9} M and 10^{-8} M (Fig. 8).

DISCUSSION

Hypertriglyceridemia was noted in 48% of the patients one year after hemodialysis treatment began, though hyper-

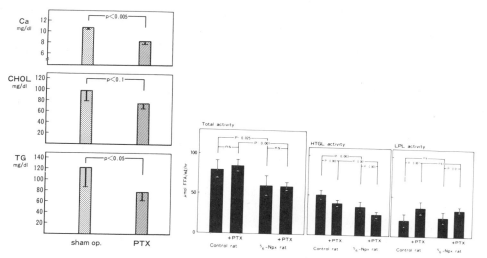

Fig. 5 Levels of serum lipids before and after PTX in uremic rats.

Fig. 6 Effect of PTX on serum levels of lipase in control and uremic rats. Total activity is for PHLA.

Table 3 Effect of PTH on the production of cholesterol
and TG in SaOS2 cells

| $1-34$PTH | Incorporation of $[^{14}C]$ into $(\times 10^3 pM/ng)$ | |
	Chol	TG
0 M	61.5 ± 8.1	74.8 ± 20.4
10^{-9} M	66.7 ± 8.0	89.6 ± 28.5
10^{-8} M	88.0 ± 21.1 *	109.0 ± 14.7 *
10^{-7} M	94.5 ± 24.4 *	133.1 ± 41.3 *

* : $p < 0.025$

cholesterolemia was present in 5% of the same patients. These
findings were compatible with Ponticelli's report, in which
55% of the hemodialysed patients had type IV hyperlipoprotei-
nemia.   The main cause of hypertriglyceridemia in end-stage
renal disease is probably peripheral impairment of the removal
of lipids from the bloodstream, probably because of the lowered metabolic turnover of VLDL caused by the suppressed LPL
(15), suppressed HTGL (16), and abnormalities in the protein
composition of apoprotein (17). Lipid metabolism in uremia
is influenced by hormonal disorders such as hypogonadism,
hypothyroidism, or diabetes mellitus (18), so secondary hyperparathyroidism may influence lipid metabolism in uremia.
    This clinical study of 30 hemodialysed patients showed
that the high level of TG may be sustained over the course of
hemodialysis by the progress of secondary hyperparathyroidism
in spite of declining cholesterol.   The serum level of TG was
positively correlated to the grade of secondary hyperparathyroidism.   The association of PTH to the deranged lipid
metabolism in uremia is compatible with results of studies
about PTX and renal transplants in hemodialysed patients (19-
21), but reports are contradictory about the effectiveness of
PTX on serum lipids in primary hyperparathyroidism (20, 22,
23).   In our study, there was no significant change in the
primary hyperparathyroidism after PTX. Hypertriglyceridemia

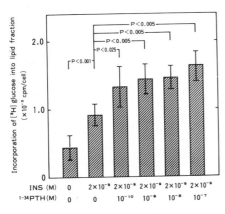

Fig. 7 Effect of PTH on lipogenesis in rat adipocytes.

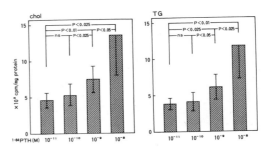

Fig. 8 Effect of PTH on synthesis
of cholesterol and TG in rat hepatocytes.

before PTX was found in only 2 of the 10 patients. In one patient, TG decreased after PTX, and in the other, TG did not change. The reason why our results could not be used to evaluate the effectiveness of PTX in decreasing serum TG in primary hyperparathyroidism is probably because the serum levels of TG were low or normal before the operation.

The decrease in PHLA found the uremic rats here was compatible with clinical findings (15). PHLA did not change after PTX, but the ratio of LPL activity to HTGL activity changed greatly after PTX, probably because of acute decreases in serum PTH and Ca ion. No definite conclusion can be made from these results yet, because we need to do experiments in which the calcium level is held steady artificially after PTX. However, the results do suggest that PTH decreased the activities of LPL and HTGL. Reciprocal regulation of LPL activity and hormone-sensitive lipase activity may be mediated by a product of lipolysis such as intracellular free fatty acids (FFA), so the decrease in PHLA may have arisen because of partial inhibition of adipose tissue LPL by excessive adipose tissue lipolysis stimulated by plasma PTH (24). HTGL activity was found to be reduced directly by PTH in the experiment on incorporation of [14 C]triolein into the hepatocytes.

PTH participates in the energy metabolism of skeletal muscle (25). Purified bovine PTH at the concentration of 10^{-6} M directly stimulates the production of glucose in isolated liver cells (2). Our study showed that lipogenesis in the hepatocytes was enhanced by PTH 1-84 but not PTH 1-34 as reported by Klahr and coworkers (26), who showed that PTH 1-84 but not PTH 1-34 increases glucose production from alanine in the perfused liver. Therefore, the C-terminal fragment of PTH or a longer chain of the mid-portion is probably essential for the actions of PTH on gluconeogenesis and lipogenesis in the hepatocytes. PTH directly stimulated lipogenesis in the liver as well as in adipose tissues, and directly suppressed HTGL activity which decreased the uptake of lipoprotein, the substrate for lipogenesis. So the actual production of lipids in the liver would be a balance between these effects.

The current general understanding of PTH effects on lipid metabolism is that 1) PTH stimulates lipolysis to increase FFA, the substrate, which may enhance lipid synthesis, 2) PTH may suppress PHLA, and a high level of FFA inhibits tissue LPL to decrease the peripheral removal of lipids, and 3) PTH accelerates peripheral insulin resistance, increases insulin secretion, and stimulates glucose production and catabolism of protein, probably to enhance lipid synthesis. From our results, the direct action of PTH in enhancing lipogenesis and suppressing HTGL activity, seems to be important in the pathogenesis of hyperlipidemia in secondary hyperparathyroidism (Fig. 10).

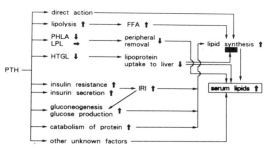

Fig. 9 Possible roles of PTH in lipid metabolism; including our concept.

209

REFERENCES

1. Landau, R.L., and Kappas, A., 1965, Anabolic hormones in hyperparathyroidism, Ann. Internal Med., 62:1223.

2. Moxley, M.A., Bell, N.H., Wagle, S.R., Allen, D.O., and Ashmore, J., 1974, Parathyroid hormone stimulation of glucose and urea production in isolated liver cells, Am. J. Physiol., 227:1058.

3. Gozariu, L., Forster, K., Faulhaber, J.D., Minne, H., and Ziegler, R., 1974, Parathyroid hormone and calcitonin: Influences upon lipolysis of human adipose tissue, Horm. Metab. Res. 6:243.

4. Sinha, T.K., Thajchayapong, P., Queener, S.F., Allen, D.O., and Bell, N.H., 1976, On the lipolytic action of parathyroid hormone in man, Metabolism 25:251.

5. Taniguchi, A., Kataoka, K., Kono, T., Oseko, F., Okuda, H., Nagata, I., and Imura, H., 1987, J. Lipid Res. 28:490.

6. Hallberg, D., and Werner, S., 1976, Circulatory and lipolytic effects of parathyroid hormone: An experimental study in dogs, Horm. Metab. Res. 9:424.

7. Bagdade, J.D., Yee, E., Wilson, D.E., and Shafrir, E., 1978, Hyperlipidemia in renal failure. Studies of plasma lipoproteins, hepatic trigliceride production, and tissue lipoprotein lipase in a chronically uremic rat model, J. Lab. Clin. Med. 91:176.

8. Boland, C.J., Fried, R.M., and Tashjian, A.H., Jr., 1986, Measurement of cytosolic free Ca^{++} concentrations in human and rat osteosarcoma cells: Actions of bone resorption-stimulating hormones, Endocrinology 118:980.

9. Gliemann, J., Østerlind, K., Vinten, J., and Gammeltoft, 1972, A procedure for measurement of distribution spaces in isolated fat cells, Biochem. Biophys. Acta 286:1.

10. Nilsson-Ehle, P., and Schotz, M.C., 1976, A stable, radioactive substrate emulsion for assay of lipoprotein lipase, J. Lipid Res. 17:536.

11. Nakamura, T., Yoshimoto, K., Aoyama, K., and Ichihara, A., 1982, Hormonal regulations of glucose-6-phosphate dehydrogenase and lipogenesis in primary cultures of rat hepatocytes, J. Biochem. 91:681.

12. Moody, A.J., Stan, M.A., Stan, M., and Gliemann, J., 1974, A simple free fat cell bioassay for insulin, Horm. Metab. Res. 6:12.

13. Paloyan, E., Kolar, J., Castle, J., Paloyan, D., and Harper, P.V., 1963, The role of the parathyroid in lipid metabolism, Fed. Proc. 22:676.

14. Cantin, M., 1965, Kidney, parathyroid, and lipemia, Lab. Invest. 14:1691.

15. Murase, T., Cattran, D.C., Rubenstein, B., and Steiner, G., 1975, Inhibition of lipoprotein lipase by uremic plasma: A possible cause of hypertriglyceridemia, Metabolism 24:1279.

16. Apprelbaum-Bowden, D., Goldberg, A.P., Hazzard, W.R., 1979, Postheparin plasma triglyceride lipase in chronic hemodialysis: Evidence for a role of hepatic lipase in lipoprotein metabolism, Metab. Clin. Exp. 28:917.

17. Staprans, I., Felts, J.M., and Zacherle, B., 1979, Apoprotein composition of plasma lipoproteins in uremic patients on hemodialysis, Clin. Chem. Acta. 93:135.

18. Brunzell, J.R., and Goldberg, A.P., 1983, Hyperlipidemia, in: "Textbook of nephrology" Vol. II, Massry, S.G., and Glassock, R.J. eds., Williams and Wilkins, Baltimore.

19. Drueke, T., and Lacour, B., 1985, Parathyroid hormone and hyperlipidemia of uremia, Contr. Nephrol. 49:12.

20. Lacour, B., Roullet, J.B., Liagre, A.M., Jorgetti, V., Beyne, Pascale, Dubost, C., and Drueke, T, 1986, Serum lipoprotein disturbances in primary and secondary hyperparathyroidism and effects of parathyroidectomy, Am. J. Kid. Dis. 8:422.

21. Lazarus, J.M., Lowrie, E.G., Hampers, C.L., and Merrill, J.P., 1975, Cardiovascular disease in uremic patients on hemodialysis, Kid. Int. 7 (suppl):167.

22. De Moor, P., Creytiens, G., Bouillon, R., and Joossens, J.V., 1973, Results obtained in 75 patients operated upon for hyperparathyroidism: low cholesterol levels in overt primary hyperparathyroidism, Annals Endocr. 34:616.

23. Ljunghall, S., Lithell, H., Vessby, B., and Wide, L., 1978, Glucose and lipoprotein metabolism in primary hyperparathyroidism. Effects of parathyroidectomy, Acta Endocr. 89:580.

24. Lacour, B., Basile, C., Drueke, T., Funck-Brentano, J.L., 1982, Parathyroid function and lipid metabolism in the rat, Mineral Electrolyte Metab. 7:157.

25. Baczynski, R., Massry, S.G., Magott, M., El-Belbessi, S., Kohan, R., and Brautbar, N., 1985, Effect of parathyroid hormone on energy metabolism of skeletal muscle, Kid. Int. 28:722.

26. Klahr, S., Hruska, K., and Martin, K., 1980, Effects of parathyroid hormone on glucose production by the liver, Contr. Nephrol. 20:129.

STUDIES ON THE PATHOGENESIS OF HYPERTRIGLYCERIDEMIA IN CHRONIC RENAL FAILURE: THE SIGNIFICANCE OF INTRAVENOUS FAT TOLERANCE TEST (IVFTT) BEFORE AND AFTER SUBTOTAL PARATHYROIDECTOMY (PTX)

Seishi Inoue, Yoshikazu Fujita, Hidetaro Mori, Oshi Inagaki Ryoichi Yorifuji and Toshiaki Hirabayashi

Dialysis Unit
Hyogo College of Medicine
Nishinomiya, Hyogo, Japan

INTRODUCTION

The majority of patients with chronic renal failure (CRF) undergoing hemodialysis treatment is shown to have hypertriglyceridemia and a high frequency of premature morbidity and mortality from cardiovascular disease[1].

Many studies of the mechanism of serum triglyceride (TG) elevation in CRF have been reported and many factors seemed to be involved among them; lately parathyroid hormone (PTH) which is increased in CRF, has also been shown to influence plasma lipid levels.

The following studies were undertaken to investigate the pathogenic role of secondary hyperparathyroidism in hypertriglyceridemia in CRF.

PATIENTS AND METHODS

Studies were undertaken in two study groups.

In the first study group, the serum levels of TG, cholesterol, β-lipoprotein and HDL-cholesterol were determined and compared before parathyroidectomy (PTX) and 2 months after, 3 months after, 4,5,6,9 and 12 months afterwards in 23 patients. Blood samples were obtained at 9 am after an overnight fast. Statistical analysis was done by Student's unpaired t test.

In the second study group, we compared fractional clearance rate (K_2 rate) of TG by means of intravenous fat tolerance test (IVFTT)[23] before and after PTX in 10 patients. IVFTT was done within 2 weeks before PTX and in 3 to 6 months afterwards. The method of IVFTT is shown Figure 1.

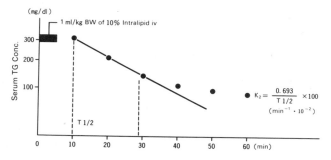

Figure 1. Method of IVFTT (Lewis)

Table 1. Clinical Summary of the First Study Group.

	N	Age	Sex m f	HD-Dur (Month)	PTG * (g)	PTH-C (ng/ml) **	
						Pre PTX	Post PTX***
1st Study Group	11	41.0 ±7.6	3 8	100.3 ±30.4	2.82 ±1.74	29.6 ±26.3	0.7 ±0.3

Mean±SD   * PTG : Parathyroid glands removed(g)
** PTH-C : Normal range < 0.5 ng/ml
*** Post PTX : 6 months after PTX

1 ml per Kg body weight of 10% Intralipid®solution was infused intravenously during 5 minutes after starting the infusion of Intralipid. Their clearance rate (K₂ rate) was calculated from the slope of disappearance rate. As a control, IVFTT was also done in 10 fasting healthy subjects.

PTX was performed subtotally by removing the largest 3 glands and all but about 50 mg of the fourth gland. The effectiveness of PTX was assessed by sequential evaluation of serum calcium, phosphate, alkaline phosphatase and PTH levels as well as by remission of clinical symptoms. In all patients, PTX was effective as judged by the aforementioned items.

Serum PTH levels were measured by Eiken PTH-C RIAKIT. Statistical analysis was done by Student's paired t test.

RESULTS

First Study Group

11 out of 23 patients showed hypertriglyceridemia above 150 mg/dl and were studied as the first study group thereafter. The clinical summary of this group is shown in Table 1. This group consisted of 3 male and 8 female patients, aged between 29 and 57 years (mean:41.0 years). They had undergone hemodialysis from 52 to 163 months (mean:100 months) at the time of study. The mean weight of parathyroid removed in 11 patients of the first study group was 2.82±1.74 gm (0.45-7.15 gm). Mean PTH-C level was 29.6±26.3 ng/ml before PTX, and 0.46±0.23 at 2 months, 0.52±0.36 at 3 months, 0.53±0.23 at 6 months and 0.72±0.45 ng/ml at 12 months after PTX.

As shown in Figure 2, preoperative mean TG concentration was 192±33 mg/dl and postoperative mean TG concentration accompanied a significant

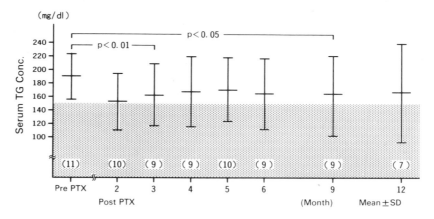

Figure 2. Changes in mean TG concentration after PTX.

Table 2. Patient Profiles of the 2nd Study Group

No.	Name	Age	Sex	Dur. of HD (M)	Parathyroid removed(g)
1	M. K.	41	f	98	2. 30
2	I. K.	45	m	148	2. 16
3	K. T.	44	m	145	3. 25
4	O. K.	33	f	114	2. 90
5	K. A.	44	f	112	0. 56
6	K. M.	47	· f	136	3. 80
7	H. H.	46	m	78	2. 60
8	T. I.	41	m	141	1. 13
9	K. M.	52	f	91	4. 49
10	T. I.	41	f	104	0. 38
Mean		43.4	m 4 f 6	116	2. 36

Table 3. Biochemical Data before and after PTX

	Before	After	P
s-Calcium, mg/dl	9. 3± 0. 3	9. 4±0. 3	NS
s-Phosphate, mg/dl	7. 4± 0. 5	5. 6±0. 5	<0. 01
Alkaline Phosphatase, KAU	60. 1±11. 7	17. 0±5. 3	<0. 001
c-PTH, ng/ml	36. 3± 6. 9	0. 8±0. 3	<0. 001

Mean±SEM

decrease from 2 to 9 months, but did not reach the normal range and
remained in slightly increased levels.

Postoperatively, serum cholesterol, β-lipoprotein and HDL-cholesterol
levels did not change significantly and HDL-cholesterol levels continued
at a decreased level after PTX as well as before PTX.

Second Study Group

Patient profiles of the second study group are shown in Table 2.
There were 4 male and 6 female patients, aged between 33 and 52 years
(mean:43.4 years). They had undergone hemodialysis from 78 to 148 months
(mean:116 months) at the time of study. Mean weight of parathyroid glands
in these 10 patients was 2.36g. Their biochemical data before and after
PTX are shown in Table 3. There is no significant difference in serum Ca
levels. Serum phosphate, alkaline phosphatase and C-PTH levels decreased
significantly, and it was clear that surgeries were effective.

In changes of postoperative TG concentration, 5 patients showed a
decrease, 2 no change and 3 an increase, and mean TG concentration decreased
from 155.9 to 136.2 mg/dl, but the changes did not reach significant
difference.(Table 4)

K_2 rate after PTX increased in all patients except one; 7 patients
who had showed lower K_2 rate before PTX showed especially remarkable

Table 4. TG and K2 rate before and after PTX

No.	Name	Triglyceride		K2 rate ($\times 10^{-2}$)	
		Pre PTX	Post PTX	Pre PTX	Post PTX
1	M. K.	94	83	1.6	2.0
2	I. K.	184	107	0.6	0.3
3	K. T.	148	90	1.0	2.2
4	O. K.	144	145	0.4	0.8
5	K. A.	171	196	1.5	1.6
6	K. M.	226	246	0.2	0.7
7	H. H.	110	61	0.7	2.0
8	T. I.	153	69	0.7	1.6
9	K. M.	179	187	0.1	1.2
10	T. I.	148	178	0.5	0.7
	Mean	155.9	136.2	0.73	1.31
	SEM	11.9	20.0	0.159	0.21

$0.1 < p < 0.2$ $p < 0.01$

increase. However, even if K2 rates increased after PTX, they stayed at abnormally low levels compared to normal K2 rate ($2.56 \pm 0.69 \times \min^{-1} \cdot 10^{-2}$). (Figure 3)

There was a slight inverse relationship between K2 rates and TG concentrations before PTX, but after PTX there was no relationship. (Figure 4)

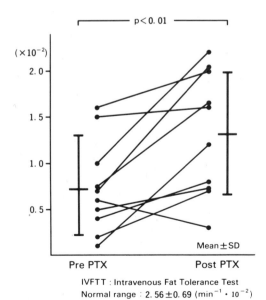

IVFTT : Intravenous Fat Tolerance Test
Normal range : 2.56 ± 0.69 ($\min^{-1} \cdot 10^{-2}$)

Figure 3. K2 rate in IVFTT before and after PTX

DISCUSSION

The pathogenesis of hypertriglyceridemia in CRF has been discussed from the viewpoint of overproduction or lack of removal capacity[4]

It seemed possible that heparin[4], acetate[5] and glucose overload[6], low protein-high carbohydrate diet and lack of exercise might be involved in part in hypertriglyceridemia in hemodialysis patients. However, in more recent years many investigators consider that such factors do not play the main role in it, but its major etiological factor is defective clearance of TG from circulation.

In support of the concept of defective clearance as a mechanism for hypertriglyceridemia in CRF, decreased clearance rate[3] of TG in IVFTT and impaired turnover of VLDL-TG[7] have been reported, and as causative factors concerning the low capacity of TG removal, decreased enzyme activity of LPL[8], TG lipase[9] and LCAT[10], and presence of LPL inhibitor were presented.

From our results that hypertriglyceridemia was improved after PTX in the first study group, we suspected that the removal of excess PTH was effective on decrease of serum TG levels.

In other experimental studies[11,12] PTX have been followed by improvement of lipid metabolism in CRF.

On the other hand, Lazarus[13] et al have presented conflicting data. The purpose of IVFTT in the second study group was to investigate in more detail the role of PTH in TG metabolism.

In the present studies, we showed that clearance rates of TG increased after PTX, and our results proved that PTH might be a component of inhibiting factors to LPL activity in CRF.

Lacour[14] et al proposed that endogenous hyperparathyroidism induced by a Ca poor diet in rats was associated with a significant increase in serum TG concentration and significant decrease in the serum clearance rate of intravenously infused Intralipid® and exogenous hyperparathyroidism by parathyroid extract injection was also accompanied by a slight increase in serum TG as well as a decrease in plasma PHLA.

About PTH as an inhibitive factor of LPL, Bagdade[15] proposed from an experiment in rats that PTH inhibits the enzymatic activity of LPL.

A multitude of clinical and experimental data point toward PTH as a major uremic toxin[16] and implicate the excess blood levels of this hormone in the genesis of many uremic manifestations.

Our present data suggested that PTH play a certain important role in lipid metabolism in CRF.

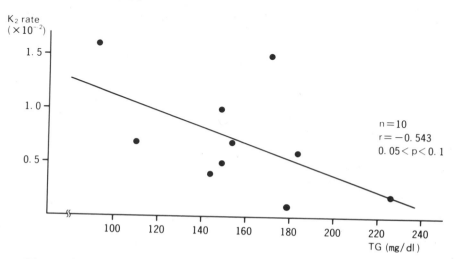

Figure 4. Correlation between preoperative TG concentrations and K_2 rates in IVFTT

SUMMARY

An investigation was carried out to determine whether serum TG concentration in patients with secondary hyperparathyroidism decrease after
PTX, and IVFTT was performed to elucidate the mechanism of reduction of TG,
and it was found that hypertriglyceridemia had improved and clearance
capacity of TG increased after PTX.

REFERENCE

1) A.Lindner,B.Charra,D.J.Sherrard and B.H.Scribner,Accelerated atherosclerosis in prolonged maintenance hemodialysis,N.Engl.J.Med.290:679(1974)
2) B.Lewis,J.Boberg,M.Mancini and L.A.Carlson,Determination of the intravenous fat tolerance test with Intralipid®by nephelometry,Atherosclerosis
   15:83(1972)
3) G.I.Russel,T.G.Davies and J.Walls,Evaluation of the intravenous fat
   tolerance in chronic renal disease,Clin.Nephrol.13:282(1980)
4) L.S.Ibels,M.F.Reardon and P.J.Neslel,Plasma post-heparin lipolytic
   activity and triglyceride clearance in uremic and hemodialysis patients
   and renal allograft recipients,J.Lab.Clin.Med.84:684(1976)
5) E.Savdie,J.E.Mahony and J.H.Stewart,Effect of acetate on serum lipids
   in maintenance hemodialysis,Trans.Amer.Soc.Artif.Int.Org.23:385(1977)
6) D.H.Dombeck,D.D.Lindholm and J.A.Vieira,Lipid metabolism in uremia and
   the effect of dialysate glucose and oral androgen therapy,Trans.Amer.
   Soc.Artif.Org.19:150(1973)
7) E.Savdie,J.C.Gibson,G.A.Crawford,L.A.Simons and L.F.Mahony,Impaired
   plasma triglyceride clearance as a feature of both uremic and posttransplant triglyceridemia,Kidney Int.18:774(1980)
8) J.K.Huttunen,A.Pasternak,T.Vänttinen,C.Ehnholm and E.A.Nikkilä,Lipo-
   protein matabolism in patients with chronic uremia,Acta Med.Scand.204
   :211(1978)
9) T.Murase,D.C.Cattran,B.Rubenstein and G.Steiner,Inhibition lipoprotein
   lipase by uremic plasma,A possible cause hypertriglyceridemia,
   Metabolism,24:2179(1975)
10) G.G.Guarneri and M.Moracchello,Lecithin cholesterol acyltransferase
    activity in chronic uremia,Kidney Int.Suppl.No.8:S26.(1983)
11) E.Poloyan,J.Kolar,J.Castles,D.Poloyan,P.V.Harper,The role of the para-
    thyroids in lipid metabolism,Fed.Proc.22:676(1963)
12) M.Cantin,Kidney,Parathyroid and lipemia,Lab.Invest.14:1691(1965)
13) J.M.Lazarus,E.G.Lowrie,C.L.Hampers and J.P.Merril,Cardiovascular disease
    in uremic patients on hemodialysis,Kidney Int.7:Suppl,pp.176(1975)
14) B.Lacour,C.Basile,T.Druek and J-L.F.Brentano,Parathyroid function
    and lipid metabolism in the rat,Mineral Electrolyte Metab.7:157(1982)
15) J.Bagdade,E.Yee and O.J.Pykälistö,Parathyroid hormone and triglyceride
    transport:Effects on triglyceride secretion rate and adipose tissue
    lipoprotein lipase in the rat,Horm.Metab.Res.10:443(1978)
16) S.G.Massry,Is parathyroid hormone a uremic toxin ?,Nephron,19:125(1977)

CARBOHYDRATE INTOLERANCE AND IMPAIRED PANCREATIC INSULIN RELEASE IN CHRONIC RENAL FAILURE: ROLE OF EXCESS BLOOD LEVELS OF PARATHYROID HORMONE

Shaul G. Massry, George Z. Fadda
and Mohammad Akmal

Division of Nephrology and Department of Medicine
University of Southern California School of
Medicine, Los Angeles, CA. 90033

Patients   with   chronic   renal   failure   display abnormalities in carbohydrate metabolism (1-5). They almost always have resistance to the peripheral action of insulin (5,6), while insulin secretion could be normal (4,7), increased (8,9) or decreased (3).   Glucose intolerance is, therefore, usually encountered in uremic patients in whom both impaired tissue sensitivity to insulin and impaired secretion of the hormone co-exist (5,10).

Certain data suggests that parathyroid hormone (PTH) may affect carbohydrate metabolism. Patients with primary hyperparathyroidism may have glucose intolerance (11,12). Elevated insulin plasma levels both in the fasting state and in response to glucose (11,12), as well as insulin resistance (12) have been reported in these patients.

It is plausible, therefore, to suggest that the state of secondary hyperparathyroidism which exists in patients with advanced renal failure (13-16) plays an important role in the genesis of the glucose intolerance of uremia.

We first examined the role of PTH in the genesis of the glucose intolerance of uremia utilizing intravenous glucose tolerance test (IVGTT) and euglycemic and hyperglycemic clamp studies   as   described   by   DeFronzo   et   al.   (17).   The investigations were performed in two groups of dogs with comparable degree and duration of chronic renal failure (CRF) produced by 5/6 nephrectomy; one group (6 dogs) with intact parathyroid   glands   (NPX)   and   hence   secondary hyperparathyroidism, and the second group (6 dogs) without the parathyroid gland (NPX-PTX) but maintained normocalcemic by high intake of calcium.   The details of the experimental procedures and the various techniques and methods utilized in the study were reported elsewhere (18).

The 5/6 nephrectomy resulted in a significant (p<0.01) decrease in creatinine clearance in both the NPX (from 56$\pm$2 to 12$\pm$4 ml/min) and the NPX-PTX (from 58$\pm$3 to 13$\pm$ 3 ml/min) dogs and in a significant increase in serum PTH levels in the NPX animals (from 1.0$\pm$0.5 to 37$\pm$0.5 pg/ml). There were no significant differences among the plasma concentrations of electrolytes before and after the induction of CRF. Plasma levels of PTH was elevated in NPX dogs and undetectable in NPX-PTX animals (Table 1).

The results of the IVGTT before and 3 months after CRF in NPX and NPX-PTX dogs are shown in figure 1. Within 3 minutes after the injection of the glucose load, the plasma concentrations of glucose reached their peak and decreased thereafter. The NPX animals with intact parathyroid glands and elevated blood levels of PTH displayed glucose intolerance with the plasma concentrations of glucose being significantly ($p<0.01$) higher at 20, 30, 40, 50 and 60 minutes than those observed before CRF (fig. 1). In contrast, there was no significant differences between the results in the IVGTT before and after CRF in the NPX-PTX (fig. 2). Thus, these latter animals did not have glucose intolerance.

The K-g rate of glucose (the rate of decline in plasma concentration of glucose) decreased significantly ($p<0.01$) after CRF in the NPX dogs (from 2.86 ± 0.48 to 1.23 ± 0.18 %/min) while K-g rate in the NPX-PTX dogs was not affected by CRF (2.41 ± 0.43 vs 2.86 ± 0.86 %/min, fig. 3).

There were significant increments in plasma insulin levels during IVGTT in all animals. In the NPX dogs insulin concentrations increased from 24 ± 2.3 uU/ml to peak of 105 uU/ml ($p<0.01$) and remained elevated throughout the study. In the NPX-PTX dogs, the maximum increment in plasma insulin concentration (from 18 ± 1.2 to 229 ± 19.4 uU/ml) was more than twice that observed in the NPX animals ($p<0.01$); the levels gradually declined but were higher than those in the NPX dogs during the first 30 minutes ($p<0.01$) and returned to baseline values by 1 hour (fig. 4). These differences in plasma insulin were not due to higher plasma glucose concentrations in NPX-PTX dogs, and for any given level of plasma glucose during IVGTT, the plasma insulin was higher in NPX-PTX than in NPX dogs (fig. 5).

The results of the studies with hyperglycemic clamp are given in figure 6. The total amount of glucose metabolized during the 20 to 120 minute period was significantly ($p<0.01$) lower by 38% in the NPX compared to the NPX-PTX group (6.64 ± 1.13 vs. 10.74 ± 1.10 mg/kg . min). The early, late and total insulin responses were greater in NPX-PTX animals than in NPX dogs. The total response gave values of 147 ± 31 vs. 72 ± 9 uU/ml ($p<0.025$). There was no significant difference between the M/I ratio, a measure of tissue sensitivity of insulin, in the NPX and NPX-PTX dogs (9.9 ± 0.66 vs. 8.9 ± 1.3 mg/kg . min per uU/ml).

The results of the studies with the euglycemic clamp are presented in figure 7. The total amount of glucose metabolized during elevated blood levels of insulin inthe NPX dogs (5.59 ± 0.71 mg/kg . min) was not different from that in the NPX-PTX animals (5.85 ± 0.47 mg/kg . min). Also the M/I ratio was not different among the two groups of dogs (5.12 ± 0.76 vs. 5.18 ± 0.57 mg/kg . min per uU/ml) but both values were significantly ($p<0.01$) lower than in normal dogs (9.98 ± 1.26 mg/kg . min per uU/ml). The metabolic clearance rate of insulin was significantly reduced in both NPX (12.1 ± 0.7 mg/kg . min, $p<0.01$) and NPX-PTX (12.1 ± 0.9 mg/kg . min, $p<0.02$) dogs as compared with control animals.

Figure 8 provides the results of the studies evaluating basal hepatic gluclose production and the response to insulin utilizing the bolus injection and the continuous infusion of [^{3}H]-glucose. Basal hepatic glucose production was similar

Table 1. Biochemical Data Before and After Induction of Uremia

Parameter		IVGTT NPX dogs (n = 6) B	A	IVGTT NPX-PTX dogs (n = 6) B	A	Clamp NPX dogs (n = 6) B	A	Clamp NPX-PTX dogs (n = 7) B	A
Weight, kg		20±0.6	20±0.6	20±0.8	20±0.8	21±0.7	21±0.7	21±1	20±0.9
Duration of uremia, wk		12	12	12	12	46±8	46±8	48±7	48±7
Creatinine clearance, ml/min		56±2	12±4*	58±3	13±3*	58±2	13±4*	56±2	13±3*
Fasting plasma glucose, mg/dl	HC	96±7	97±10	106±5	97±3	96±2	95±2	93±1	95±1
	EC					96±2	100±4	93±1	91±3
Fasting plasma insulin, uU/ml	HC	14±1	25±2‡	14±1	18±1	15±1	24±3	16±1	23±3
	EC					15±1	26±4	16±1	25±4
Plasma sodium, meq/liter		149±1	150±1	150±1	149±1	149±1	148±1	149±1	149±1
Plasma bicarbonate, meq/liter		21±0.6	19±0.5	21±0.3	20±0.4	29±0.6	19±0.5	22±0.5	21±0.5
Plasma total calcium, mg/dl		10.3±0.3	9.8±0.2	10.6±0.2	9.9±0.2	10.0±0.3	9.8±0.2	10.4±0.2	10.0±0.2
Plasma ionized calcium, mg/dl		2.3±0.04	2.2±0.1	2.6±0.1	2.4±0.1	2.5±0.1	2.3±0.1	2.4±0.1	2.2±0.1
Plasma inorganic phosphorus, mg/dl		4.1±0.3	4.0±0.6	4.4±0.2	4.7±0.2	4.0±0.2	4.0±0.3	4.5±0.3	4.7±0.2
Plasma magnesium, mg/dl		1.9±0.1	2.0±0.1	1.9±0.1	2.0±0.1	1.9±0.03	2.0±0.04	1.9±0.1	2.0±0.1
Serum PTH, uleq/ml		1.0±0.5	37±0.5‡	1.0±0.5	UD	UD	36±0.1‡	1.1±0.5	UD
Serum-free thyroxine index		2.0±0.1	2.0±0.1	2.0±0.1	1.9±0.04	2.0±0.1	2.0±0.1	1.9±0.05	2.0±0.04
Plasma potassium, meq/liter		4.5±0.1	4.5±0.1	4.4±0.1	4.4±0.1	4.4±0.1	4.3±0.1	4.4±0.1	4.5±0.1

Data are presented as mean ± SE. NPX, 5/6 nephrectomy but intact parathyroid glands; NPX-PTX, 5/6 nephrectomy and thyroparathyrodecomy; B, before CRF; A, after CRF; HC, hyperglycemic clamp; EC = euglycemic clamp. * Significant difference (P <0.01) from data obtained before induction of uremia. ‡ Significant difference (P <0.01) between NPX and NPX-PTX after induction of uremia. Reproduced by permission from Akmal et al (18).

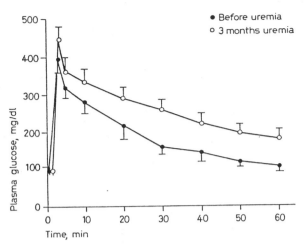

Figure 1. The changes in plasma glucose concentrations during intravenous glucose tolerance tests performed before (●) and after
(○) 3 months of CRF in dogs with intact parathyroid glands.
Each data point represents the mean value of 6 dogs and the
brackets denote 1 SE. Plasma glucose levels in dogs with CRF
were significantly higher ($p < 0.01$) at 20-60 min. With permission from Akmal et al (18).

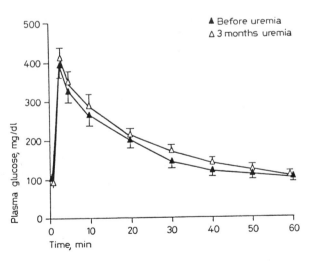

Figure 2. The changes in plasma glucose concentrations during intravenous glucose tolerance tests performed before (▲) and after
(△) 3 months of CRF in parathyroidectomized dogs. Each data
point represents the mean value of 6 dogs and the brackets
denote 1 SE. There was no significant differences in plasma
glucose concentration before and after CRF at all times.
With permission from Akmal et al (18).

222

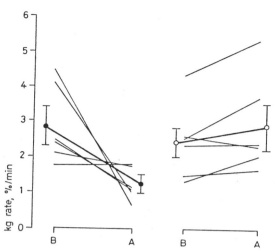

Figure 3. The kg rate before and 3 months after the CRF in NPX (left panel) and NPX-PTX (right panel). B denotes before CRF and A denotes CRF. Each line represents 1 animal and the heavy lines depict the mean values with brackets denoting 1 SE. The kg rate after CRF was significantly (p 0.01) lower than before CRF in NPX dogs. With permission from Akmal et al (18).

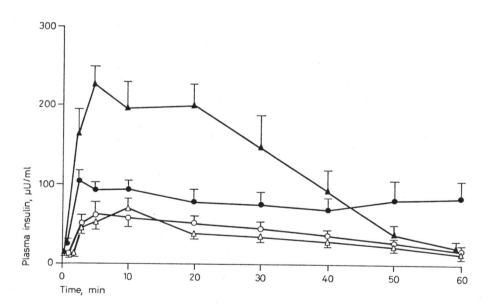

Figure 4. The changes in plasma insulin concentrations during intravenous glucose tolerance tests performed before (open symbols) and after 3 months of CRF (closed symbols) in NPX (o ●) and NPX-PTX (△ ▲). With permission from Akmal et al (18).

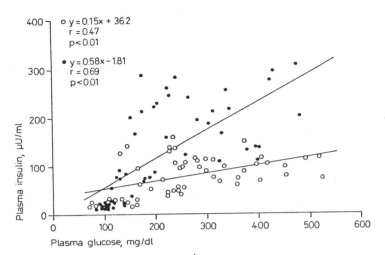

Figure 5. The relationship between plasma insulin and glucose concentrations observed during intravenous glucose tolerance performed in NPX (○) and NPX-PTX (●). With permission from Akmal et al (18).

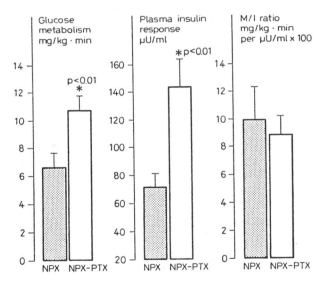

Figure 6. Glucose metabolism, total insulin response and M/I ratio (total amount of glucose metabolized [M] divided by the total insulin response [I]) observed during the hyperglycemic clamp in NPX and NPX-PTX dogs. Each column represents the mean of data from 6 NPX and 7 NPX-PTX dogs. The brackets denote 1 SE. Asterisks indicate significant difference from NPX with p 0.01. with permission from Akmal et al (18).

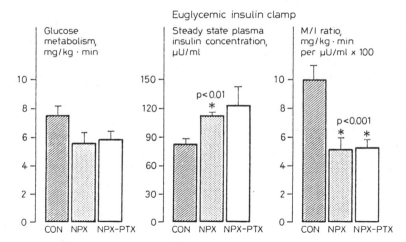

Euglycemic insulin clamp

Figure 7. Glucose metabolism, steady state plasma insulin concentrations and M/I ratio (total amount of glucose metabolized [M] divided by total insulin response [I] observed during euglycemic insulin clamp in normal dogs and in NPX and NPX-PTX dogs. Each column represents the mean of data from 6 NPX and 7 NPX-PTX dogs. The brackets denote 1 SE. CON = Control. Asterisks denote significant difference (p<0.01) from control. With permission from Akmal et al (18).

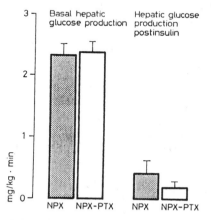

Figure 8. Basal and postinsulin hepatic glucose production observed during euglycemic insulin clamp in 3 NPX and 3 NPX-PTX dogs. The columns represent the mean data and the brackets denote 1 SE. With permission from Akmal et al (18).

in NPX and NPX-PTX dogs (2.33+0.32 vs. 2.38+0.35 mg/kg . min), and the values were not different from those previously reported in normal dogs (2.80+0.20 mg/kg . min) (19).

We also studied the binding affinity, binding sites concentration and binding capacity of monocytes to insulin in the NPX, NPX-PTX and normal dogs. There were no signifcant differences in these parameters among the three groups of animals.

The results of these studies demonstrate that the state of secondary hyperparathyroidism in CRF plays a major role in the genesis of the glucose intolerance in uremia. However, the excess PTH does not affect insulin action on peripheral tissues since the M/I ratio is significantly lower than normal in both NPX and NPX-PTX animals and there is no significant difference in M/I ratio between these two groups of animals. The normalizatin of the glucose tolerance in the NPX-PTX dogs must, therefore, be due to improvement in insulin secretion by the β-cells as both the IVGTT and the clamp studies demonstrated. It should also be noted that since both the early and late phases of insulin secretion were enhanced by parathyroidectomy, one must assume that the release of both the stores as well as the newly synthesized insulin is enchanced in the NPX-PTX animals. Finally, it should be mentioned that the effect of parathyroidectomy on plasma insulin concentration during herperglycemia is independent of the state of CRF inasmuch as plasma insulin levels during IVGTT in chronic normocalcemic-normophosphatemic-thyroparathyroidectomized dogs were twice (p<0.01) the levels of normocalcemic dogs with intact parathyroid glands (fig. 9).

In summary, our results indicate that (a) glucose intolerance does not develop with CRF in the absence of PTH; (b) PTH does not affect the metabolic clearance of insulin in CFR, and (c) the normalization of glucose intolerance in CRF in the absence of PTH is due to increased insulin secretion. Thus, the data are consistent with the notion that excess PTH in CRF interferes with the ability of the β-cells to augment the insulin secretion appropriately in response to the insulin-resistant state.

The observations of Mak et al. (20) in 8 children with CRF before and after medical suppression of the secondary hyperparathyroidism are consistent with our results. They demonstrated that the glucose intolerance in these children disappeared after the normalization of the blood levels of PTH, and the improvement was due to increased insulin response to hyperglycemia after the treatment of the secondary hyperparathyroidism. They concluded that the higher plasma insulin levels overcame the insulin-resistant state, which was affected by the suppression of the parathyroid gland activity.

Although the studies described above strongly suggest that secondary hyperparathyrodism of chronic renal failure (CRF) may impair insulin release from the pancreas, there is no direct evidence that the high blood levels of PTH indeed impair insulin release. Further, in the intact organism many other factors such as serum levels of calcium, phosphorus, magnesium or potassium may modulate the response of the pancreas to hyperglycemia. To further elucidate the interaction between CRF, PTH and insulin release, we examined insulin secretion by islets of Langerhans isolated from CRF rats with intact parathyroid glands, parathyroidectomized CRF

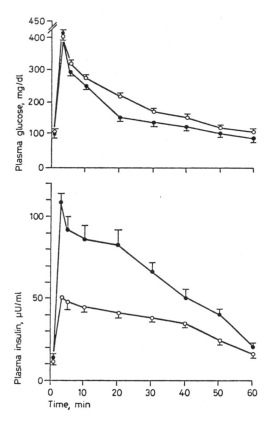

Figure 9. The changes in plasma glucose and insulin concentrations during intravenous glucose tolerance tests performed in 6 normal dogs (○) and 6 normocalcemic-normophosphatemic chronic (6 weeks) thryoparathyroidectomized dogs with normal renal function (●). Each data point is the mean of 6 animals and the brackets denote 1 SE. Plasma insulin levels were significantly higher (p<0.01) at all points between 3 and 50 min. With permission from Akmal et al (18).

rats, rats with normal renal function and a state of hyperparathyroidism produced by prolonged administration of PTH and control animals.

Sprague-Dawley rats weighing 320-375 g were studied. They were fed normal rat chow diet (ICN Nutritional Biochemical, Cleveland, OH) throughout the study and allowed to drink ad libitum.

Two types of protocols were used. In the first protocol, the rats were studied after 42 days of chronic renal failure in the presence and absence of the parathyroid glands. Parathyroidectomy was performed by electrocautary, and the success of the procedure was ascertained by a decrease in serum levels of calcium of at least 2 mg/dl. The PTX rats were allowed to freely drink water containing 5% of calcium gluconate. This procedure is adequate to normalize plasma calcium in the PTX rats. Seven days after PTX, the animals underwent a right nephrectomy through a flank incision; four days later, a partial left nephrectomy was performed. The nephrectomy procedure was also done in rats with intact parathyroid glands. This protocol, therfore, provided two groups of animals with CRF: one with intact parathyroid glands (CRF-control) and the other without parathyroid glands (CRF-PTX).

In the second protocol, normal rats received intraperitoneal injections of 1-84 PTH (Sigma Chemical Company, St. Louis, MO) for 42 days. The hormone was dissolved in normal saline and 50 ug was injected in the morning and another 50 ug in the late afternoon. The control animals received sham injections of the vehicle only.

The animals were sarificed by decapitation and the pancreas was removed, dissected free of adipose tissue and lymph nodes. Islets of Langerhans were isolated by the collagenase digestion method of Lacy and Kostianovsky (21) and picked free of exocrine tissue under a dissecting microscope. With every study of CRF-control or PTH-treated rats a simultaneous study was performed in a normal animal when it was technically feasible. The insulin release from islets of CRF-control and CRF-PTX were evaluated under static and dynamic conditions, the dynamic studies were done according to methods previously reported by others (22,23) and from our laboratory as well (24).

Briefly, in the static studies the islets were preincubated for a period of 30 minutes at 37°C in a modified Krebs-Ringer bicarbonate buffer (pH 7.4) containing 10 mM HEPES and 0.5 mg/dl bovine serum albumin (incubation media) and 2.8 mM D-glucose. The islets were then matched for size by visual inspesction and groups of 10 islets were incubated in tubes containing 1.0 ml of the incubation media and were studied with the following secretagogues: 1) 2.8 mM D-glucose, b) 16.7 mM D-glucose, c) 100 uM isobutyl-1-methylxanthine (IBMX) and 16.7 mM D-glucose, and d) 10 uM for forskolin and 16.7 mM D-glucose. After 30 minutes of incubation in a shaker bath at $37\,^\circ$C, the supernatants were aspirated for determination of insulin.

The dynamic studies were conducted in a four channel perifusion apparatus utilizing previously described methods (23). Twenty five size-matched islets were placed in each of the four concical chambers of 0.07 ml capacity and were perifused at a rate of 0.8 ml/min with the incubation media containing 2.8 mM D-glucose at a temperature at 37°C and a gas mixture of 95% of O_2 and 5% CP_2 being continuously bubbled into the perifusate. After leaving the chambers, the perifusate was filtered through 8.0 um pore size filter (Sartorius, Burlingame, CA) and was collected. Each study was performed in duplicates. After 39 minutes of per-incubation, the collection of the effluent was started and continued at a 1 minute interval for 41 minutes. The first six collections (6 minutes) represents the basal level of insulin release during perifusion with 2.8 mM D-glucose. Thereafter, the D-glucose concentration in the perifusate was increased to 16.7 mM and an additional 35 samples were collected and insulin concentrations were determined in various samples of effluent.

Calcium content of the pancreas was measured. About 0.5-1.0 g of pancreas was placed in tared porcelain crucibles and weighed to 0.01 mg. All samples were dried at 105 °C for 48 hours and then reweighed to determine water content. Samples were then ashed for 12 hours in an oven with 700 ° C. The samples were then extracted in 0.75N HNO_3 for 24 hours and calcium concentration was determined.

One hour intravenous glucose tolerance test was also done in control, CRF-control and in CRF-PTX rats. The animals were not fasted before the test. The jugular vein and carotid artery were cannulated with PE 10 tubing under general anesthesia with Ketamine-HCl 25 mg/kg (Bristol Laboratories, Syracuse, NY). The animals were allowed to recover from the surgical procedure and were studied 8 hours later and in the awake state. The rats received 0.3 g of D-glucose/kg body wt in a bolus intravenous injection. A total of 8 blood samples of 60 ul were collected serially from the arterial line for the measurement of glucose.

In the dynamic study of insulin release, the changes from baseline with time were examined by calculating the area under the curve for each study. Insulin release started to increase 4 minutes after the change of the concentration of D-glucose in the perifusate to 16.7 mM. Therefore, the average values of insulin release during the 6 minute prior to the change in glucose concentration and of the 4 minutes immediately thereafter were used as a baseline level. The calculation of area under the curve allowed us to estimate insulin release during the initial phase (5 min. between min. 4-9) and the total insulin release (31 min. between min. 4-35).

The choice to perform the study after six weeks of PTH administration or of CRF was based on results of experiments carried out to determine the time relationship between the duration of CRF or PTH treatment and insulin release from pancreatic islets. We found that PTH treatment of 4,10 and 21 days did not produced significant reduction in insulin release and that the effects of 21 days of CRF were variable with only the mean value of total insulin release being modestly (p<0.05) lower than control. These data are shown in Table 2. We therefore used the six weeks protocol where the effects on insulin release was consistent and marked. Insulin was determined by charcoal-coated radioimmunoassay (25) using rat insulin as standard.

Statistical analysis was done with the Clinfo computer system. The data are presented as mean ± SE. Changes from baseline in parameters with multiple measurements with time (glucose tolerance and dynamic insulin release) were evaluated by calculating area under the curve for each experiment utilizing the trapezoidal rule. The areas under

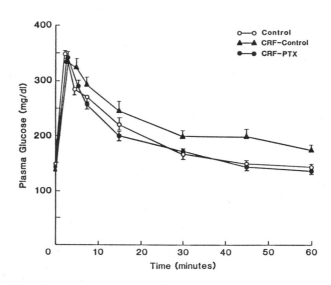

Figure 10. The changes in plasma glucose concentration during intravenous glucose tolerance test performed in 4 control rats, 5 CRF-control rats and 5 CRF-PTX animals. Each data point represents the mean value and the bracket 1 SE. Reproduced by permission from Fadda et al (24).

Table 2. Early and Total Insulin Release From Pancreatic Islets after Various Periods of Parathyroid Hormone Treatment and Chronic Renal Failure

	Serum creatine mg/dl	Insulin Release (pg/islet)	
		Early (6 min)	Total (31 min)
4 day			
Control	0.53±0.03	249±36	3777±479
PTH-Treated	0.56±0.04	279±27	3077±274
P	NS	NS	NS
10 day			
Control	0.51±0.06	201±87	3376±201
PTH-Treated	0.47±0.02	287±98	4490±333
P	NS	NS	<0.05
21 day			
Control	0.52±0.04	275±62	3421±261
PTH-Treated	0.40±0.05	208±35	3152±317
P	NS	NS	NS
Control	0.43±.03	305±80	3581±261
CRF-control	1.28±.12	243±99	2345±499
P	<0.01	NS	<0.05

Data are presented as mean ± SE of 4 studies
Data of insulin release represent area under the curve ± SE
Reproduced by permission from Fadda et al (24).

the curve as well as the data from studies from static insulin release were analyzed by one way analysis of variance and compared with each other using the Duncan multiple range test. Non-parametric analysis was also done using Wilcox non-paired rank sum tests adjusted for multiple comparison. The area under the curve for the studies form control and PTH-treated rats were compared by unpaired t-test.

The results of the IVGTT in the rats are similar to those obtained in dogs and described above. The CRF-control animals demonstrated glucose intolerance with the area under the curve being significantly grater (p<0.05) than in contorl rats. In contrast, glucose tolerance perserved in CRF-PTX rats with an area under the curve not different from normal (fig. 10). Also blood glucose concentration at 45, and 60 minutes of CRF-control rats was significantly higher (p<0.01) than corresponding values in both normal and CRF-PTX rats. These observations clearly demonstrate that the rat is an appropriate animal model to study the glucose intolerance of CRF.

There were no significant differences in the body weight and in the blood levels of calcium and phosphorus among the three groups. The 5/6 nephrectomy resulted in a significant rise in the blood concentrations of creatinine and magnesium but the latter two parameters were not significantly different among the two CRF groups of animals. Insulin release during static studies, and calcium content of the pancreas in control, CRF-control and CRF-PTX rats were given in Table 3 and figure 11. Calcium content of the pancreas in CRF-control (11.2±0.7 g/kg dry wt) was significantly higher (p<0.01) than in normal (5.9±0.9 g/kg dry wt) or CRF-PTX rats (6.7±0.7 g/kg dry wt). The calcium content of the later animals were not different from that of normal rats.

Insulin release induced by 16.7 mM glucose during static studies in CRF-control rats was significantly lower (p<0.01) than that in normal or CRF-PTX rats and insulin release in the latter two groups were not significantly different. In presence of 16.7 mM glucose, both IBMX and forskolin significantly (p>0.01) stimulated insulin release in all three groups of animals but insulin release was significantly lower in CRF-control than in normal and CRF-PTX. However, the increments in insulin release induced by IBMX and forskolin were not different among the three groups of animals.

Insulin release during the dynamic studies is shown in Figure 12. It is evident that insulin release in CRF-control rats was lower than in control or CRF-PTX animals. Early insulin release (5 minutes) calculated from area under the curve in CRF-control rats (59±31 pg/islet) was significantly lower (p<0.01) than in control (209±20 pg/islet) or CRF-PTX (187±26 pg/islet). Total insulin release (31 minutes) was also significantly lower (p<0.01) in the CRF-control (1082±104 pg/islet) than in control (3196±216 pg/islet) or in CRF-PTX (2856±356 pg/islet) rats. There were no significant differences between early or total insulin relase between control and CRF-PTX rats.

The long term administration of 1-84 PTH to rats did not cause significant changes in their weight (355±15 vs. 360±g), blood creatinine (0.7±0.09 vs, 0.6±0.10 mg/dl) or blood magnesium (1.87±0.4 vs. 1.71±0.1 mg/dl). The blood levels of phosphorus decreased modestly but significantly after PTH administration (6.7±0.3 vs. 7.6±0.3 mg/dl, p<0.01).

Table 3. Insulin Release During Static Studies and Calcium Content of Pancreas in Control, CRF-Control and CRF-PTX Rats

	INSULIN RELEASE (pg/islet/min)						Total Pancreatic Calcium* (g/kg dry weight)
	2.8 mM glucose	16.7 mM glucose	IBMX 16.7 mM glucose	Δ 1	Forskolin 16.7 mM glucose	Δ 2	
a. Control	5.6±0.7	86±9	148±14	62±12	131±12	45±7	5.0±0.9
b. CRF-Control	3.3±0.5	56±5	93±6	37±13	87±7	31±9	11.2±0.7
c. CRF-PTX	6.2±1.6	91±9	141±12	50±11	142±9	51±15	6.4±0.7
P Values							
a vs. b	NS	<0.01	<0.01	NS	0.01	NS	<0.01
a vs. c	NS	NS	NS	NS	NS	NS	NS
b vs. c	NS	<0.01	<0.01	NS	0.01	NS	<0.01

Data are presented as mean ± SE. The n for control is 6, for CRF-control is 5 and for CRF-PTX is 6, Δ1 = increment of IBMX-induced insulin release above 16.7 mM glucose induced insulin release, Δ2 = increment of forskolin-induced insulin release above 16.7 mM glucose release. Reproduced by permission from Fadda et al (24).

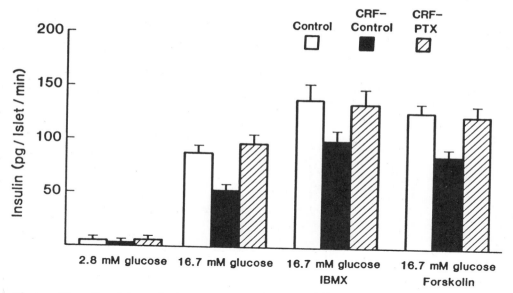

Figure 11. Insulin release from pancreatic islet during studies with static incubation 13 normal rats, 6 CRF-control rats and 6 CRF-PTX rats. Each column represents mean value and brackets 1 SE. Reproduced by permission from Fadda et al (24).

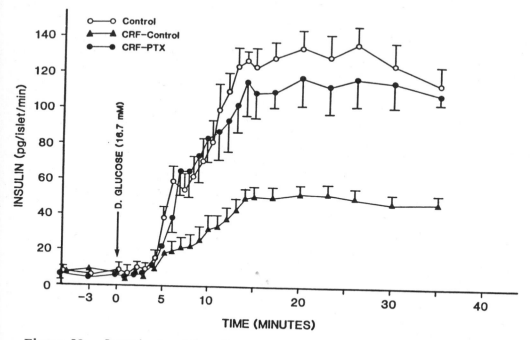

Figure 12. Dynamic insulin release from perifused pancreatic islets in 5 control rats, 5 CRF-control animal and 5 CRF-PTX rats. Each data point represents the mean value and bracket 1 SE. Reproduced by permission from Fadda et al (24).

The calcium content of the pancreas was significantly higher (p<0.05) in PTH-treated animals (7.4±0.6 g/Kg dry wt) as compared to control rats (5.9±0.9 g/kg dry wt).

Figure 13 depicts insulin release during dynamic studies in 4 control rats and 5 PTH-treated rats. The initial insulin release (5 minutes) in the PTH-treated animals (140±12 pg/islet) was significantly lower (p<0.01) than in control (208±28 pg/islet). Also total insulin release (31 minutes) in PTH-treated rats (1979±82 pg/islet) was significantly lower (p<0.01) than control rats (3220±82 pg/islet).

The results of these studies show that rats with six weeks of CRF developed glucose intolerance, with decrease in insulin secetion from their islets and that these abnormalities were reversed by prior parathyroidectomy. These data are similar to those reported in dogs (18) and in humans (20, 26). Exogenous administration of PTH to rats also resulted in marked suppression of insulin secretion from the islets.

The blood levels of PTH were not measured in our animals since the assay of PTH in the rat is not widely available and is done in very few laboratories. However, current data indicate that chronic renal failure in humans (14-16) and in dogs (18) is associated with secondary hyperparathyroidism, and increased activity of the parathyroid glands develops in rats within hours after the induction of renal failure (27). We can, therefore, assume with high degree of confidence that our CRF rats did have secondary hyperparathyroidism.

Thus, the defect in insulin release by pancreatic islets obtained from CRF-control rats appears to be due to the state of secondary hyperparathyroidism of CRF. Two observations in our study support this conclusion. First, both early and total insulin release from islets of normocalcemic parathyroidectomized rats with similar degree and duration of CRF were not different from results obtained in normal rats. Second, insulin release by islets from rats with normal renal function and a state of hyperparathyroidism produced by PTH administration for six weeks was also significantly lower than insulin release from islets of normal rats. Thus, insulin release is impaired in the presence of hyperparathyroidism independent of the presence of absence of CRF.

Available data indicate that stimulation of insulin release by glucose is mediated by a rise in cytosolic calcium concentration during the early phase of insulin release is brought about by mobilization of calcium from intracellular stores (29, 30) and this process may require energy (31). On the other hand, the rise in cytosolic calcium during the second phase of insulin release is due to an increase in calcium influx into the β-cells (28, 32, 33). Many other agents that act as insulin secretogogues such as amino acids or acetylcholine also increase cytosolic calcium (33,34).

The mechanism through which excess PTH may blunt glucose-induced insulin release is not as yet delineated. Several possibilities should be considered. PTH has been shown to acutely stimulate calcium influx into many cells (35-40), and one would, therefore, expect that this hormone should stimulate rather than blunt insulin release. However, it is possible that the effect of a chronic excess of PTH on the β-cells is different from an acute effect. A corollary to a different effect of acute or chronic excess of

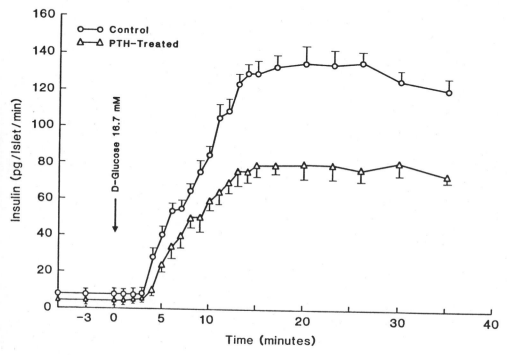

Figure 13. Dynamic insulin release from perifused pancreatic islets in 4 control animal and 6 PTH-treated rats. Each data point represents the mean value and brackets 1 SE. Reproduced by permission from Fadda et al (24).

PTH is found in observations in other systems. Excess amount of the hormone acutely stimulates chronotropic (41) and inotropic (42) properties of the heart cells and enhances random motility of polymorphonuclear leucocytes (42), but chronic exposure to excess PTH decreased or stops the beating of heart cells (41), impairs the metabolism and function of the heart (44) and reduced random motility of the leukocytes (43). The available data on insulin response to hyperglycemia with primary hyperparathyroidism (a state of chronic excess of PTH) do not help resolve these issues in that these patients have hypercalcemia and/or hypophosphatemia, both of which affects insulin release.

It is possible that the effects of changes in cytosolic calcium of the β-cells on insulin release depends on the magnitude of the change and its duration. One may speculate that chronic exposure to PTH may lead to sustained rise in cytosolic calcium. Direct evidence for such a notion is not available but, the calcium content of the pancreas was significantly increased in the rats with hyperparathyroidism with and without CRF. If this change in calcium content is equally distributed in the pancreas, one may assume that calcium overloading of the islet cells is present. Under such circumstances the capacity of cellular oganelles to sequester calcium may approach saturation and a new steady state with higher cytosolic calcium may develop. This proposition requires confiramtion with direct measurements of cytosolic calcium.

Frankel et al (45) have shown that higher cytocolic calcium may activate potassium permeability, cause repolarization of cell membranes and blunt insulin release. Also, it is known that glucose-induced insulin release plateaus as cytosolic calcium reaches a certain level (28). If the β-cells during states of chronic hyperparathyroidism have high concentration of calcium than normal, the critical level of cytosloic calcium at which glucose-induced insulin secretion plateaus would be reached earlier and insulin release would be blunted.

Chronic exposure to PTH in rats caused impairment in energy production, shutle and utilization by the myocardium (44) and skeletal muscle (45). It is, therefore, possible that a similar effect on β-cells of the pancreatic islet may reduce energy availability necessary for calcium mobilization during the initial phase of insulin release. Such an effect may blunt or abolish the glucose-induced early insulin release and provide an explanation for the observed reduction in insulin release in CRF-control and PTH-treated rats.

It also appears that the reduction in insulin release in our rats with excess PTH does not seem to be related to derangement in the adenylate cyclase-cyclic AMP system. Indeed, an increase in islet cyclic-AMP produced either by forskolin which stimulates adenylate cyclase activity (47) or by IBMX which inhibits phosphodiesterase activity caused a similar increments in insulin secretion in the normal rats and in CRF animals with and without excess PTH.

In summary, the studies in rat show that 1)CRF impairs insulin release from pancreatic islets, 2)This abnormality is reversed by prior parathyroidectomy, 3)Secondary hyperparathyroidism induced by PTH-treatment in normal rats impairs insulin release from pancreatic islets. The data provide a direct evidence for the role of secondary hyperparathyroidism in the genesis of abnormal carbohydrate metabolism in CRF. This effect of excess PTH is not related to alterations in cAMP production but may potentially be due to calcium accumulation in the pancreas.

If the effect of chronic exposure to PTH on insulin secretion by the pancreatic islets is indeed due to accumulation of calcium in the islets, the treatment with a calcium channel blocker should prevent the increase in pancreatic islets calcium, normalize insulin secretion and reverse the glucose intolerance of CRF. The third part of our studies examined the effects of treatment of CRF rats with verapamil for 42 days on glucose intolerance and on calcium content of and insulin secretion from pancreatic islets (48).

Four groups of rats were studied including: a)normal rats, b)normal rats treated with verapamil 0.1 ug/g body weight given subcutaneously twice per day (normal-VER), c) CRF rats, and d)CRF rats treated with verapamil (CRF-VER). The techniques for the production of CRF, isolation of pancreatic islets, and the methods for the study of insulin secretion have already been described above.

The nephrectomy procedure resulted in a significant (p<0.01) rise in the plasma levels of creatinine with the values being 3 times higher than in normal or normal-VER rats. There were no significant differences in the plasma levels of calcium and phosphorus among the various groups of rats. The plasma levels of potassium in CRF rats were significantly (p<0.01) higher than those of the other three groups.

Within 5 minutes after the injection of glucose load, the plasma concentration of glucose reached their peak and decreased thereafter. The rats with CRF displayed glucose intolerance (fig. 14) with the area under the curve for plasma glucose (9065$\pm$199 mg/dl. 60 minutes) significantly (p<0.01) higher than that of the other three groups of animals (normal: 6528$\pm$468; normal-VER: 6143$\pm$144; CRF-VER: 6990$\pm$350 mg/dl. 60 minutes). The treatment of CRF rats with verapamil was associated with a normal glucose tolerance test and the area under the curve for plasma glucose in the CRF-VER is not different from that in normal or normal-VER rats. Verapamil did not affect glucose tolerance in normal animals.

There were significant increments in plasma insulin levels in all groups of animals (fig. 15). There was no significant difference in the changes in the plasma insulin levels between normal and normal-VER rats. The area under the curve in normal rats was (75$\pm$5 pg/ml. 60 minutes) and normal rats treated with verapamil was (79$\pm$1 pg/ml. 60 minutes). In the CRF animals, plasma insulin concentrations increased from 0.9$\pm$0.06 pg/ml to a peak of 4.0$\pm$0.67 pg/ml and remained elevated to a lesser degree throughout the study. In the CRF-VER rats, the maximum increment in plasma insulin concentration (from 0.8$\pm$0.06 to 5.80$\pm$0.41 pg/ml) was significantly (p<0.01) higher than that observed in CRF rats. The levels then gradually decreased but there always higher than those in CRF rats. The area under the curve for plasma insulin in the studies in CRF-VER (185$\pm$18 pg/ml. 60 minutes) was also significantly (p<0.01) higher than in CRF rats (118$\pm$16 pg/ml. 60 minutes).

Insulin release induced by 16.7 mM D-glucose during static studies in CRF rats (51$\pm$2 pg/islet/min) was significantly (p<0.01) lower than that in normal (148$\pm$13 pg/islet/min), normal-VER (151$\pm$14 pg/islet/min) and CRF-VER

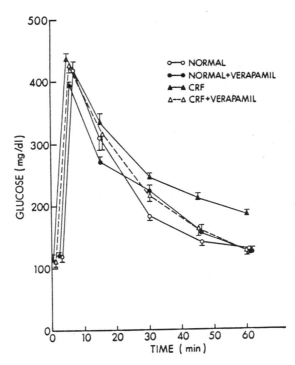

Figure 14. The changes in plasma glucose concentration during intravenous glucose tolerance tests. Each data point represents
mean value and brackets denote 1 SE. Reproduced by permission from Fadda et al (48).

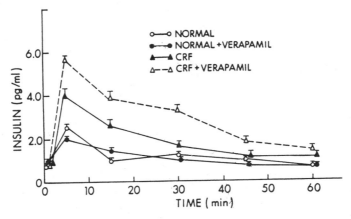

Figure 15. The changes in plasma levels of insulin during intravenous
glucose tolerance tests. Each data point represents mean
value and brackets denote 1 SE. Reproduced by permission
from Fadda et al (48).

(115±4 pg/islet/min) (fig 16). Both IBMX and Forskolin produced significant (p<0.01) rise in insulin secretion and the increment over that produced by 16.7 mM glucose alone were not significantly different (fig. 16) in the four groups of rats.

Insulin release during the dynamic studies is shown in figure 17. It is evident that insulin release in CRF rats was lower than normal, normal-VER , and CRF-VER rats. Indeed, the areas under the curve for both the early and total insulin release in CRF rats were significantly (p<0.01) lower than those in the other three groups of animals. Although treatment of CRF rats with verapamil was associated with a significantly higher first phase insulin release, the values were still significantly (p<0.01) lower than those in normal or normal-VER animals; however, total insulin release in CRF-VER rats was not different from normal or normal-VER animals.

The calcium content of the pancreas in CRF rats was (10.8±0.90 g/Kg dry weight) significantly (p<0.01) higher than that of normal (4.7±0.15 g/kg dry weight), normal-VER (4.5±0.28 g/Kg dry weight), CRF-VER animals (5.1±0.44 g/Kg dry weight). There were no significant differences in the calcium content of the pancreas among the latter three groups of animals. Thus, verapamil treatment of CRF animal prevented the accumulation of calcium in the pancreas.

The results of this part of our study demonstrate that treatment of CRF rats for six weeks with verapamil corrected the glucose intolerance. This was most likely due to the higher blood levels of insulin after the intravenous glucose injection. These observations are similar to those reported by us in parathyroidectomized CRF dogs (18) and in CRF humans in who the activity of the parathyroid glands was suppressed medically or in those subjected to PTX (20,26). Thus, it appears that reduction of PTH levels in animals or humans with CRF by medical or surgical means (20,26) or that the chronic treatment of CRF rats with verapamil which does not affect serum levels of PTH (49) permits the pancreas to produce more insulin, and such a response is sufficient to overcome the resistance to the peripheral action of insulin and results in normal glucose tolerance.

These data provide further support for the notion that the impaired insulin release in CRF is mediated through increased calcium content of the pancreatic islets. Again, the calcium content of the pancreas from CRF rats with intact parathyroid glands was significantly higher than normal and insulin release from the islets of these animals was markedly impaired. Chronic treatment of the CRF rats with verapamil which does not affect PTH levels (49) prevented the PTH-induced calcium accumulation in the pancreas by blocking calcium entry and normalized the glucose-induced insulin release from the pancreatic islets.

The results of the static studies with forskolin and IBMX indicate that the reduction in insulin secretion from islets of CRF rats and the correction of this defect by treatment with verapamil is not related to an effect on the adenylate cyclase-cyclic AMP system. An increase in cyclic AMP produced either by forskolin which stimulates adenylate cyclase activity (47) or by IBMX which inhibits phosphodiesterase activity (28) from normal, normal-VER, CRF and CRF-VER rats.

The plasma levels of insulin during IGVTT in CRF rats

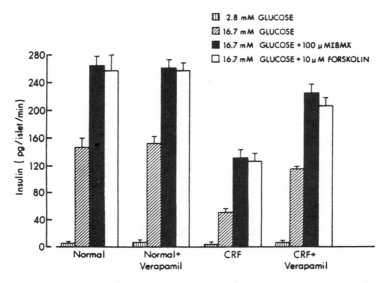

Figure 16. Insulin release from pancreatic islets during studies with static incubation. Each column represents mean value and brackets denote 1 SE. Reproduced by permission from Fadda et al (48).

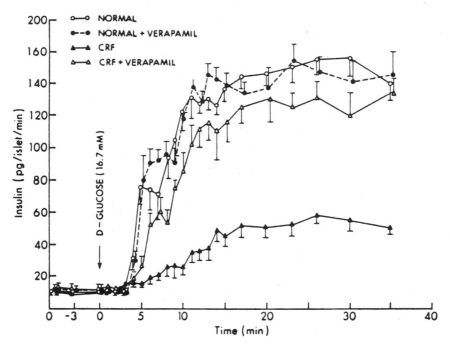

Figure 17. Dynamic insulin release from perifused pancreatic islets. Each data point depicts mean value and brackets represents 1 SE. Reproduced by permission from Fadda et al (48).

were higher than that in the normal animals while insulin release from islets was lower in the former than in the later group. This observation seems contradictory. However, it must be emphasized that plasma insulin levels represent the balance between the rate of secretion and that of degradation. Thus, the decreased degradation of insulin in CRF (50) is responsible for the higher insulin levels despite low insulin secretion. In CRF-VER rats, the higher insulin secretion from the islets combined with decreased degradation secondary to CRF are responsible for the significantly higher plasma insulin levels observed in these rats compared to the untreated CRF animals. It is, theorectically, possible that verapamil may alter insulin degradation but neither our study nor others refute or confirm such a possibility.

It is well established that verapamil added in vitro to pancreatic islets inhibits insulin release by these structures (29,51). However, the effects of the in vivo administration of the drug may differ from those observed in the in vitro experiments. Indeed, several studies have shown that acute intravenous infusion of verapamil or oral administration of the drug for several days did not affect blood levels of insulin during glucose tolerance tests (52-54). Others reported a decrease in blood insulin levels during intravenous infusion of verapamil in humans (55), dogs (56), or rats (46). It is very difficult to compare these data describing the effects of acute in vivo administration of verapamil with our studies which evaluated the chronic in vivo effect of the drug in animals with CRF. Further, our results showed that the chronic administration of verapamil to normal rats does not affect glucose tolerance, blood levels of insulin or insulin release from the islets of these animals.

The observations of the studies with verapamil may provide a therapeutic approach for the control of glucose intolerance of CRF. However, it must be mentioned that in our study verapamil was given simultaneously with the induction of CRF. It is possible that verapamil may not correct glucose intolerance if it is given to animals or humans with established CRF. In such a situation, it may not be possible to reverse the changes in pancreatic calcium. However, Mak et al. (20, 26) were able to normalize glucose intolerance in CRF patients after six months of medical suppression of hyperparathyroidism or PTX suggesting that reversal of the pancreatic abnormality is possible. We know of one study in which dialysis patients were treated for 9 weeks with another calcium channel blocker, nifedipine (57). Blood levels of insulin during oral glucose tolerance test were higher than in the patients receiving placebo but the difference did not reach statistical significance. It is possible that a longer period of treatment with the drug is needed to achieve complete correction of the glucose intolerance by normalization of the pancreatic response to glucose.

In summary this last part of our studies show that the calcium channel blocker, verapamil, by preventing calcium accumulation in the pancreas, reversed the abnormalities in insulin release that occur in CRF. This effect allowed a greater rise in blood levels of insulin during infusion of glucose to CRF rats. These higher levels of insulin over came the peripheral resistance to its action, and hence normalized glucose tolerance in CRF.

REFERENCES

1. Neubauer, E.: Uber Hyperglykamie bei Hochdrucknephritis und die Beziehungen zwischen Glykamie and Glucosuire beim Diabetes mellitus. Biochem. Z. 25:284-295, 1910.

2. Westervelt, F.G.; Schreiner, G.E.: The carbohydrate intolerance of uremic patients. Ann. Intern. Med. 57:266-275 1962.

3. Hampers, C.L.; Soeldoner, J.S.; Doak, P.B.; Merrill, J.P.: Effect of chronic renal failure and hemodialysis on corbohydrate metabolism. J. Clin. Invest. 45:1719-1931 1966.

4. Horton, E.S.; Johnson, C.; Lebovitz, H.E.: Carbohydrate metabolism in uremia. Ann. Intern. Med. 68:63-74, 1968.

5. DeFronzo, R.A.; Andres, R.; Edgar, P.; Walker, W.G.: Carbohydrate metabolism in uremia. A review. Medicine 52:469-481, 1973.

6. DeFronzo, R.A.; Alverstrand, A.; Smith, D.; Hendler, R.; Hendler, E.; Wahren, J.: Insulin resistance in uremia. J. clin. Invest. 67:563-568, 1981.

7. Samaan, N.A.; Freeman, R.M.: Growth hormone levels in severe renal failure. Metabolism 19:102-113, 1970.

8. Lowrie, E.G.; Soeldner, J.S.; Hampers, C.L.; Merrill, J.P.: Glucose metabolism and insulin secretion in uremic, prediabetic, and normal subjects. J. Lab. Clin. Med. 76:603-615, 1970.

9. Hutching, R.H.; Hagstrom, R.M.; Scribner, B.H.: Glucose intolerance in patients on long-term intermittent dialysis. Ann. Intern. Med. 65:275-285, 1966.

10. DeFronzo, R.A.: Pathogenesis of glucose intolerance in uremia. Metabolism 27:1866-1880, 1978.

11. Ginsberg, H.; Olefsky, J.M.; Reaven, G.M.: Evaluation of insulin resistance in patients with primary hyperparathyroidism. Proc. Exp. Biol. Med. 148:942-945, 1975.

12. Kim, H.; Kalkhoff, R.K.; Costrini, N.V.; Cerletty, J.M.; Jacobson, M.: Plasma insulin distrubances in primary hyperparathyroidism. J. Clin. Invest. 50:2596-2605, 1971.

13. Pappenheimer, A.M.; Wilens, S.L.: Enlargement of the parathyroid glands in renal disease. Am. J. Path. 11:73-91, 1935.

14. Roth, S.I.; Marshall, R.B.: Pathology and ultrastructure of the human parathyroid glands in chronic renal failure. Arch. Intern. Med. 124:390-407, 1969.

15. Berson, S.A.; Yalow, R.: Parathyroid hormone in plasma in adenomatous hyperparathyroidism, uremia, and bronchogenic carcinoma. Science 154:907-909, 196.

16. Massry, S.G.; Coburn, J.W.; Peacock, M.; Kleeman, C.R.: Turnover of endogenous parathyroid hormone in uremic patients and those undergoing hemodialysis. Trans. Am. Soc. Artif. Internal Organs 8:422-426-422, 1972.

17. DeFronzo, R.A.; Tobin, J.D.; Andres, R.: Glucose clamp technique. A method for qualifying insulin secretion and resistance. Am. J. Physiol. 237:E214-E223, 1979.

18. Akmal, M.; Massry, S.G.; Goldstein, A.D.; Fanti, P.; Weisz, A.; DeFronzo, R.: Role of parathyroid hormone in the glucose intolerance of chronic renal failure. J. Clin. Invest. 75:1037-1044, 1985.

19. Bevilacqua, S.; Barrett, E.; Farranini, E.; Gusberg, R.; Stewart, A.; Richardson, L.; Smith, D.; DeFronzo, R.: Lack of effect of parathyroid hormone on hepatic glucose metabolism in the dog. Metabolism 30:469-475, 1981.

20. Mak, R.H.; Turner, C.; Haycock, G.B.; Chantler, C.: Secondary hyperparathyroidism and glucose intolerance in children with uremia. Kidney Int. 24:5123-5133.

21. Lacey, P.E.; Kostianovsky, M.: Method for the isolation of intact islets of Langerhans from the rat pancreas. Diabetes 16:35-39, 1967.

22. Molina, J.M.; Premdas, F.H.; Lipson, L.G.: Insulin release in aging: Dynamic response of isolated islets of Langerhans of the rat to D-glucose and D-glyceraldehyde. Endocrinology 116:821-826, 1985.

23. Molina, J.M.; Premdas, F.H.; Klenck, R.E.; Eddlestone, G.; Oldham, S.B.; Lipson, L.G.: The dynamic insulin secretory response of isolated pancreatic islets of the diabetic mouse. Diabetes 33:1120-1123, 1984.

24. Fadda, G.Z.; Akmal, M.; Premdas, F.H.; Lipson, L.G.; Massry, S.G.: Insulin release from pancreatic islets: Effect of CRF and excess PTH. Kidney Int. 33:1066-1072, 1988.

25. Herbert, .; Lau, K.S.; Gottlieb, C.W.; Bleicher, S.J.: Coated charcoal immunoassay for insulin. J. Clin. Endocrinol. Metabolism 25:1375-1384, 1965.

26. Mak, R.H.K.; Bettinelli, A.; Turner, C.; Haycock, G.B.; Chantler, C.: The influence of hyperparathyroidism on glucose metabolism in uremia. J. Clin. Endocronol. Metbolism 60:229-233, 1985.

27. Jastak, J.T.; Morrison, A.B.; Raisz, G.L.: Effect of renal insufficiency on parathyroid gland and calcium homeostasis. Am. J. Physiology 215:84-89, 1968.

28. Wollheim, C.B.; Sharp, G.W.G.: Regulation of insulin release by calcium. Physiol. Review 61:914-973, 1981.

29. Wollheim, C.B.; Kikuchi, M.; Renold, A.E.; Sharp, G.W.G.: The roles of intracellular and extracellular Ca^{++} in glucose-stimulated biphasic insulin release by rat islets. J. Clin. Investigation 62:451-458, 1978.

30. Wollheim, C.B.; Siegel, E.G.; Kikuchi, M.; Renold, A.E.; Sharp, G.W.G.: The role of extracellular Ca^{++} and islet calcium stores in the regulation of biphasic insulin release. Horm. Metab. Res (Supp) 10:108-115, 1980.

31. Hellman, B.: Calcium and pancreatic -cell function. Mobilization of a glucose-stimulated pool of intracellular ^{45}Ca by metabolic inhibitors and the ionophore A-23187. Acta, Endocriniol. Copenhagen 90:624-636, 1979.

32. Hellman, B.; Sehlin, J.; Taljedal, I.B.: Calcium uptake by pancreatic -cells as measured with the aid of ^{45}Ca and mannitol-^{3}H. Am. J. Physiology 221:1795-1801, 1971.

33. Malaisse, W.J.; Hutton, J.C.; Carpinelli, A.R.; Herchuelz, A.; Valverde, I.; Sener, A.: The stimulus-secretion coupling of amino acid-induced insulin release. Metabolism and cationic effects of leucine. Diabetes 29:431-437, 1980.

34. Wollheim, C.B.; Siegel, E.G.; Sharp, G.W.G.: Dependency of acetylcholine-induced insulin release on Ca^{++} uptake by rat pancreatic islets. Endocrinology 107:924-929, 1980.

35. Wallach, S.; Bellavia, J.V.; Schorr, J.; Schaffers, J.: Tissue distribution of electrolytes, Ca^{42} and Mg^{28} in experimental hyper- and hypoparathyroidism. Endocrinology 78:16-28, 1966.

36. Borle, A.B.: Calcium metabolism in Hella cells and the effect of parathyroid hormone. J. Cell Biology 36:567-582, 1968.

37. Borle, A.B.: Effects of purified parathyroid hormone on

the calcium metabolism of monkey kidney cells. Endocrinology 83:1316-1322, 1968.

38. Chausmer, A.B.; Sherman, B.S.; Wallach, S.: The effect of parathyroid hormone on hepatic cell transport of calcium. Endocrinology, 90:663-672, 1972.

39. Borle, A.B.: Calcium metabolism at the cellular level. Fed. Proc. 30:1944-1950, 1973.

40. Bogin, E.; Massry, S.G.; Levy, J.; Djaldeti, M.; Bristol, G.; Smith, J.: Effect of parathyroid hormone on osmotic fragility of human erythrocyte. J. Clin. Invest. 69:1017-1025, 1982.

41. Bogin, E.; Massry, S.G.; Harary, I.: Effect of parathyroid hormone on rat heart cells. J. Clin. Investigation 67:1215-1227, 1981.

42. Kohot, J.; Klein, K.L.; Kaplan, R.A.; Sanborn, W.G.; Kurokawa, K.: Parathyroid hormone has a positive inotropic action on the heart. Endocrinology 109:2252-2254, 1981.

43. Massry, S.G.; Doherty, C.C.; Kimball, P.; Moyer, D.; Brautbar, N.: Effect of intact parathyroid hormone (PTH) and its amino-terminal fragment on human polymorphonuclear leukocyte: Implications in urema. Proc. Amer. Soc. Nephrology 15:12A, 1982.

44. Baczynski, R.; Massry, S.G.; Kohan, R.; Saglikes, Y.; Brautbar, N.: Effect of parathyroid hormone on myocardial energy metabolism in the rat. Kidney Int. 27:718-725, 1985.

45. Frankel, J.J.; Atwater, I.; Grodsky, G.M.: Calcium affects insulin release and membrane potential in islet — cells. Am. J. Physiology 240:C64-C72, 1981.

46. Baczynski, R.; Massry, S.G.; Magott, M.; El-Belbessi, S.; Kohan, R.; Brautbar, N.: Effect of parathyroid hormone on energy metabolism of skeletal muscle. Kidney Int. 28:722-727, 1985

47. Seamon, K.B.; Padgett, W.; Daly, J.W.: Forskolin: Unique diterpene activator of adenylate cyclase in membranes and intact cells. Proc. Natl. Acad. Science (USA) 78:3363-3367, 1981.

48. Fadda, G.Z.; Akmal, M.; Soliman, A.R.; Lipson, L.G.; Massry, S.G.: Correction of glucose intolerance and the impaired insulin release of chronic renal failure by verapamil. Kidney Int. (In Press).

49. Nicolov, N.T.; Todorova, M.; Ileva, T.; Velkov, Z.; Lolov, R.; Petkova, M.; Ancov, V.; Skeitanova, S.; Tzoncheva, A.; Grigorova, R.: Effect of calcium blocking agent verapamil on blood pressure, ventricular contractibility, parathyroid hormone, calcium and phosphorus in plasma, catecholamine and plasma renin activity in spontaneously hypertensive rats. Clin. Exp. Hypertension (A) 10:273-288, 1988.

50. DeFronzo, R.A.; Alverstrand, A.; Smith, D.J.: Insulin, glucose, amino acid, and lipid metabolism in chronic renal insufficiency. Nephrology Volume II, Springer-Verlag: 1334-1348, 1984.

51. Devis, G.; Somers, G.; VanObberghen, E.; Malaisse, W.J.: Calcium antagonists and islet function. I. inhibition of insulin release by verapamil. Diabetes 24:547-551, 1975.

52. Rojdmark, S.; Anderson, D.E.H.; Hed, R.; Sundblad, L.: Effect of verapamil on glucose response of intravenous infecting glucose and insulin in health subjects. Horm. Metab. Res. 12:285-290, 1980.

53. Anderson, D.E.H.; Rojdmark, S.: Improvement of glucose intolerance by verapamil in patient with non-insulin-

dependent diabetes mellitus. Acta. Med. Scand. 210:27-33, 1981.

54. Rojdmark, S.; Anderson, D.E.H.; Hed, R.; Norlund, A.; Sundblad, L.; Wiechel, K.L.: Does verapamil influence glucose-induced insulin release in man? Acta. Med. Scand. 210:501-505, 1981.

55. DeMarinis, L.; Barbarino, A.: Calcium antagonists and hormone release. I. Effect of verapamil on insulin release in normal subjects and patients with islet-cell tumor. Metabolism 29 (7):599-604, 1980.

56. Dominic, A.J.; Miller, R.E.; Anderson, J.; McAllister, R.G.: Pharmacology of verapamil. II Impairment of glucose tolerance by verapamil in the conscious dog. Pharmacology 20:196-202, 1980.

57. Ledercq-Meyer, V.; Marchand, J.; Malaisse, W.J.: The role of calcium in glucagon release studies with verapamil. Diabetes 27 (10):996-1004, 1978.

58. Reigel, W.; Horl, W.H.; Heidland A.: Long-sterm effect of niphidipine on carbohydrate and lipid metabolism in hypertensive hemodialyzed patients. Klin. Wochensch. 64:1124-1130, 1986.

PTH AND ACID-BASE REGULATION

Neil A. Kurtzman

Department of Internal Medicine
Texas Tech University Health Sciences Center
Lubbock, Texas

INTRODUCTION

PTH exerts effects on both the renal and extrarenal regulation of acid-base homeostasis. This brief revue will highlight the effects of the hormone on urinary acidification and on the whole body buffering of acid loads. Several balance studies will be cited to illustrate the integration of the renal and extrarenal effects of the peptide in the whole animal. Finally, I will discuss the modulating effect of metabolic acidosis on the anticalciuric action of PTH.

EFFECTS ON URINARY ACIDIFICATION

Interest in the renal effects of PTH arose with the report of hyper-chloremic metabolic acidosis in patients with primary hyperparathyroidism.[1] The presumption inherent in this observation was that PTH depressed proximal bicarbonate reabsorption and caused a mild proximal renal tubular acidosis. Clearance studies infusing either PTH or its second messenger cyclic AMP showed that, while bicarbonate excretion increased, bicarbonate reabsorption was not sufficiently depressed to cause metabolic acidosis.[2] Thyroparathyroidectomy increased bicarbonate reabsorption to a level significantly greater than normal (Figure 1). Under this condition PTH infusion lowered bicarbonate reabsorption back to its usual level. Similar results were observed with cyclic AMP.

More recently, micropuncture studies have shown that PTH transiently depresses renal bicarbonate reabsorption.[3] Proximal bicarbonate reabsorption remains depressed but enhanced loop reabsorption results in distal delivery no greater than seen under baseline conditions. Distal acidification is not depressed by PTH.[4] There is one study which shows enhanced distal acidification following PTH administration using the urinary pCO_2 technique.[5] This technique, however, has never been validated to detect enhanced acidification.

The molecular mechanism whereby PTH depresses proximal reabsorption recently has been delineated. The hormone inhibits the Na/H antiporter of cultured renal proximal tubular cells.[6] The effect is mediated by cyclic AMP.

New Actions of Parathyroid Hormone
Edited by S. G. Massry and T. Fujita
Plenum Press, New York

EXTRARENAL EFFECTS OF PTH

Considerable evidence suggests that PTH plays a role in the buffering of acid loads through a mechanism independent of the kidney.[7] The absence of PTH does not impair extrarenal buffering,[8,9] but the presence of increased amounts of the peptide markedly enhance buffering (Figure 2).[9] This enhanced capacity to buffer acid results whether the PTH is exogenous or endogenous. For example, either EDTA induced PTH release or the secondary hyperparathyroidism of chronic renal failure increases the buffering capacity of the organism.

The source of the buffer released under the influence of PTH is not certain, though bone seems a likely candidate. Regardless of its etiology, PTH releases buffer only when carbonic anhydrase activity is intact.[9] Acetazolamide completely blocks the buffering effect of PTH when given to anephric rats.

Phosphate depletion also enhances extrarenal buffering (Figure 3).[10] This effect is likely mediated by a mechanism different from that of PTH, since the buffering action of the two maneuvers is additive.

WHOLE ANIMAL STUDIES

Carefully controlled studies of the effect of chronic hyperparathyroidism in both dogs and human show that, rather than inducing metabolic

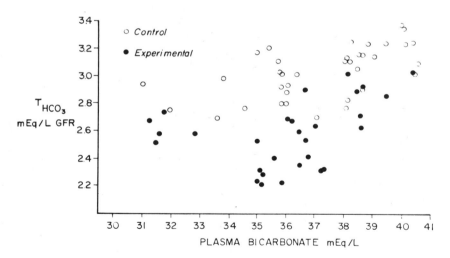

Fig. 1. Bicarbonate reabsorption is plotted against plasma bicarbonate concentration in TPTX controls (o) and TPTX animals receiving highly purified PTH (•). Bicarbonate reabsorption is increased before PTH administration and decreased to the normal range after administration of the hormone. (Reprinted from Karlinsky et al, Amer J Physiol 227:1226, 1974, with permission.)

acidosis, metabolic alkalosis ensues.[11-13] Interestingly, hyperparathyroidism has no effect on acid-base homeostasis.[14] The metabolic alkalosis of hyperparathyroidism is of both renal and extrarenal origin. The
extrarenal component is revealed by the failure of net acid excretion to
rise enough to account for the generation of the alkalosis. Since bicarbonate excretion does not rise to correct the alkalosis, the set point at
which the kidney maintains the plasma bicarbonate concentration must have
increased. The site in the nephron responsible for this change in set point
cannot be determined by balance studies, but the micropuncture data cited
above suggest a locus beyond the proximal tubule.

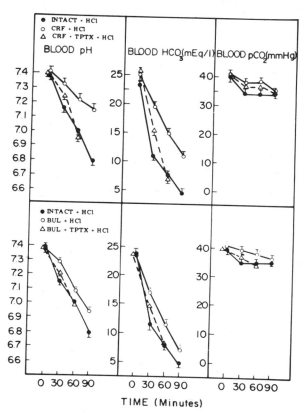

Fig. 2. The upper panel shows acid-base data
from rats with CRF with (o) and without
(Δ) parathyroid glands. Data from
control animals is shown for comparison
(●). CRF rats with parathyroid glands
have significantly higher blood pH and
bicarbonate than TPTX plus CRF rats and
controls. The lower panel displays the
same data from rats with bilateral
ureteral ligation in the presence (o)
and absence (●) of parathyroid glands.
Blood pH and bicarbonate is significantly higher in rats with bilateral
ureteral ligation and parathyroid glands
with the control rats and TPTX rats with
bilateral ureteral ligation. (Reprinted
from Arruda et al, Amer J Physiol
239:F533, 1980, with permission.)

TPTX dogs with metabolic acidosis excrete more calcium in their urine at any one level of fractional sodium excretion than do TPTX dogs who are not acidotic.[15],[16] There is debate as to whether this increase in calcium excretion is due to the absence of PTH. Data from our laboratory suggests that it is not.[15] PTH did not exert its usual anticalciuric effect when given to animals with ammonium chloride induced metabolic acidosis (Figure 4). This effect was independent of alterations in filtered calcium or changes in sodium transport.

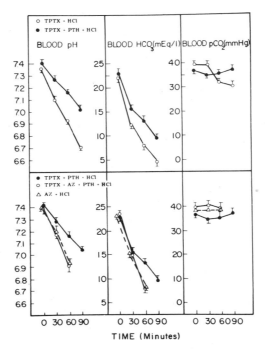

Fig. 3. The upper panel shows acid-base data during HCl infusion in TPTX rats (o) and TPTX rats infused with PTH (●). TPTX rats infused with PTH have significantly higher blood pH and bicarbonate than TPTX rats in infused with PTH. The lower panel depicts data from TPTX rats infused with PTH and acetazolamide (o). Data from TPTX rats infused with PTH from the upper panel are displayed for comparison. Data from intact rats infused with acetazolamide (Δ) are also shown. Observe that blood pH and bicarbonate are significantly higher in TPTX rats infused with PTH than in TPTX rats infused with PTH and acetazolamide. (Reprinted from Arruda et al, Amer J Physiol 239:F533, 1980, with permission.)

The alkalosis seems to be mediated by PTH or vitamin D rather than hypercalcemia. Either PTH or vitamin D causes metabolic alkalosis, while hypercalcemia unassociated with excess of either of these two agents cause metabolic acidosis.[12]

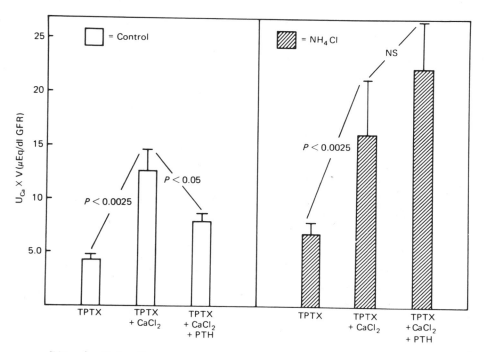

Fig. 4. This figure summarizes calcium excretion corrected for GFR in control TPTX dogs (left panel) and acidotic TPTX dogs (right panel). PTH infusion to control TPTX dogs receiving CaCl to prevent a fall in filtered calcium secondary to hypothyroidism lowered calcium excretion without a change in filtered calcium. In contrast, PTH infusion to acidotic TPTX dogs failed to decrease calcium excretion. Again, there was no change in filtered calcium. (Reprinted from Batlle et al, Kidney Internat 22:264, 1982, with permission.)

SUMMARY

1. PTH decreases proximal bicarbonate reabsorption.

2. PTH likely enhances distal bicarbonate reabsorption.

3. PTH enhances extrarenal buffering through a mechanism requiring intact carbonic anhydrase activity.

4. When given chronically PTH causes metabolic alkalosis which is of both renal and extrarenal origin.

5. PTH is not anticalciuric during metabolic acidosis.

REFERENCES

1. F. P. Muldowney, D. V. Carroll, J. F. Donohoe, and R. F. Freaney, Correction of renal bicarbonate wastage by parathyroidectomy, Quart J Med. 40:487 (1971).
2. M. L. Karlinsky, D. S. Sager, N. A. Kurtzman, and V. P. G. Pillay, Effect of parathormone and cyclic adenosine monophosphate on renal bicarbonate reabsorption, Amer J Physiol. 227:1226 (1974).
3. M. Bichara, O. Mercier, M. Paillard, and F. Leviel, Effects of parathyroid hormone on urinary acidification, Amer J Physiol. 251:F444 (1986).
4. J. A. L. Arruda, L. Nascimento, C. Westenfelder, and N. A. Kurtzman, Effect of parathyroid hormone on urinary acidification, Amer J Physiol. 232:F429 (1977).
5. O. Mercier, M. Bichara, M. Paillard, and A. Prigent, Effects of parathyroid hormone on collecting duct hydrogen secretion, Amer J Physiol. 251:F802 (1986).
6. A. S. Pollock, D. G. Warnock, and G. J. Strewler, Parathyroid hormone inhibition of Na^+-H^+ antiporter activity in a cultured renal cell line, Amer J Physiol. 250:F217 (1986).
7. D. S. Fraley and S. Adler, An extrarenal role for parathyroid hormone in the disposal of acute acid loads in rats and dogs, J Clin Invest. 63:985 (1979).
8. N. E. Madias, C. A. Johns, and S. M. Homer, Independence of the acute acid-buffering response from endogenous parathyroid hormone, Amer J Physiol. 243:F141 (1982.
9. J. A. L. Arruda, V. Alla, H. Rubenstein, M. Cruz-Soto, S. Sabatini, D. C. Batlle, and N. A. Kurtzman, Parathyroid hormone and extrarenal acid buffering, Amer J Physiol. 239:F533, 1980.
10. J. A. L. Arruda, V. Alla, H. Rubenstein, M. Cruz0Soto, S. Sabatini, D. C. Batlle, and N. A. Kurtzman, Metabolic and hormonal factors influencing extrarenal buffering of an acute acid load, Mineral Electrolyte Metab. 8:36 (1982).
11. J. H. Licht and K. McVicker, Parathyroid-hormone-induced metabolic alkalosis in dogs, Mineral Electrolyte Metab. 8:78 (1982).
12. H. N. Hulter, A. Sebastian, R. D. Toto, E. L. Bonner, Jr., and L. P. Ilnicki, Renal and systemic acid-base effects of the chronic administration of hypercalcemia-producing agents: Calcitriol, PTH, and intravenous calcium, Kidney Internat. 21:445 (1982).
13. H. N. Hulter and J. C. Peterson, Acid-base homeostasis during chronic PTH excess in humans. Kidney Internat. 28:187 (1985).
14. H. N. Hulter, R. D. Toto, E. L. Bonner, Jr., L. P. Ilnicki, and A. Sebastian, Renal and systemic acid-base effects of chronic hypoparathyroidism in dogs, Amer J Physiol. 241:F495 (1981).
15. D. Batlle, K. Itsarayoungyuen, S. Hays, J. A. L. Arruda, and N. A. Kurtzman, Parathyroid hormone is not anticalciuric during chronic metabolic acidosis, Kidney Internat. 22:264 (1982).
16. A. Goulding and D. R. Campbell, Thyroparathyroidectomy exaggerates calciuric action of ammonium chloride in rats, Amer J Physiol. 246:F54 (1984).

THE EFFECT OF PARATHYROID HORMONE ON WATER METABOLISM

Sandra Sabatini

Department of Internal Medicine
Texas Tech University Health Sciences Center
Lubbock, Texas

INTRODUCTION

Numerous reports exist showing that humans with primary hyperpara-thyroidism are unable to concentrate the urine normally (1-3). These patients develop polyuria, and when challenged with vasopressin do not respond by increasing urine osmolality. Usually all have hypercalcemia, hypercalciuria, and nephrocalcinosis.

In these patients there are a variety of factors which could contrib-ute to the polyuria. They include a decreased glomerular filtration rate, an increase in medullary blood flow, decreased solute delivery to the distal tubule, and resistance to the effects of vasopressin (AVP).

PTH AND WATER FLOW IN VIVO

Many species have been studied to better understand the abnormalities of water balance seen in patients with primary hyperparathyroidism. In dogs and rats, for example, PTH, Vitamin D, and calcium have been given acutely and chronically to mimic the hypercalcemia which is virtually universal in humans with primary hyperparathyroidism. These agents have been given orally and parenterally. Table 1 summarizes some of the results obtained. Recognizing that there may be differences in the models studied, most show that maximum urine osmolality is decreased. An interesting exception is that seen with high dose PTH (acute). Winaver et al (4) showed that U OSM in TPTX dogs varies depending on the dose of PTH given. At "physiologic" PTH infusion, U OSM decreases, whereas at "pharmacologic" PTH infusion U OSM increases. The differences are also reflected in free water clearance (C H_2O). These findings suggest that PTH has effects independent of activation of adenylate cyclase, as in both instances it is activated. While the authors did not study whether this was mediated by a calcium mechanism, work from our laboratory, using a different model, shows that it may be.

Most of the studies in Table 1 show that PTH decreases C H_2O and $T^C H_2O$. These observations suggest that the hormone (or hypercalcemia) affect thick ascending limb function. Bennett (7) however, showed that dogs given oral calcium for 5 weeks have normal (or supernormal) C H_2O when corrected for solute delivery to the thick ascending limb. Other

New Actions of Parathyroid Hormone
Edited by S. G. Massry and T. Fujita
Plenum Press, New York

Table 1. Effect of PTH, Calcium, and Vitamin D on Water Metabolism *In Vivo*

Species	U_{OSM}	C_{H2O}	$T^C_{H_2O}$	(Ref)
HUMAN				
(I° Hyperpara)	↓		↓	(1)
DOG				
(Low dose PTH)	↓	↑		(4)
(High dose PTH)	↑	↓		(4)
(24 hr PTH)	↓	↓	↓	(5)
(Oral Ca, wk)	↓	NL,↑	NL	(6)
(Acute Ca iv)	↓	↓	↓	(7)
(Vit D, 5 d)	↓	↓	↓	(8)
RAT				
(PTH)	↑ (in the presence of AVP)			(9)
(Vit D, 5 d)	↓	NL	↓	(10)

studies have shown abnormalities in C H_2O despite correction for solute delivery (Table 1).

In most of the studies cited in Table 1 GFR is decreased. This is true, as well, in many patients with primary hyperparathyroidism. Suki et al (7) carefully studied the role of GFR on C H_2O and $T^C_{H_2O}$ in dogs following an acute calcium infusion. Acute hypercalcemia decreased GFR, C H_2O, and $T^C_{H_2O}$ at any given solute load. The abnormalities in water handling were not present when GFR was decreased by aortic constriction. These results suggest that calcium exerts a direct effect on water handling independent of effects on GFR. Furthermore, they suggest that the abnormalities of water handling in humans with PTH excess may be mediated via a calcium mechanism.

It is not known if PTH affects medullary blood flow. Acute hypercalcemia increases medullary blood flow. This increase, thus, makes the medullary interstitium less hypertonic. Consequently, less water diffuses from the collecting duct into the interstitium. Whether this mechanism accounts for the polyuria and abnormal concentrating ability of hyperparathyroidism is not known.

Vasopressin resistance has been reported in PTH excess states. Cell calcium critically affects AVP responsiveness of the collecting duct (or nonmammalian collecting duct analogues). Renal medullary cell calcium concentration was markedly elevated in dogs following 24 hr PTH administration (5), whereas cortical cell calcium was unchanged as compared to control. This observation alone could explain the mechanism of AVP resistance. If the high tissue calcium is prolonged, as it likely is in patients with primary hyperparathryoidism, interstitial calcification with distortion of the normal anatomic architecture will eventually develop.

PTH AND WATER FLOW *IN VITRO*

We have studied the effect of PTH (intact hormone and a number of fragments) on water flow in toad bladder. Without AVP the toad bladder transports only minute quantities of water (basal water flow). In the presence of serosal AVP (or cyclic AMP) large quantities of water move across the epithelium from the mucosa to the serosa (maximal water flow). The purpose of our experiments was to examine the effect of PTH (and some of the fragments) on water flow in toad bladder. Further studies were designed using isolated toad bladder epithelial cells to elucidate the cellular mechanism of action of PTH.

Basal Water Flow

Intact (1-84) PTH (1μg/ml) significantly stimulates basal water flow (11). Water flow increases from 7.8 ± 0.8 $\mu l/cm^2/hr$ to 11.7 ± 1.7 $\mu l/cm^2/hr$ (N=12, P<0.05). This increase, while small in magnitude, is similar to effects seen following incubation of the toad bladder with carbachol and the calcium ionophore, A23187 (12). In contrast to these observations, PTH fragments 1-34, 44-68, 53-84, and 68-84 (1 μg/ml) have no effect on basal water flow (13).

AVP-and Cyclic AMP-Stimulated Water Flow

When AVP (20 mU/ml) or cyclic AMP (10 mM) is added to the serosal fluid of toad bladder, water flow markedly increases. Water flow increases 20 to 25 fold above basal levels. Serosal addition of PTH (1-84), in concentrations as low as 1 ng/ml, inhibits the water flow response to AVP (11). This inhibition occurs over a wide concentration range (1 ng/ml to 10 μg/ml). The 1-34 PTH fragment also inhibits AVP-stimulated water flow, but only at a high concentration (1 μg/ml). The other PTH fragments tested (44-68, 53-84, 68-84) have no effect on AVP-stimulated water flow (13).

Since AVP and PTH are both polypeptides, PTH theoretically could be competing for the vasopressin receptor on the basolateral membrane of toad bladder, thus preventing its action. To examine this possibility, we studied the effect of PTH on cyclic AMP-mediated water flow. PTH (1 ng/ml to 100 μg/ml) significantly inhibits the response of toad bladder to the hydroosmotic response elicited by exogenous 10 mM cyclic AMP. The 1-34 PTH fragment inhibits cyclic AMP-stimulated water flow, but the other fragments were without effect. These results suggest that the effect of PTH on water flow in toad bladder is specific for the intact hormone and occurs independent of the generation of cyclic AMP.

There are in vivo studies showing that PTH enhances U OSM in response to AVP (9). When studied directly as we did in the isolated bladder, PTH inhibits, not potentiates, the AVP water flow response. The in vivo findings, thus, may be be related to an effect of PTH on solute transport in thick ascending limb or in some other segment of the nephron. Regardless, they are likely not due to an effect on vasopressin mediated water flow.

To further investigate the role of calcium on the PTH effect, water flow in toad hemibladders was studied in the presence of low, but not zero, extracellular calcium (Table 2). Low calcium abolishes the effect of PTH on water flow. Similar results were obtained if hemibladders were pretreated with indomethacin to prevent toad bladder prostaglandin synthesis (Table 2).

Prostaglandins inhibit water flow in toad urinary bladder, and the calcium ionophore stimulates prostaglandin synthesis in renal tissue (cited in Refs 11, 13). If toad bladders are pretreated with indomethacin and then challenged with AVP and PTH, the effect of PTH on water flow is abolished. Lanthanum displaces membrane bound calcium and prevents the effect of A23187 on water transport (12). Lanthanum pretreatment also

Table 2. Effect of Low Extracellular Ca, Indomethacin $(10^{-6}M)$, Lanthanum $(5 \times 10^{-5}M)$, and Verapamil $(10^{-4}M)$ on the Hydroosmotic Effect of PTH

Maneuver	AVP Stimulated H_2O Flow $(\mu l/cm^2/hr)$	
	Control	+PTH
Control	105 ± 6	77 ± 7*
Low Ca (0.1mM)	139 ± 13	115 ± 15
Indomethacin $(10^{-6}M)$	175 ± 20	188 ± 31
Lanthanum $(5 \times 10^{-5}M)$	109 ± 7	119 ± 9
Verapamil $(10^{-4}M)$	23 ± 5	28 ± 7

N=8-17 hemibladders per group; AVP (20 mU/ml)
*P<0.01 from paired hemibladder
(Ref 11 and unpublished data)

abolishes the inhibitory effect of PTH on AVP-stimulated water flow (Table 2).

Verapamil inhibits "slow" calcium channels in some tissues. If the effect of PTH were mediated by a rise in cytosolic calcium from the extracellular fluid, verapamil pretreatment should prevent this. As shown in Table 2, verapamil pretreatment alone causes AVP-stimulated water flow to fall markedly. This decrease in water flow occurs virtually immediately and the addition of PTH has no effect. This finding strongly suggests that in toad bladder, a maximal water flow response is seen when cell calcium concentration is maintained within a very narrow range. Values above or below this yield an abnormal response. Verapamil, by inhibiting calcium entry, likely results in decreased cytosolic calcium levels, and PTH cannot augment this sufficiently.

PTH AND CALCIUM TRANSPORT

Because PTH has been shown to affect calcium transport in a number of tissues (14-16), we designed experiments to examine the role of the hormone on calcium homeostasis in dispersed toad bladder epithelial cells. In these studies the effect of PTH was examined on radioisotopic Ca^{45} uptake and efflux. The effect of PTH was also studied using dual wave spectrophotometry so that the onset of action and temporal relationship could be followed continuously. As shown in Table 3, PTH (1-84) significantly stimulates Ca^{45} uptake in isolated toad bladder epithelial cells. This increase is similar to that seen with A23187 and carbachol (Table 3). In contrast to these findings, PTH has no effect on Ca^{45} efflux from preloaded epithelial cells (11). Cumulative Ca^{45} efflux from control cells was 2.4 ± 0.5 nmol/mg protein/30 min; following 1.5 µg/ml PTH cumulative Ca^{45} efflux was 3.0 ± 0.6 (N=11, NS).

To examine the temporal relationship of the effect of PTH, the hormone was added to a suspension of toad bladder cells, and calcium

Table 3.   Effect of Agents on Ca^{45} Uptake in Toad
Bladder Epithelial Cells

Agent	N	Ca^{45} Uptake (nmol/mg protein/5 min)
1-84 PTH (1.5 µg/ml)	7	10.1 ± 0.9*
A23187 (1 X 10^{-5}M)	5	10.3 ± 0.8*
Carbachol (1 X 10^{-4}M)	5	8.8 ± 0.6*
Control	7	4.9 ± 0.5

*$P<0.01$ above control
(Refs 11, 12)

transport was measured for 10-15 minutes using differential light absorbance (Δ507-540 nm) in the presence of the calcium sensitive dye murexide (11). PTH increased calcium uptake within 15 seconds and the increase in calcium uptake was sustained. Unlike other agents, PTH does not cause oscillatory changes in calcium transport. Using this technique a 2 fold increase in calcium above basal was seen over the time period studied (16 to 36 nmol/mg protein, $P<0.02$).

The results, taken together, strongly suggest that PTH exerts a direct effect on water flow in toad bladder. The intact hormone stimulates basal water flow and inhibits maximal water flow. Both effects appear to be mediated via a calcium mechanism. Cytosolic calcium in all tissues is precisely regulated within a very narrow range ($\approx10^{-7}$M). Values above or below this range are likely associated with an altered water flow response in toad bladder. We postulate that the stimulation in basal water flow is due to a small increase in cytosolic calcium. The inhibition of maximal water flow seen following PTH may be due to a marked increase in cytosolic calcium, however, we did not systematically examine whether both hormones will increase cytosolic calcium above that seen with PTH alone.

Increasing cell calcium concentration seems to affect water transport by stimulating prostaglandin synthesis or release. This mechanism is suggested by the observation that pretreatment of the bladders with prostaglandin inhibitors abolishes the effect of PTH on water flow.

That the intact hormone is more potent than the 1-34 fragment suggests that full hormone configuration must be present in order for an effect on water flow to be seen. The midregion and carboxy terminal fragments alone have no effect on water flow in toad bladder.

ACKNOWLEDGEMENTS

Dr. Sabatini is the recipient of a National Institutes of Health Research Career Development Award, #KO4-DK-01527. This work was supported in part by National Institutes of Health grant RO1-DK-36119.

The author would like to thank Ms Sondra Rogers for her excellent typographical assistance.

REFERENCES

1. Fourman, P., McConkey, B., and Smith, J.W.G. Lancet 3/19, 619, 1960.
2. Cohen, S.I., Fitzgerald, M.G., Fourman, P., and Griffiths, W.J. Q. J. Med. 26:423, 1957.
3. Gill, J.R. and Bartter, F.C. J. Clin. Invest. 40:716, 1961.
4. Winaver, J., Chen, T.C., Fragola, J., Robertson, G., Slatopolsky, E. and Puschett, J.B. J. Lab. Clin. Med. 99:457, 1982.
5. Epstein, F.H., Beck, D., Carone, F.A., Levitin, H., and Manitius, A. J. Clin. Invest. 38:1214, 1959.
6. Bennett, C. J. Clin. Invest. 49:1447, 1970.
7. Suki, W. N., Eknoyan, G., Rector, F.C. Jr., and Seldin, D.W. Nephron 6:50, 1969.
8. Manitius, A., Levitin, H., Beck, D., and Epstein, F.H. J. Clin. Invest. 39:693, 1960.
9. Humes, D., Simmons, C.F. Jr., and Brenner, B.M. Am. J. Physiol. 239:F244, 1980.
10. Bank, N. and Aynedjian, H.S. J. Clin. Invest. 44:681, 1965.
11. Sabatini, S. Am. J. Physiol. 250:F532, 1986.
12. Sabatini, S. and Arruda, J.A.L. in: Calcium in Normal and Pathophysiological Biological Systems, CRC Press, Inc., Boca Raton, FL, 2:31, 1982.
13. Sabatini, S., Yang, W., and Kurtzman, N. J. Pharmacol. Exp. Ther. 241:448, 1987.
14. Borle, A.B., J. Cell Biol. 36:567, 1968.
15. Goldstein, D.A., Chui, L.A., and Massry, S.G. J. Clin. Invest 62:88, 1978.
16. Bogin, E., Massry, S.G., Levi, J., Djaldeti, M., Bristol, G., and Smith, J. J. Clin. Invest. 69:1017, 1982.

MECHANISM OF EFFECT OF PTH ON $(Ca^{2+}+Mg^{2+})$-ATPase ACTIVITY OF RENAL BASOLATERAL MEMBRANES

Kazuyuki Itoh, Shigeto Morimoto, Tsunehito Shiraishi, Kazuhisa Taniguchi, Toshio Onishi, and Yuichi Kumahara

Department of Medicine and Geriatrics
Osaka University Medical School, Osaka, Japan

INTRODUCTION

Parathyroid hormone (PTH) has important regulatory effects on biological processes in its target organs. In renal proximal tubular cells, the physiological actions of PTH are known to be mediated, at least in part, by adenyl cyclase, which catalyzes conversion of adenosine triphosphate (ATP) to adenosine 3',5'-cyclic monophosphate (cyclic AMP, cAMP).[1] Recently Levy, et al.[2] reported that PTH stimulated the activity of $(Ca^{2+}+Mg^{2+})$-ATPase, a membrane bound Ca^{2+}-extrusion pump enzyme in the basolateral membranes (BLM) of renal proximal tubular cells, which have receptors for this hormone.[3,4] We examined the intracellular mechanism of the action of PTH on the receptor-Ca^{2+}-pump interaction.

MATERIALS AND METHODS

Human PTH (1-84) was obtained from Toyojozo Co. (Shizuoka, Japan). cAMP-dependent protein kinase inhibitor (H-8) was purchased from Seikagaku Kogyo Co. (Tokyo, Japan). $[\gamma-^{32}P]$ ATP (2000-3000 Ci/mmol) was obtained from Amersham Co. (Arlington Heights, IL). Trifluoperazine (calmodulin antagonist) and cAMP were from Sigma Chemical Co. (St. Louis, MO). Proximal tubular BLM from canine kidney were prepared by the method of Windus, et al..[5]

$(Ca^{2+}+Mg^{2+})$-ATPase activity was measured by a modification of the method of Pershadsingh and McDonald.[6] The reaction mixture contained BLM (7.2 μg of protein), 50 mM Tris·HCl (pH 7.2), 20 mM NaN_3 [as mitochondrial ATPase inhibitor], 0.1 mM ouabain [as (Na^++K^+)-ATPase inhibitor], 1 mM ATP and the required submicromolar free Ca^{2+} concentration obtained with Ca^{2+}-EGTA buffer. The association constants of Ca^{2+}-EGTA and Ca^{2+}-ATP at pH 7.2 were taken as 6.8×10^7 and 8.5×10^3, respectively.[7] The reaction was started by addition of ATP and after incubation at 37°C for 30 min, it was stopped by addition of ice-cold trichloroacetic acid. The mixture was centrifuged, and the released phosphate (Pi) in the supernatant was determined by the method of Youngberg and Youngberg.[8] $(Ca^{2+}+Mg^{2+})$-ATPase activity was calculated by subtracting values with EGTA alone from those with Ca^{2+} and EGTA. The BLM were phosphorylated by incubation at 30°C of 50 μl of medium containing 50 mM Tris HCl (pH 7.2), 20 mM NaN_3, 0.1 mM ouabain, 1 mM EGTA and 1 mM [$\gamma-^{32}P$] ATP. After the reaction, the extent of phosphorylation of membrane was determined by a reported method[9], and samples were submitted to SDS polyacrylamide gel electrophoresis and autoradiography. SDS polyacrylamide gel electrophoresis was carried out in the buffer system of Laemmli.[10] Protein concentrations were determined by the method of Lowry et al.[11] with bovine serum albumin as a standard.

RESULTS

As shown in the Table 1, our BLM preparation had higher activities of plasma membrane marker enzymes and lower activities of endoplasmic reticulum and mitochondrial marker enzymes than the homogenate. We used this BLM preparation in following experiments.

First, we demonstrated high affinity $(Ca^{2+}+Mg^{2+})$-ATPase activity on the BLM (Fig. 1A). A double reciprocal plot (inset) showed that the Km of the enzyme for free Ca^{2+} was 1.3×10^{-7} M and the maximal velocity was 200 nmol Pi/mg/min at 37 °C. As shown in Fig. 1B, trifluoperazine (calmodulin antagonist) inhibited the enzyme activity dose dependently ($IC50 = 40$ μM). These characteristics showed that the high affinity $(Ca^{2+}+Mg^{2+})$-ATPase activity in the BLM was identical with that reported previously.[3,4,16] Next, we examined the effects of PTH and cAMP on the $(Ca^{2+}+Mg^{2+})$-ATPase activity at a Ca^{2+} concentration of 0.1 μM, which was in the linear range of the Ca^{2+} dependence curve (Fig. 1A). As shown in Fig. 2, both PTH (10^{-7}-10^{-6} M) and cAMP (10^{-6}-10^{-4} M) stimulated the $(Ca^{2+}+Mg^{2+})$-ATPase activity significantly and dose-dependently. However, at 2 μM free Ca^{2+}, which gave the maximal velocity, neither PTH nor cAMP had any effect on the enzyme activity (data not shown). The stimulatory effects of PTH and cAMP were completely inhibited by 5 μM H-8, an inhibitor of cAMP dependent protein kinase, to the reaction medium.

Table 1. Specific Activities of Marker Enzymes in Renal Cortex Homogenate and the BLM Preparations

Enzyme (marker)	Homogenate	BLM	Enrichment
$(Ca^{2+}+Mg^{2+})$-ATPase (plasma membrane)	13.59 ± 0.97^a	164.2 ± 12.1^a	12.1 ± 1.9
Ouabain sensitive $(Na^{+}+K^{+})$-ATPase (plasma membrane)	92.9 ± 7.7^a	785.7 ± 55.2^a	8.5 ± 1.4
NADPH cytochrome c reductase (endoplasmic reticulum)	16.6 ± 0.16^b	12.2 ± 0.38^b	0.73 ± 0.04
Cytochrome c oxidase (mitochondria)	154 ± 4.3^b	10.2 ± 0.54^b	0.066 ± 0.007

Marker enzymes were assayed by reported methods.[12–15] Specific activities are shown as nmol/mg/min (a) or pmol/mg/min (b), respectively, and are means ± SE for four separate determinants.

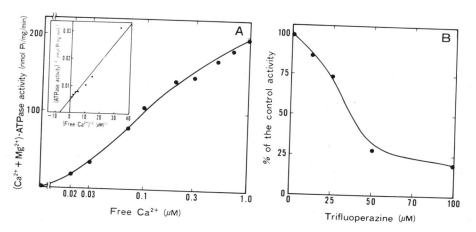

Fig. 1. A. Dependence of $(Ca^{2+}+Mg^{2+})$-ATPase Activity in the BLM on free Ca^{2+}.

Enzyme activity was determined at free Ca^{2+} concentrations of 0.02 to 1 uM. Inset showed the double reciprocal plot.

B. Effect of Trifluoperazine (Calmodulin Antagonist) on $(Ca^{2+}+Mg^{2+})$-ATPase Activity.

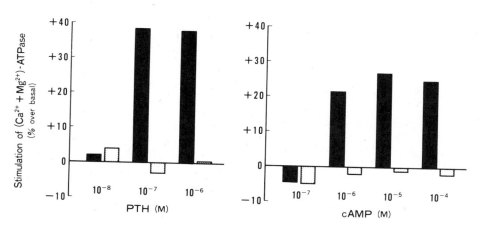

Fig. 2. Effects of Human PTH(1-84) and cAMP on $(Ca^{2+}+Mg^{2+})$-ATPase Activity in Canine Kidney BLM.

Enzyme activity was estimated at 0.1 µM free Ca^{2+} concentration in the absence (solid bars) or presence (shaded bars) of 5 µM cAMP dependent protein kinase inhibitor (H-8). Activities were calculated as percentage of the control activity without additions.

Table 2. Effects of Human–PTH(1–84) on Phosphorylation of BLM.

Addition	Amount of phosphorylation (% of control)	
	30 sec incubation	2 min incubation
None	1.52 ± 0.06 (100)	3.09 ± 0.04 (100)
PTH (10^{-7} M)	2.35 ± 0.07 (155)	4.14 ± 0.12 (134)
PTH (10^{-7} M) + H–8 (5 µM)	1.38 ± 0.01 (91)	2.98 ± 0.06 (96)

BLM (37 µg) were phosphorylated at 30°C in 50 µl of reaction medium consisting of 50 mM Tris·HCl (pH 7.2), 20 mM NaN_3, 0.1 mM ouabain, 1 mM EGTA and 1 mM [γ-^{32}P] ATP without or with 10^{-7}M PTH or with 10^{-7}M PTH plus 5 µM H–8 (cAMP dependent protein kinase inhibitor). Values for phosphorylation (nmol of Pi/mg of BLM protein) are means $\pm$ SE for three separate determinants.

These results suggest that PTH stimulated the cAMP–dependent phosphorylation of BLM. Therefore, we next examined the effect of PTH on the phosphorylation of the membranes. As shown in Table 2, 10^{-7} M PTH stimulated the phosphorylation of BLM (1.34–fold the basal level at 2 min) and this stimulatory effect was completely inhibited by 5 µM H–8.

Finally to identify the substrate protein for cAMP–dependent protein kinase, that was activated by PTH, we examined ^{32}P incorporation into proteins by SDS polyacrylamide gel electrophoresis followed by autoradiography. As shown in Fig. 3, a major band of Mr 9000 and the other minor bands were autophosphorylated. PTH (10^{-7} M), stimulated the phosphorylation of this Mr 9000 band and this stimulatory effect was blocked by H–8. Therefore, PTH stimulated the phosphorylation of a protein of Mr 9000 by activating the cyclic AMP–dependent protein kinase present in the BLM preparation.

Fig. 3. Autoradiograms of cAMP–dependent Phosphorylation of Proteins in Canine Kidney BLM.

BLM (37 µg) were incubated at 30°C in the same reaction medium as for Table 2 with the following additions: lane (b), none; lane (c), 10^{-7} M PTH + 5 µM H–8; lane (d), 10^{-7} M PTH. Samples were separated by 15% SDS polyacrylamide gel electrophoresis and subjected to autoradiography. Gel stained with Coomassie brilliant blue is shown in lane (a).

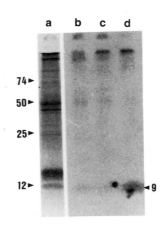

DISCUSSION

In the present study, we showed that in BLM prepared from canine kidney, PTH stimulated $(Ca^{2+}+Mg^{2+})$-ATPase activity _via_ cAMP-dependent phosphorylation, and that cAMP-dependent protein kinase mainly phosphorylated a protein of Mr 9000. These findings indicated an intracellular cascade of events induced by PTH for a physiological response. $(Ca^{2+}+Mg^{2+})$-ATPase is a Ca^{2+}-extrusion pump in the plasma membrane of variety of cells and tissues[17,18] This enzyme is Ca^{2+}-calmodulin dependent, and Niggli, _et al._[17] purified erythrocyte $(Ca^{2+}+Mg^{2+})$-ATPase by calmodulin affinity column chromatography. Furthermore, Lamers, _et al._[12] reported that $(Ca^{2+}+Mg^{2+})$-ATPase in the cardiac salcolemma is regulated by cAMP through protein kinase as well as Ca^{2+}-calmodulin. They also showed that a cardiac sarcolemma protein of about Mr 9000 is a substrate for both Ca^{2+}-calmodulin dependent kinase and cAMP-dependent protein kinase, and that cAMP-dependent phosphorylation causes 1.6-fold increase in affinity of the Ca^{2+}-pump enzyme for Ca^{2+} without changing its maximal velocity. In human blood platelets also, stimulation of Ca^{2+} uptake was found to be associated with cAMP dependent phosphorylation of a membrane protein with an apparent Mr of 22000.[19,20] Thus like cardiac sarcolemma and platelets, renal tubular BLM responds to cAMP by increase in activity of the Ca^{2+}-extrusion pump.

Further we obtained evidence that PTH stimulated cAMP-dependent phosphorylation of BLM through protein kinase and also activated $(Ca^{2+}+Mg^{2+})$-ATPase activity. This result indicated that PTH regulated Ca^{2+}-pump activity through its receptor. In fact, recently both PTH and cAMP were reported to decreased the intracellular Ca^{2+} concentration in kidney proximal tubular cells.[21] Therefore we conclude that PTH mediates its cellular effect in part by regulating the intracellular calcium concentration. Studies are required on whether PTH stimulates phosphorylation of BLM in vivo.

ACKNOWLEDGMENTS

This work was supported by grants from "the Research Program on Cell Calcium Signals in the Cardiovascular System" and from the Ministry of Education, Science and Culture of Japan (No. 62570393). We thank Miss Chiaki Nishi for technical assistance in $(Ca^{2+}+Mg^{2+})$-ATPase assay.

REFERENCES

1. G. L. Melson, L. R. Chase, and G. D. Aurbach, Parathyroid hormone-sensitive adenyl cyclase in isolated renal tubules, _Endocrinology_ 86:511 (1970).
2. J. Levy, J. R. Gavin III, S. Morimoto, M. R. Hammerman, and L. V. Avioli, Hormonal regulation of $(Ca^{2+}+Mg^{2+})$-ATPase activity in canine renal basolateral membrane, _Endocrinology_ 119: 2405 (1986).
3. M. P. E. Heeswijk, J. A. M. Geersten, and C. H. Os, Kinetic properties of the ATP-dependent Ca^{2+} pump and the Na^{+}/Ca^{2+} pump and the Na^{+}/Ca^{2+} exchange system in basolateral membrane from rat kidney cortex, _J. Membr. Biol._ 79: 19 (1984).
4. P. Gmaj, H. Murver, and R. Kinne, Calcium ion transport across plasma membrane isolated from rat kidney cortex, _Biochem. j._ 178: 549 (1979).
5. D. W. Windus, D. E. Cohn, S. Klahr, and M. R. Hammerman,

Glutamine transport in renal basolateral vesicles from dog with metabolic acidosis, Am. J. Physiol. 246: F78 (1984).

6. H. A. Pershadsingh, and J. M. McDonald, A High Affinity Calcium-stimulated magnesium-dependent adenosine triphosphatase in rat adipocyte plasma membranes, J. Biol. Chem. 255: 4087 (1980).

7. H. A. Pershadsingh, M. L. McDaniel, M. Landt, C. G. Bry, P. E. Lacy, and J. M. McDonald, Ca^{2+}-activated ATPase and ATP-dependent calmodulin-stimulated Ca^{2+} transport in islet cell plasma membrane, Nature 288: 492 (1980).

8. G. E. Youngberg, and M. V. Youngberg, Phosphorus metabolism: A system of blood phosphorus analysis, J. Lab. Clin.Med. 16: 158 (1930).

9. R. S. Adelstein, and C. B. Klee, Purification and characterization of smooth muscle myosin light chain kinase, J. Biol. Chem. 256: 7501 (1981).

10. U. K. Laemmli, Cleavage of structural proteins during the assembly of the head of bacteriophage T4, Nature 227: 680 (1970).

11. O. H. Lowry, N. J. Rosebraugh, A. L. Farr, and R. J. Randall, Protein measurement with the Folin phenol reagent, J. Biol. Chem. 36: 265 (1951).

12. J. J. Lamers, H. T. Stinis, and H. R. De Jongl, On the role of cyclic AMP and Ca^{2+}-calmodulin dependent phosphorylation in the control of $(Ca^{2+}+Mg^{2+})$-ATPase of cardiac sarcolemma, FEBS Lett. 127: 139 (1981).

13. B. M. Schoot, A. F. M. Schoots, J. J. H. H. M. De Pont, I. M. A. H. Schurumans, Stekhoven, and S. L. Bonting, Studies on $(Na^{+}+K^{+})$activated ATPase. XL1, Biochim. Biophys. Acta, 483: 181 (1977).

14. G. L. Sottosava, B. Kuylenstierna, L. Ernster, and A. Bergstrand, An electron-transport system associated with outer membrane of liver mitochondria, J. Cell. Biol. 32: 415 (1967).

15. D. C. Wharton, and A. Tzagoloff, Cytochrome oxidase from beef heart mitochondria, Meth. Enzymol. 10: 245 (1967).

16. H. A. Pershadsingh, and J. M. McDonald, $(Ca^{2+}+Mg^{2+})$-ATPase in adipocyte plasmalemma: inhibition by insulin and concanavalin A in the intact cell, Biochem. Int. 2: 243 (1981).

17. V. Niggli, J. T. Penniston, and E. Carafoli, Purification of the $(Ca^{2+}-Mg^{2+})$-ATPase from human erythrocyte membrane using a calmodulin affinity column, J. Biol. Chem. 254: 9955 (1979).

18. P. Caroni, and E. Carafoli, The Ca^{2+}-pumping ATPase of heart sarcolemma, J. Biol. Chem. 256: 3263 (1981).

19. R. Kaser-Glanzmann, M. Jakabova, J. N. George, and E. F. Luscher, Stimulation of calcium uptake in platelet membrane vesicles by adenosine 3',5'-cyclic monophosphate and protein kinase, Biochim.Biophys.Acta.466:429(1977).

20. R. Kaser-Glanzmann, E. Gerber, and E. F. Luscher, Regulation of the intracellular calcium level in human blood platelets: cyclic adenosine 3',5'-monophosphate dependent phosphorylation of a 22,000 dalton component in isolated Ca^{2+}-accumulating vesicles, Biochim. Biophys. Acta. 558: 344 (1979).

21. G. M. Dolson, M. K. Hise, and E. J. Weinman, Relationship among parathyroid hormone, cAMP, and calcium on proximal tubule sodium transport, Am. J. Physiol. 249: F409 (1985)

ENHANCEMENT OF THE STIMULATORY EFFECT OF

Ca^{++} ON ALDOSTERONE SECRETION BY PTH

Klaus Olgaard, Henrik Daugaard, and Martin Egfjord
Technical assistance: Vibeke Pless and Merete Holm

Medical Department P, Division of Nephrology
Rigshospitalet, Copenhagen
Denmark

ABSTRACT

In previous clinical investigations we found a stimulatory effect of the presence of hyperparathyroidism on the Ca^{++} induced secretion of aldosterone and vasopressin. The present investigation, therefore, examined the possible effect of PTH on the Ca^{++} mediated aldosterone secretion from purified rat zona glomerulosa cells.

Ca^{++} was added to the preparations from 0.5 to 2.0 mM and PTH 1-84 or 1-34 were added at concentrations from 10^{-7} to 10^{-10} M. The cells were then incubated for 120 min and aldosterone measured in the supernatant. The aldosterone response to Ca^{++} stimulation (without PTH added) served as baseline controls, while cell preparations with ACTH 10^{-6} M added secured the viability and responsiveness of the cells. In all cell preparations with PTH (1-84 as well as 1-34) added the aldosterone responses to a certain Ca^{++} concentration increased by up to 200 per cent above baseline values.

It is suggested that PTH may act as a Ca^{++} ionophore on endocrine systems which are not normally related to PTH and thus enhance the calcium stimulated secretion. It is further suggested that this phenomenon may take place in uremia during the state of secondary hyperparathyroidism (HPT).

INTRODUCTION

A significant effect of calcium has previously been demonstrated in our laboratory on the aldosterone and vasopressin secretion (1, 2) in patients on chronic dialysis. However, a similar calcium stimulus to normal subjects did not affect aldosterone or vasopressin secretion. In patients with normal kidney function and secondary HPT a calcium infusion resulted in a significant increase of the aldosterone and vasopressin levels in plasma, while no change was seen during or following calcium infusion after normalization of the secondary HPT. Thus, indirect evidence was provided for an effect of PTH on

the stimulatory effect of calcium on hormone secretion from
endocrine systems, which are not normally considered to be
influenced by PTH. As such a possible effect of PTH might be
of importance to our understanding of some of the endocrine
disturbancies which take place in uremia, the present investigation examined the possible effect of PTH 1-84 and 1-34 on
the calcium stimulated aldosterone secretion from isolated zona
glomerulosa cells obtained from the rat.

EXPERIMENTAL DESIGN

All experiments were performed in triplicates with 10^5
zona glomerulosa cells (obtained according to a modification
of the method described by Fakunding et al. (3)) in each vial
during an incubation period of 2 hours under 95% O_2 and 5% CO_2.
As the PTH 1-84 and 1-34 (kindly supplied by Jerry Morrisey,
Ph.D., Washington University, St. Louis) added was dissolved
in 8M urea, control experiments were performed with different
molar concentrations of urea, but no hormone added.

To secure the viability and the responsiveness of the aldosterone secretion from the zona glomerulosa cells, experiments were performed with ACTH 1-24 added to the medium at 10^{-8}
to 10^{-4}M. Similar experiments were performed with the ionophore
A 23187 added from 10^{-8} to 10^{-4}M.

After a pilot study to find the appropriate conc. of PTH,
a final protocol was chosen with b-PTH 1-84 added from 10^{-10}
to 10^{-7}M. All experiments were performed at three different
calcium conc. in the medium (0.5; 1.0; 2.0 mM Ca^{++}). In each
experiment the basal non-hormonal stimulated aldosterone secretion was measured and the response to ACTH stimulation (10^{-6}M)
used as a "positive control". Similar experiments were performed with b-PTH 1-34 added to the medium. After 2 hours of incubation and centrifugation the supernatant was aspirated and
kept at -20° C until the aldosterone measurements were performed. All supernatants from one single experiment were measured
in the same assay.

The secretion of aldosterone was measured by a modification of a previously published method (4). The aldosterone antiserum (SB-ALDO-H) had in our laboratory a high specificity
with no crossreaction to cortisone, cortisol or corticosterone.
Intra-assay variation was 9% and inter-assay variation was 11%.
The sensivity was 10 pg/ml.

RESULTS

The basal aldosterone secretion was stable and not influenced by the concentration of urea in the medium.

Response to ACTH 1-24

Basal aldosterone concentration was 1100 pg/10^5 cells and
at a concentration of 10^{-6}M ACTH 1-24 aldosterone increased
more than 10 times (Figure 1). The aldosterone response to ACTH
1-24 10^{-6}M was used as an indication of the responsiveness of
the zona glomerulosa cells in order to compare responses of
different cell populations with different non-stimulated basal
aldosterone levels.

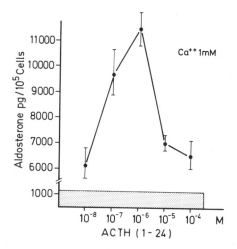

Fig. 1.   The aldosterone response per lo^5 zona glomerulosa
cells to two hours of incubation in the presence
of ACTH 1-24 in different molar concentrations.
The hatched bar at the bottom indicates the basal
non-stimulated aldosterone levels. Ca^{++} concentration of the medium 1 mM.
Mean $\pm$ SEM.   N = 4 sets of triplicates.

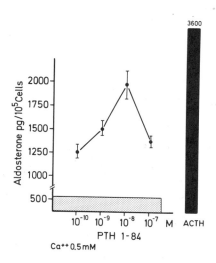

Fig. 2.   The aldosterone response per lo^5 zona glomerulosa
cells to two hours of incubation in the presence
of a Ca^{++} concentration of 0.5 mM and b-PTH 1-84
at concentrations from 10^{-10}M to 10^{-7}M. The hatched
bar at the bottom indicates the basal non-stimulated aldosterone levels, while the block bar to the
right demonstrates the aldosterone response to two
hours of incubation in the presence of ACTH 1-25
lo^{-6}M.
Mean $\pm$ SEM.   N = 7 sets of triplicates.

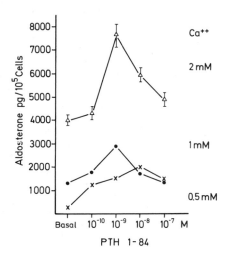

Fig. 3.   The aldosterone response per lo^5 zona glomerulosa
cells to two hours of incubation in the presence
of different calcium concentrations in the medium
(0.5; 1,0; 2.0 mM) and different concentrations of
b-PTH 1-84 (10^{-10}M to 10^{-7}M). The upper curve shows
means ± SEM of 4 sets of triplicates, while the two
curves at the bottom illustrate representative experiments (means of triplicates).

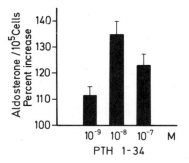

Fig. 4.   The percentage increase above basal levels of aldosterone per lo^5 zona glomerulosa cells in response
to two hours of incubation in the presence of b-PTH
1-34 at three different molar concentrations.
Mean ± SEM.   N = 7 sets of triplicates.

Response to A 23187

The aldosterone response to 1 mM Ca^{++} was tested with the ionophore A 23187 added at $10^{-8}M$ to $10^{-4}M$. Basal aldosterone levels were 1100 pg/10^5 cells and a significant increase to more than 2500 pg/lo^5 cells ($p < 0.01$) was found with A 23187 added from $10^{-7}M$ to $10^{-6}M$.

Response to b-PTH 1-84

Figure 2 demonstrates that the aldosterone response to 0.5 mM Ca^{++} increased from 600 pg to 1950 pg/10^5 cells when b-PTH 1-84 $lo^{-8}M$ was added to the medium. A significant increase of the aldosterone concentration was seen at PTH concentrations from $10^{-10}M$ to $10^{-7}M$.

The effect of PTH on the calcium stimulated aldosterone secretion did depend upon the calcium concentration in the medium, as shown in Figure 3, where all concentrations of PTH ($10^{-10}M$ to $10^{-7}M$) increased the aldosterone response above basal levels.

Response to b-PTH 1-34

Figure 4 demonstrates the effect of b-PTH 1-34 $10^{-9}M$ to $10^{-7}M$. The response is given as percentage increase above basal aldosterone levels. A clear increase was seen after b-PTH 1-34 $10^{-8}M$ and $10^{-7}M$.

COMMENTS

The present investigation demonstrates that zona glomerulosa cells at a given calcium concentration increased the aldosterone concentration in the medium when b-PTH 1-84 as well as 1-34 were added. This is in clear agreement with our previous clinical results (1, 2) and may suggest that some of the endocrine disturbances, which are described in patients with secondary hyperparathyroidism - mainly uremic patients - might be due to the high circulating levels of PTH. This would be in accordance with the many investigations demonstrating that PTH might be "one of the uremic toxins" (5-lo).

ACKNOWLEDGEMENTS

The present investigation was kindly supported by grants from The Danish Medical Research Council.

REFERENCES

1. K. Olgaard, S. Madsen, M. Hammer, and J. Ladefoged, Calcium dependent aldosterone secretion in anephric and non-nephrectomized patients on regular hemodialysis, J. Clin. Endocrin. Metab. 46:74o (1978).
2. M. Hammer, J. Ladefoged, S. Madsen, K. Olgaard, and E. Tvedegaard, Calcium stimulated vasopressin secretion in uremic patients. An effect mediated via PTH? J. Clin. Endocrin. Metab. 51:lo78 (198o).

3. J. L. Fakunding, R. Chow, and K. J. Catt, The role of calcium in the stimulation of aldosterone production by adrenocorticotropin, angiotensin II, and potassium in isolated glomerulosa cells, Endocrinology lo5:327 (1979).

4. K. Olgaard, Plasma aldosterone by radioimmunoassay determination in normal man and in patients on maintenance haemodialysis, Scand. J. Clin. Lab. Invest. 35:31 (1975).

5. S. G. Massry and D. A. Goldstein, Role of parathyroid hormone in uremic toxicity, Kidney Int. 13 (Suppl. 8):39 (1978).

6. M. M. Avram, D. A. Feinfeld, and A. H. Huatuco, Search for the uremic toxin, New Engl. J. Med. 298:looo (1978).

7. D. A. Goldstein and S. G. Massry, Effect of parathyroid hormone administration and its withdrawal on brain calcium and electroencephalogram, Mineral Electrolyte Metab. 1:84 (1978).

8. E. Bogin, S. G. Massry, J. Levi, M. Djaldeti, G. Bristol, and J. Smith, Effect of parathyroid hormone on osmotic fragility of human erythrocytes, J. Clin. Invest. 69:lol7 (1982).

9. K. Olgaard, M. Arbelaez, J. Schwartz, S. Klahr, and E. Slatopolsky, Abnormal skeletal response to parathyroid hormone in dogs with chronic uremia. Calcif. Tissue Int. 34:4o3 (1982).

lo. K. Olgaard, J. Schwartz, D. Finco, M. Arbelaez, A. Korkor, K. Martin, S. Klahr, and E. Slatopolsky, Extraction of parathyroid hormone and release of adenosine 3',5'-monophosphate by isolated perfused bones obtained from dogs with acute uremia, Endocrinology 111:1678 (1982).

ROLE OF HYPERPARATHYROIDISM IN HORMONAL DISORDERS OF

PATIENTS WITH CHRONIC RENAL INSUFFICIENCY

K. Lindenau, K. Vetter, J. Pfitzner, L. Meyer
I. Kaschube, W. Dutz, F. Kokot, and P.T. Fröhling

District Hospital, Research Clinic of Nutrition
St. Josefs Hospital, Potsdam, GDR
Silesian School of Medicine, Katowice, Poland

Introduction

Endocrine disorders are a typical feature in chronic renal
failure. The consequences of these disorders are several
clinical syndromes such as renal osteodystrophy, hypogonadism,
renal anaemia, disturbances of the central and peripheral
nervous system and disturbed carbohydrate-, protein- and
lipid metabolism. Optimum nutritional treatment (i.e. low
protein diet supplemented with a keto acid - amino acid mixture) can reduce the hyperparathyroidism in the pre-dialysis
period. This phenomenon was reported independently by the
Pisa-Group (1) and ourselves (2). Dialysis treatment can
replace all excretorial renal function, but the effect on the
hormonal derangements remained questionable. After kidney
transplantation three types of hormonal disturbances were
described (3):
  1. inherited from uremia,
  2. steroid induced,
  3. graft function related.
This paper aims at investigating the behaviour of PTH and
its relation to other endocrine disorders under different
kinds of renal replacement therapy.

Patients and methods

Composition of the patient groups and the characteristics
of special treatment are given in Table I.

Tab. I Patient characteristics

	AGE (years)	SEX ♂	SEX ♀	DIA-GNOSIS	DURATION OF TREATMENT (months)	CREATININE (μmol/l)	PROTEIN INTAKE (g/kgb.w.)	CHARACTERISTICS OF SPECIAL TREATMENT
ONT n=109	49.1 ±12.1	59	50	GN 24 PN 60 OTHERS 25	28.0 (6-84)	950 ± 233	0.4 g/kg b.w. per day	AMINO ACID/KETO ACID SUBSTITUTED DIET. PART OF THEM RECEIVED VIT. D_2
RDT n=127	42.2 ±11.6	61	66	GN 40 PN 48 OTHERS 39	36.0 (2-120)	1115 ± 242	~1.2 g/kg b.w. per day	15 h DIAL./WEEK HOLLOW FIBRE DIALYZER Q_b 150-200 ml/min Q_d 500 ml/min PART REC. VIT D_2
KT n=42	37.0 ± 6.0	20	22	GN 24 PN 12 OTHERS 06	RDT 19.4 (2-62) TRANSPLAN. 58.7 (12-158)	189 ± 145	1.0 g/kg b.w. per day	IMMUNOSUPPRES-SION: AZATHIOPRIN~75-150mg CORTICOID 75-20mg CYCLOSPORIN ∅ PART REC. VIT. D_2

ONT = OPTMUM NUTRITIONAL TREATMENT ; RDT = REGUL. DIALYSIS TREATMENT
KT = KIDNEY TRANSPLANTATION

Under optimum nutritional treatment (ONT), (i.e. mixed low protein diet substituted with an amino acid - keto acid mixture) the analysis of the hormonal spectrum was carried out in 109 patients. In 30 cases a direct comparison of hormonal levels was performed before and 2 weeks after adding ketoanalogues under clinical balance conditions. Patients under regular dialysis treatment (RDT) were treated with conventional hemodialysis three times a week for about 15 hours with a hollow fibre dialyser with an average duration of 36 months. High protein intake was ordered but the real protein intake was about 1.2 g / kg body weight per day. After kidney transplantation all patients were on long-term successful treatment (at least 12 months), and most of them developed only mild renal insufficiency. The immunosuppression therapy was based on Azathioprin and small doses of corticosteroids.
In all three groups part of the patients were treated with vitamin D_2.
The determination of PTH (including the total hormone resp. its N-terminal fraction), 25-OH-D, calcitonin (CT), prolactin (PRL), human growth hormone (HGH), insulin (IRI), gastrin (GA), and testosterone (TE) were carried out by radioimmunological methods. The estimation of the other parameters was carried out by standard methods. The data were given as median values, the statistical analysis was performed by the MANN- WHITNEY - U - test.

Results and discussion

Table II gives the normal range and the results (given as median values) of the hormonal analysis of patients under different kinds of renal replacement therapy in comparison with a group of untreated uremics.

Tab. II Hormonal analysis of patients under different kinds of renal replacement therapy

	CREAT. μmol/l	PTH ng/ml	CT pg/ml	TE ng/ml	PRL ng/ml	GA pg/ml	IRI μu/l	HGH ng/ml
NORMAL RANGE	71-106	<0.6	94.0 ± 7.9	4.0-7.0	<5.0	50.0 ± 5.4	15.0 ± 5.0	7.0
UNTREATED CONTROLS n=20	835	4.35	228	2.35	42.8	144.0	23.2	15.5
ONT n=109	916	0.70	345	5.10	23.0	60.0	20.0	8.3
RDT n=127	1,116	2.53	450	2.30	39.5	131.0	25.5	10.7
KT n=42	131	1.28	515	3.90	9.0	80.0	29.0	9.0

ONT-OPTIMUM NUTRITIONAL TREATMENT;
RDT-REG.DIALYSIS TREATMENT, KT–KIDNEY TRANSPLANTATION

The untreated controls show the typical constellation of uremics – excessive hyperparathyroidism, hyperprolactinaemia, hypergastrinaemia, slightly increased levels of CT, IRI and HGH, and decreased TE levels in male patients. Patients under ONT revealed well controlled hyperparathyroidism; testosterone levels into the normal range; HGH, IRI and gastrin are only slightly increased. PTH levels are significantly lower compared with those of patients on RDT. Hyperparathyroidism persists in many patients after kidney transplantation in spite of the relatively good renal function.

Hyperinsulinaemia was found in most patients of all three groups but the levels were significantly higher in patients on dialysis treatment. Human growth hormone was slightly increased in all three groups. Prolactin showed a highly significant tendency towards normalization in transplanted patients. No difference in hyperprolactinaemia was found in patients under ONT and on RDT.

Gastrin levels were elevated independently of the kind of treatment, but less increased in ONT treated patients. Testosterone was significantly decreased in male patients on RDT.

We can see that dialysis treatment can not improve the hormonal disorders in endstage renal failure. Most endocrine disturbances are less pronounced under optimum nutritional treatment. Surprisingly many endocrine disorders persist in spite of successful kidney transplantation.

Because of the important role of PTH as uremic toxin we looked for the relation between BTH and the other investigated hormones under the different kinds of renal replacement therapy.

Tab. III   Behaviour of hormonal status in relation of different stages of HPT in patients under ONT

	n	CREAT, µmol/l	PTH ng/ml	CT pg/ml	HGH ng/ml	GA pg/ml	PRL ng/ml	IRI µU/l	TE ng/ml
ONT PTH< 0.7	53	916	0.4	390	7.5	60.0	23.0	19.0	5.90
PTH 0.7–2.4	50	893	1.34	372	8.8	59.0	23.1	19.2	7.06
PTH >2.4	06	1,123	3.40	265	9.6	34.0	35.0	26.0	2.20

＊ $p < 0.05$

Markedly increased PTH levels were not frequently found under ONT.
Insulin and HGH behaviour were independent of PTH. The contraregulary increase of calcitonin to severe hyperparathyroidism was insufficient, also in other patient groups. In contrast to the groups mentioned, patients under ONT did not reveal an increase of the gastrin levels depending on the markedly elevated PTH levels. This can be interpreted as a special effect of keto acid administration in these patients.
Hyperparathyroidism can aggravate the hypogonadism in male patients. These results confirm the hypothesis by MASSRY about the role of PTH in the development of hypogonadism (4).

Tab. IV   Behaviour of hormonal status in relation of different stages of HPT in patients on RDT

	n	CREAT. µmol/l	PTH ng/ml	CT pg/ml	HGH ng/ml	GA pg/ml	PRL ng/ml	IRI µU/l	TE ng/ml
RDT PTH<0.7	06	1,189	0.45	750	8.75	196.3	6.5	114.0	3.25
PTH 0.7 – 2.4	63	1,122	1.80	390	12.75	122.8	33.6	30.0	2.10
PTH >2.4	58	1,202	3.30	350	10.00	195.7	55.5	22.0	2.25

＊ $p < 0.05$

Most of the patients on hemodialysis revealed markedly
elevated PTH levels. The contraregulatory increase of calcitonin in response to hyperparathyroidism was insufficient, too.
Levels of HGH and gastrin were increased independently of the
stage of hyperparathyroidism, but prolactin was found increased depending on the stage of elevated PTH levels, and
the testosterone levels were lower in male patients on RDT
with hyperparathyroidism.

Tab. V Behaviour of hormonal status in relation of different
stages of HPT in patients after KT

	n	CREAT. μmol/l	PTH ng/ml	CT pg/ml	HGH ng/ml	GA pg/ml	PRL ng/ml	IRI μU/l	TE ng/ml
KT PTH<0.7	06	123	0.53	720	14.8	68.0	9.0	33.7	4.65
PTH 0.7–2.4	30	179	1.33	711	7.9	93.0	9.0	31.9	4.47
PTH >2.4	06	307	5.28	520	8.0	164.0	19.6	25.5	3.63

＊ $p < 0.05$

After kidney transplantation the excretory function of
kidneys went back to normal, but some of the endocrine parameters persisted in pathological ranges.
PTH levels were found elevated in most of the patients. The
adequate response of calcitonin to hyperparathyroidism was
missing, and testosterone was decreased in male patients
with elevated PTH levels.
The elevation of gastrin was more pronounced in the group
of patients with marked increased PTH levels, the elevation
of insulin was independent of PTH corresponding the behaviour of insulin in patients on RDT.
Increased PTH levels generally lead to higher release of
prolactin. In transplantated patients the prolactin levels
were normalized if hyperparathyroidism was well controlled,
but corresponding to the behaviour in the other groups a
higher release of prolactin was observed if PTH levels were
markedly increased.

In the light of our results we can make the following
conclusion:

- Optimum nutritional treatment can control hyperparathyroidism and prevent hypogonadism in the majority of the
patients.

- Patients on hemodialysis continued suffering from endocrine disorders.

- After kidney transplantation prolactin takes a significant tendency towards normalization but hyperinsulinaemia, hypergastrinaemia and increased calcitonin levels are common findings. Hyperparathyroidism persists in many cases and can be followed by hypogonadism in male patients.

- Hyperparathyroidism plays a key role in hormonal disorders of chronic renal failure.

References

1. G. Barsotti; E. Morelli; A. Guiducci; F. Ciardella; A. Giannoni; S. Lupetti; S. Giovannetti: Reversal of hyperparathyroidism in severe uremics following very low-protein and low-phosphorus diet. Nephron 30 : 310 (1982)

2. P. T. Fröhling; F. Kokot; R. Schmicker; K. Lindenau; I. Kaschube; K. Vetter: Influence of ketoacids on serum parathyroid hormone levels in patients with chronic renal failure. Clin. Nephrol. 20 : 212 (1983)

3. V. Bonomini; C. Campieri; C. Feletti; G. Orsoni; A. Vangelista: Hormonal abnormalities in renal transplantation: in Contr. Nephrol. vol. 49, p. 70 (Karger Basel 1985)

4. S. G. Massry; D. A. Goldstein; W. R. Procci; O. A.Kletzky: Impotence in patients with uremia: a possible role for parathyroid hormone. Nephron 19 : 305 (1977)

5. G. Barsotti; F. Ciardella; E. Morelli; P. Fioretti: Restoration of blood levels of testosterone in male uremics following a low protein diet supplemented with essential amino acids and keto-analogues: in Contr. Nephrol. vol. 49, p. 63 (Karger Basel 1985)

ROLE OF PTH IN THE PROGRESSION OF CHRONIC RENAL FAILURE

P.T. Fröhling, F. Kokot, K. Vetter, F. Krupki
and K. Lindenau

St. Josefs-Hospital, Research Clinic of Nutrition
District Hospital, Potsdam, GDR, Dept. of Nephrol.
Sil. School of Medicine, Katowice, Poland

Progression in chronic renal failure is a multifactorial
process. The different causes which accelerate the progression rate are summarized in Table I.

Tab. I

Cause of progression in chronic renal failure

1. Activity of the underlying renal disease
2. Hyperfiltration
3. Uremic toxins
4. Catabolism
5. Others
    a) exogenous toxins
    b) hypertension
    c) Acidosis
    d) salt and water depletion
    e) hyperuricaemia
    f) hypercalcaemia
    g) hyperparathyroidism

The underlying renal disease plays an important role for the
progression in the early and moderate stages of renal insufficiency. The rate of the progression was described as significantly higher in patients with glomerulonephritis (1). In
patients with GFR lower than 10 ml/min no differences of the
progression were found between patients with glomerulonephritis, pyelonephritis and polycystic diseases. Only the activity of the underlying disease can modify the rate of the progression. In recent years hyperfiltration has been discussed
as the main cause for the progression and was convincingly
demonstrated in animal experiments (2, 3). The evaluation of
the other factors is quite different in the opinion of the
experts (4). Hypertension was reported as a main cause for

New Actions of Parathyroid Hormone
Edited by S. G. Massry and T. Fujita
Plenum Press, New York

the progression by Alvestrand et al (5). Following our own experience we are convinced that hypertension is overrated in its importance for progression especially in advanced renal failure (6). Hyperparathyroidism is responsible for many syndromes in uremia (7-9), but its influence on the progression rate in patients with renal failure has not been sufficiently investigated. In an earlier retrospective study of 100 uremics we found the greatest retardation of the progression in patients with the best control of hyperparathyroidism and vice versa. These data are given in Table II.

Tab. II Relation between PTH and progression
(Given as median values of slopes
1/Creatinine over time)

PTH [ng/ml]	n	SLOPE
> 1.5	30	0.007
PTH [ng/ml] 0.9 - 1.5	35	0.004
PTH [ng/ml] < 0.9	35	0.002

$*$ $p < 0.05$

The rate of the progression was expressed as the slope of the reciprocal of creatinine. According to the same method we compared patients with and without keto acid supplementation to their low protein diet with regard to their progression rate behaviour (10). The superiority of keto acid supplementation was revealed in this investigation, and the

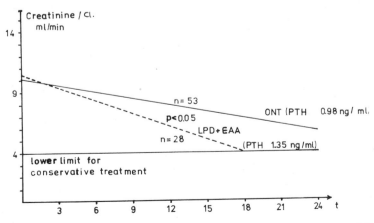

Fig. 1 Slope of Cl. creatinine depending on different kinds of treatment

PTH-levels were significantly lower in this group. This result was confirmed in a preliminary prospective study based on the comparison of the slope of creatinine-clearance.

Figure 1 shows significant differences in the slope of creatinine-clearance and also in the mean values of PTH in patients who were treated with EAA resp. KA as supplementation to a low protein diet. The effect of keto acids on PTH-levels in uremic patients was described independently by us and others (11 - 13). The change of some biochemical parameters before and after keto acid administration is represented in Table III.

Tab. III   Biochemical parameters before and after keto acid administration (paired t-test)

	n	CREATININE μmol/l	BUN mmol/l	CALCIUM mmol/l	INORGAN. PHOSPHATE SERUM mmol/l	PTH ng/ml	1.25(OH)$_2$D$_3$ pmol/l
BEFORE KA-TREATMENT	30	813 ± 221	30.3 ±8.9	2.3 ±0.3	1.74 ±0.56 *	1.71 ±0.79 *	25.1 ± 13.7 (n=12)
2 WEEKS AFTER KA-TREATMENT	30	804 ±212	26.0 ±8.8	2.3 ±0.3	1.42 ±0.36	0.84 ±0.50	30.2 ± 11.8 (n=12)

$* = p < 0.05$

It can be seen that under clinical balance conditions (with unchanged dietary treatment) a marked decrease of PTH and inorganic phosphorus was observed two weeks after the administration of keto acids. 1.25 (OH)$_2$D takes a slight but significant increase. Creatinine and calcium do not change. This is the biochemical background of the significantly greater influence of a keto acid substituted diet on the progression.

To reveal the exact role of PTH in the progression of chronic renal failure an analysis of the relation between PTH and the slope of creatinine-clearance was performed in a current prospective study about the effect of amino acid resp. keto acid substituted low protein diets on the progression.

Patients and methods

106 patients with advanced chronic renal failure (GFR lower than 15 ml/min) were treated with a low protein diet (protein intake 0.4 g/kg; energy intake at least 35 kcal/kg) supplemented with essential amino acids (EAA) resp. their ketoanalogues (KA) between 6 and 69 months. The distribution of the patient groups is given in Table IV.

Tab. IV   Characteristics of patient groups

	n=	DIAGNOSIS		SEX		AGE YEARS	DURATION OF TREATMENT MONTHS	INITIAL CREATININE μmol/l
				F	M			
KA	66	GN PN CD	14 40 12	32	34	46.3 (19-77)	14.9 (6-69)	725
EAA	36	GN PN CD	09 18 09	20	16	49.4 (20-69)	12.1 (6-36)	601

The total intake of calcium, phosphorus, sodium, potassium, protein and energy did not differ between the two groups. The composition of the keto acid mixtures which were used is depicted in Table V.

Tab. V   Composition of keto-acid mixtures

	KETOSTERIL[R]	ULTRAMIN[R]
Keto-Val	1.29	2.00
Keto-Leu	1.52	1.94
Keto-Ile	1.01	1.55
Keto-Phe	1.02	1.01
Hydroxy-Meth	0.89	1.06
Threo	0.80	0.34
Lys	1.13	0.45
Trypt	0.35	0.17
Hist	0.57	0.27
Ty	0.45	-

PTH was estimated every three months by radioimmunoassay which includes intact PTH and N-terminal fragments. Creatinine-clearance, too, was determined under clinical balance conditions every three months over a 24 hour period. Under out-patient-conditions the creatinine-clearance was carried out every 4 weeks. The progression rate was calculated as the slope of creatinine-clearance over 3 months (per trimenon). For the analysis of the relation between PTH and the progression the data were divided into three groups (PTH lower than 1.0 ng/ml, 1.0 - 2.4 ng/ml and more than 2.4 ng/ml). All data are given as median values and the

statistical analysis was performed by MANN-WHITNEY U-test.
An analysis between the correlation of PTH and the slope
of creatinine-clearance was also carried out.

Results

A total of 102 patients were observed over 471 trimenons.
Table VI gives the division into the three groups according
to their PTH -levels and the median values of the slope of
clearance creatinine and PTH.

Tab. VI   Results of slope of Cl. creatinine and PTH distri-
          buted to the different underlying diseases

	n =	OBSERVATION PERIOD TOTAL NUMB. OF TRIMEN.	MEAN PTH-LEVEL ng/ml	NUMBER OF TRIMENON ACCORDING TO PTH LEVELS (ng/ml)			SLOPE OF Cl/Creatinine per TRIMENON
				< 1.0	1.0-2.4	> 2.4	
TOTAL	102	471	1.07	263	165	43	0.93
GN	23	81	1.38	37	34	10	1.18
PN	58	319	1.03	185	110	24	0.91
CN	21	71	0.92	41	21	09	0.74

It can be seen that in 50 % of the patients hyperparathyroidism was well controlled a marked elevation of PTH was found
only in 9 %. Hyperparathyroid situations were more pronounced
in patients with glomerulonephritis (13 % showed uncontrolled
and only 45 % well controlled hyperparathyroidism). The rate
of progression was, as a rule, relatively lower (0.93 per
trimenon resp. 0.31 per month) and was expectedly slightly
higher in glomerulonephritic patients. An analysis of the
control of hyperparathyroidism depending from the kind of
treatment is shown in Table VII.

In about 60 % of the observed trimenons in the KA group the
hyperparathyroidism was well controlled, but this was only
the case in 48 % of the EAA group. On the other hand, only
in 6 % of the KA treated patients PTH was markedly increased,
whereas the amount was 15 % in the EAA group. Patients
without any nutritional treatment showed a marked increase
of PTH in more than 50 % in this stage of renal insufficiency. The relation between PTH and the slope of clearance
creatinine is depicted in Fig. 2.

Patients with well controlled hyperparathyroidism showed a
very low slope, and the group with markedly increased PTH
levels had the significantly highest rate of progression.
The same relation was found if we only took the patients
with glomerulonephritis into consideration.

Tab. VII Distribution of the PTH-groups under different kind of treatment

	NUMBER OF PAT.	NUMBER OF TRIMENON	PTH (ng / ml)		
			< 1.0	1.0 - 2.4	> 2.4
KA	66	326	193 (59.2%)	112 (34.4%)	21 (6.4%)
EAA	36	145	70 (48.2%)	53 (36.6%)	22 (15.2%)

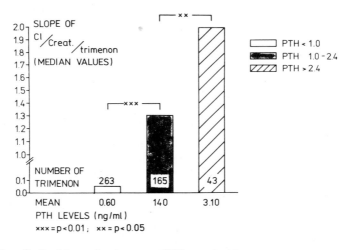

Fig. 2 Relation between PTH and the progression rate (total group, n = 471)

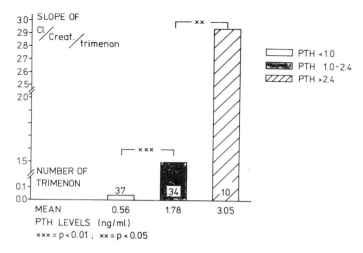

Fig. 3   Relation between PTH and the progression rate in
          patients with GN (n = 81)

The dominant influence of well controlled hyperparathyroidism
on the progression was independent of the underlying disease.
The difference of the progression rate between patients with
markedly and moderately increased PTH was less pronounced in
patients with interstitial nephritis and was not significant
for patients with polycystic diseases.

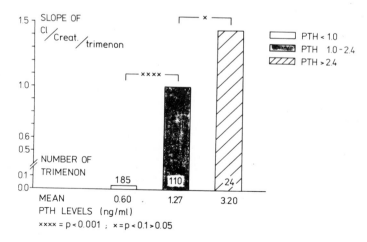

Fig. 4   Relation between PTH and the progression rate in
          patients with pyelonephritis (n = 319)

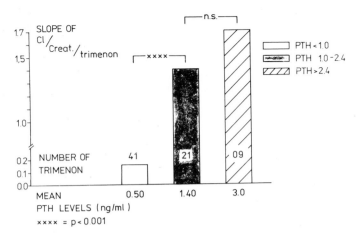

Fig. 5 Relation between PTH and the progression rate in patients with polycystic disease (n = 71)

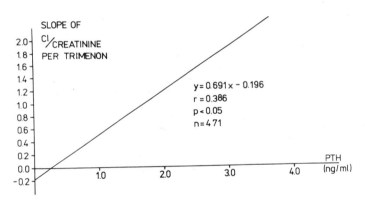

Fig. 6 Correlation between PTH and slope of Cl. creatinine

An analysis of the correlation is given in Fig. 6.

In spite of the relatively weak correlation quotient (r = 0.386) the relation is significant. This is quite clear as PTH is only one of many factors which influence the progression in renal failure. But we can conclude that this factor is very important. The correlation was more pronounced in patients with glomerulonephritis (r = 0.520) compared with the other underlying diseases (PN r = 0.329 and CK r = 0.318). The influence of the kind of treatment on the progression is represented in Fig. 7.

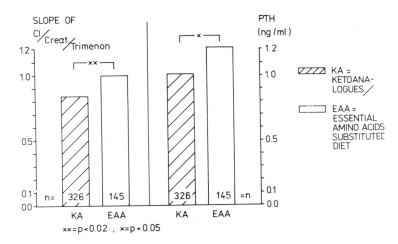

Fig. 7   Progression rate and PTH depending on the kind
         of treatment

Under keto acid treatment the slope of clearance creatinine
as well as PTH levels were significantly lower in comparison
with the results of the EAA group. This result confirms
earlier data by our own group (10) which are in good agreement with Mitch (14) and Barsotti et al (15) in stating that
keto acid supplement low protein diets have a much better
effect on the delaying of the progression as compared with
other forms of nutritional treatment in the predialysis
period. These data give the evidence that the PTH lowering
effect of keto acids is responsible for the superiority of
keto acid treatment with regard to the progression. How can
the effect of PTH on the progression be explained?

Tab. VIII

Possible mechanisms of the influence of PTH on progression
in renal failure

1. Increasing concentration of calcium in the kidney

   a) direct effect
   b) by rising of calcium phosphorus product

2. Increase of other "toxic products" (middle molecules)
   in blood.

3. Stimulation of protein catabolism.

The attempt of an explanation is given in Table VIII. It is well known that the calcium content of chronic uremic patients is much higher compared with the calcium content of kidneys with normal renal function. The enhancement is proved of intracellular calcium concentration by higher PTH-levels. Some years ago, together with Dzurik (9), we described a positive correlation between middle molecular fraction 2 (according to peak 7 by Fürst) and PTH. Probably also other potentially "nephrotoxic" compounds are more increased in the hyperparathyroid stage. The argumentation of protein catabolism as a consequence of higher PTH-levels was stressed by Massry (8) and is in a full agreement with our clinical and scientific experience over the last years.

Regardless of the mechanism the control of hyperparathyroidism is an important factor for the delay of the progression in chronic renal failure.

Conclusions

1. PTH is not only an important factor in uremic toxicity and for the development of renal osteodystrophy - it is also involved in the pathogenesis of the progression in chronic renal failure.

2. Protein restriction supplemented with keto acids (socalled optimum nutritional treatment, ONT) is the safest way of treating hyperparathyroidism in patients with moderately and advanced chronic renal insufficiency.

References

1. N. Gretz, E. Korb, M. Strauch: Low protein diets supplemented by keto acids in chronic renal failure: A prospective controlled study; Kidney International 24, Suppl. 16 : 263 (1983)

2. B. M. Brenner, T. W. Meyer, Th. H. Hostetter: Dietary protein intake and the progressive nature of kidney disease; New Eng. J. Med. 307: 652 (1982)

3. B. M. Brenner, T. W. Meyer: Mechanism of progression of renal disease, in "Nephrology II" R. R. Robinson ed., Springer, New York - Berlin - Heidelberg - Tokyo (1984)

4. W. E. Mitch: The progressive nature of renal disease; Churchil Livingstone, New York - Edinburgh - London - Melbourne (1986)

5. A. Alvestrand, P. Stenvinkel, J. Bergström: Factors influencing the progression rate of chronic renal failure. Xth Intern. Congress of Nephrol. London (1987) Abstr. p. 35

6. K. Lindenau, K. Vetter, F. Krupki, H. Sperschneider, P.T. Fröhling: Role of hypertension in the progression of chronic renal failure; Scand. J. Nephrol. (in press)

7. S. G. Massry: Is parathyroid hormone an uremic toxin? Nephron 19: 125 (1977)

8. S. G. Massry: Current status of the role of parathyroid hormone in uremic toxicity; Cont. Nephrol. 49: 1 (1985)

9. P. T. Fröhling, F. Kokot, P. Cernacek, K. Vetter, J. Kuska, V. Spustova, I. Kaschube, R. Dzurik: Relation between middle molecule and parathyroid hormone in patients with chronic renal failure; Mineral Electrolyte Metabol. 7: 48 (1982)

0. P. T. Fröhling, R. Schmicker, F. Kokot, K. Vetter, I. Kaschube, K.-H. Götz, M. Jacopian, K. Lindenau: Influence of phosphate restriction, keto-acids and vitamin D on the progression of chronic renal failure; Proc. E.D.T.A. 21: 561 (1985)

1. G. Barsotti, E. Morelli, A. Guiducci, F. Ciardella, A. Giannoni, S. Lupetti, S. Giovannetti: Reversal of hyperparathyroidism in severe uremics following very low-protein and low-phosphorus diet; Nephron 30: 310 (1982)

2. P. T. Fröhling, F. Kokot, R. Schmicker, I. Kaschube, K. Lindenau, K. Vetter: Influence of keto-acids on serum parathyroid hormone levels in patients with chronic renal failure; Clin. Nephrol. 20: 212 (1983)

3. P. A. Lucas, R. C. Brown, J. S. Woodhead, G. A. Coles: 1,25-dihydroxycholecalciferol and parathyroid hormone in advanced chronic renal failure: effects of simultaneous protein and phosphorus restriction; Clin. Nephrol. 27: 7 (1986)

4. W. E. Mitch, M. Walser, T. I. Steinman, S. Hill, S. Zeger, K. Tungsanga: The effect of a keto acid-amino-acid supplement to a restricted diet on the progression of chronic renal failure; New Engl. J. Med. 311: 623 (1984)

15. G. Barsotti, A. Guiducci, F. Ciardella, S. Giovannetti: Effects on renal function of a low-nitrogen diet supplemented with essential amino acids and ketoanalogues and of hemodialysis an free protein supply in patients with chronic renal failure; Nephron 21: 113 (1981)

HUMAN PARATHYROID HORMONE INHIBITS RENAL 24,25-DIHYDROXYVITAMIN D₃ SYNTHESIS BY A MECHANISM INVOLVING ADENOSINE 3',5'-MONOPHOSPHATE IN RATS

Takashi Shigematsu, Yoshindo Kawaguchi, Yoosuke Ogura, Tatsuo Suda*, and Tadashi Miyahara

Second Division, Department of Internal Medicine, Jikei University School of Medicine, and Department of Biochemistry, School of Dentistry, Showa University*, Tokyo Japan

INTRODUCTION

It is well-known that parathyroid hormone [PTH] and vitamin D serve critical roles in divalent ion homeostasis through their actions on kidney and bone. On the other hand, renal production of two dihydroxy metabolites of 25-hydroxyvitamin D₃ [25(OH)D₃], 1,25-dihydroxyvitamin D₃ [1,25(OH)₂D₃] and 24,25-dihydroxyvitamin D₃ [24,25(OH)₂D₃], is tightly and reciprocally regulated by a number of factors. Of several factors involved in inducing renal 1,25(OH)₂D₃ production, the most important one is PTH physiologically. This hormone stimulates renal production of 1,25(OH)₂D₃ through a mechanism involving adenosine 3',5'-monophosphate [cAMP]. In contrast, 1,25(OH)₂D₃ is known to be the sole physiological factors in enhancing renal 24,25(OH)₂D₃ production. Whether PTH regulates renal 24,25(OH)₂D₃ production as an independent action besides its stimulatory effect on renal 1,25(OH)₂D₃ production is still not clear.

We examined the effect on 24,25(OH)₂D₃ production of PTH active fragment, human PTH(1-34), and cAMP continuously infused into thyroparathyroidectomized (TPTX) rats. Low doses of PTH and cAMP similarly inhibit 24,25(OH)₂D₃ production without enhancing 1,25(OH)₂D₃ production. This effects of PTH and cAMP determined by in vitro assay using kidney homogenates and an in vivo assay measuring the accumulation of tritiated metabolites in plasma after injection of 25(OH)[³H]D₃. We report here that besides its well-known action to stimulate 1,25(OH)₂D₃, PTH inhibits renal 24,25(OH)₂D₃ synthesis by a mechanism involving cAMP.

MATERIALS AND METHODS

Animals and Assays of 25(OH)[³H]D₃ Metabolism

Male weanling rats (Sprague-Dawley strain), weighing 50g, were given a synthetic vitamin D-deficient diet (0.47% Calcium and 0.30% phosphorus). After feeding for 7 weeks, they were either sham under anesthesia with ketamine chloride (100mg/kg BW, ip). The left femoral vein was cannulated with heparinized polyethylene tube. The animals were infused

New Actions of Parathyroid Hormone
Edited by S. G. Massry and T. Fujita
Plenum Press, New York

at a rate of 3ml/h via the cannulated vein with a nutrient solution composed of 5mM $CaCl_2$, 5mM $MgCl_2$, 20mM NaCl, 2.5mM KCl, and 4% dextrose throughout the experiment.

Five hours after the operation, TPTX rats were given iv graded amounts (1.25-125ng) of $1,25(OH)_2D_3$ dissolved in 25μl ethanol to induce $24,25(OH)_2D_3$ synthesis. The TPTX rats treated with 125ng $1,25(OH)_2D_3$ were constantly infused with synthetic human PTH(1-34)(25-800 pmol/h), cAMP(10-500 nmol/h), and/or theophylline(1.0μmol/h) for the last 20-hours.

Some of the vitamin D-deficient TPTX rats were injected with 0.5μCi $25(OH)$-$[26(27)$-methyl-$^3H]D_3$ in the in vivo assay of $25(OH)_2D_3$ metabolism. The animals were killed 5 hours later, and their blood was collected. Plasma (0.5ml) was extracted by the method of Bligh and Dyer [1]. The tritiated metabolites of $25(OH)[^3H]D_3$ appearing in the plasma were separated by HPLC and measured as described below.

On the other hand, rats were anesthesized with ether and completely exsanginated from the aorta with a syringe in the in vitro assay. After the perfusing with 50 ml calcium- and magnesium-free PBS. The kidneys were removed and placed in an ice-cold 15mM Tris-acetate buffer(pH 7.4) containing 0.19M sucrose, 2mM magnesium acetate, and 25mM sodium succinate. A 10%(wt/vol) kidney homogenate was prepared in the Tris-acetate buffer. 500 ng $25(OH)[^3H]D_3$(80000cpm) dissolved in 40μl ethanol were added to 3ml 10%(wt/vol) homogenates. Oxygen gas was flashed for 1 min into each flask on ice. Then, the homogenates were incubated at 37C for 20 min. The reaction was stopped by adding 10ml methanol/ chloroform (2:1,vol/vol). Extraction was performed by the method of Bligh and Dyer [1].

Identification of $25(OH)[^3H]D_3$ metabolites

Lipid extracts of plasma and kidney homogenate mixed with 100ng authentic $1,25(OH)_2D_3$ and $24,25(OH)_2D_3$ to identify the elution positions of respective metabolites and applied to a straight phase HPLC using a Finepak-SIL column (4.6mm$\times$25cm, JASCO,Tokyo, Japan). The column was eluted at a flow rate of 1.5ml/min using a mixed solvent of n-hexane-isopropanol-methanol(88:6:6, vol/vol). Forty 30-sec fractions were collected, and the radioactivity was counted with a liquid scintillation counter. For identification of $1,25(OH)_2D_3$ and $24,25(OH)_2D_3$, the putative $1,25(OH)_2D_3$ and $24,25(OH)_2D_3$ fractions from the straight phase HPLC were separately applied to a reverse phase HPLC using a μ-Bondapak C_{18} column (4.6mm$\times$25cm, Waters). The column was eluted at a flow rate of 1.5ml/min with a solvent of methanol-water (75:25, vol/vol), and fifty 30-sec fractions were collected. The resulting radioactive peaks were subjected to a periodate cleavage test and mass spectrometry. Production of $25(OH)[^3H]D_3$ metabolites the in vitro assay was expressed as nanograms per 3ml 10% (vol/vol) kidney homogenates in vitro. In the in vivo assay, accumulation of $25(OH)[^3H]D_3$ metabolites in plasma was calculated as picomoles per 100ml plasma.

Others. Plasma calcium concentration was measured with atomic absorption spectrophotometry. Plasma phosphorus was measured by modified Fiske-Subbarow's method. Statistical significance was determined by analysis of variance or Student's t test.

RESULT

A marked increase in $24,25(OH)_2D_3$ production occurred in TPTX rats treated with 125ng $1,25(OH)_2D_3$ in both assays, whereas the production remained within a very low level in rats treated with less than 12.5ng $1,25(OH)_2D_3$. $1,25(OH)_2D_3$ production did not change within a low level in

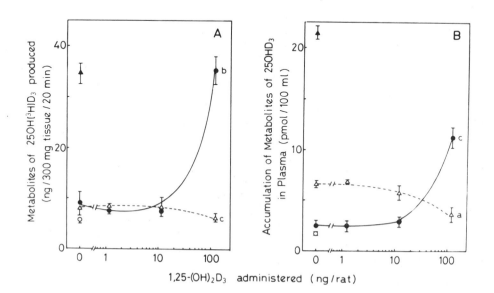

Figure 1

Effect of 1,25(OH)₂D₃(1.25-125ng) administration on 1,25-
(OH)₂D₃ and 24,25(OH)₂D₃ production in vitamin D deficient
TPTX rats into the in vitro(A) and in vivo(B) assays.
The productions of 1,25(OH)₂D₃ and 24,25(OH)₂D₃ in TPTX rats
is displayed with open triangle and closed circle, respectively. Closed triangle and open circle show the 1,25(OH)₂D₃
and 24,25(OH)₂D₃ production in sham-operated rats, respectively.
Value are means ± SEM.
  a   Significantly different from control, P<0.05
  b   Significantly different from control, P<0.01
  c   Significantly different from control, P<0.001

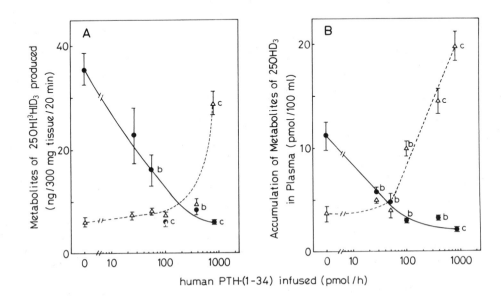

Figure 2

Dose-response effects of human PTH(1-34) [25-800pmol/h] on productions of 1,25(OH)₂D₃ and 24,25(OH)₂D₃ in TPTX rats treated with 125ng 1,25(OH)₂D₃ into the in vitro(A) and in vivo(B) assays. The open triangle shows the 1,25(OH)₂D₃ production. The 24,25(OH)₂D₃ production is shown with the closed circle.

Value are means ± SEM.

- [a] Significantly different from control, $P < 0.05$
- [b] Significantly different from control, $P < 0.01$
- [c] Significantly different from control, $P < 0.001$

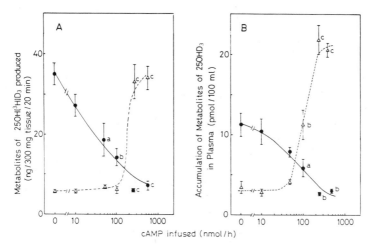

Figure 3

Dose-response effects of cAMP[10-500nmol/h] on productions
of 1,25(OH)₂D₃ and 24,25(OH)₂D₃ in TPTX rats treated with
125ng 1,25(OH)₂D₃ in the in vitro(A) and in vivo(B) assays.
The 1,25(OH)₂D₃ production is shown with the open triangle.
The 24,25(OH)₂D₃ production is displayed with the closed
circle.
Value are means ± SEM
 ᵃ Significantly different from control, P<0.05
 ᵇ Significantly different from control, P<0.01
 ᶜ Significantly different from control, P<0.001

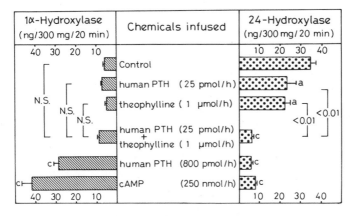

Figure 4

Effects of human PTH(1-34)PTH, cAMP and theophylline infused
on productions of 1,25(OH)₂D₃ and 24,25(OH)₂D₃ in TPTX rats
treated with 125ng 1,25(OH)₂D₃. The production rates were
measured by the in vitro assay.
Value are means ± SEM
 ᵃ Significantly different from control, P<0.05
 ᶜ Significantly different from control, P<0.001
 NS, No significant difference between the two groups.
 P<0.01, Significant difference between the two groups.

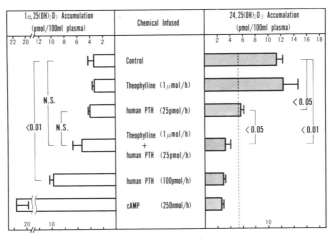

Figure 5

Effects of human PTH(1-34)PTH, cAMP and theophylline infused
on productions of $1,25(OH)_2D_3$ and $24,25(OH)_2D_3$ in TPTX rats
treated with 125ng $1,25(OH)_2D_3$. The production rates were
measured by the in vivo assay.
Value are means $\pm$ SEM
    NS, No significant difference between the two groups.
    $P < 0.01$, $P < 0.05$, Significant difference between the two groups.

TPTX rats in either assay (Fig.1). From these results, the predose of
$1,25(OH)_2D_3$ to induce $24,25(OH)_2D_3$ production in TPTX rats was fixed at
125ng in the following experiments.
    It was shown in Figure 2. that the dose-response effects were present
in the two assays of human PTH(1-34) on $25(OH)[^3H]D_3$ metabolism in TPTX
rats treated with 125ng $1,25(OH)_2D_3$. The dose-response curves were very
similar in the in vitro and the in vivo assays. In both assays, less
than 100pmol/h human PTH(1-34) dose dependently inhibited $24,25(OH)_2D_3$
production without any appreciable enhancement of $1,25(OH)_2D_3$ production.
Human PTH(1-34) stimulated $1,25(OH)_2D_3$ production at 800pmol/h in the in
vitro assay(Fig.2-A) and at 100pmol/h or more in the in vivo assay
(Fig.2-B).
    It was shown in Figure 3. that the dose-response effects of cAMP were
also present on $1,25(OH)_2D_3$ and $24,25(OH)_2D_3$ production in TPTX-rats
treated with 125ng $1,25(OH)_2D_3$ in the in vitro and in vivo assays. Like
PTH, less than 100nmol/h cAMP dosedependently suppressed $24,25(OH)_2D_3$
production in both assays without enhancing $1,25(OH)_2D_3$ production.
Stimulation of $1,25(OH)_2D_3$ production by cAMP was obtained at 250nmol/h or
more in the in vitro assay (Fig.3-A) and at 100nmol/h or more in the in
vivo assay   (Fig.3-B).
    To evaluate whether cAMP plays an inhibitory role in the PTH effect
on $24,25(OH)_2D_3$ production, the effect of theophylline was examined in the
in vitro (Fig.4) and the in vivo (Fig.5) assays. A submaximal dose of
human PTH(1-34)(25pmol/h) alone inhibited $24,25(OH)_2D_3$ production
slightly, but significantly($P < 0.05$). When 1.0 μmol/h theophylline was
constantly infused concomitantly with 25 pmol/h human PTH(1-34), $24,25$-
$(OH)_2D_3$ production was markedly inhibited without any appreciable
enhancement of $1,25(OH)_2D_3$ production.
    Plasma levels of calcium and phosphorus after infusion for 20h of
graded concentrations of human PTH(1-34) and cAMP into TPTX rats treated
with vehicle or 125ng $1,25(OH)_2D_3$ was shown in Table 1. Compared with the
plasma levels of calcium and phosphorus in TPTX rats given 125ng $1,25$-

Table 1. Plasma Levels of Calcium and Phosphorus in TPTX Rats Treated with 125ng/rat of $1,25(OH)_2D_3$

Chemical infused		Plasma Level	
		Calcium (mg/dl)	Phosphorus (mg/dl)
Control		7.3 ± 0.9	9.9 ± 0.6
Human PTH (1-34) [pmol/h]	25	6.2 ± 0.4	10.3 ± 0.9
	50	6.9 ± 0.5	11.6 ± 0.5
	100	7.1 ± 0.3	9.3 ± 0.2
	400	7.7 ± 0.7	9.7 ± 1.2
cAMP [nmol/h]	10	6.5 ± 1.3	10.7 ± 0.9
	50	5.4 ± 0.3	10.7 ± 0.2
	100	5.9 ± 0.2	11.3 ± 0.6
	250	7.9 ± 0.5	8.7 ± 0.8 [a]

Deta are means ± SEM.
[a] Significantly different from TPTX rats treated with 125ng $1,25(OH)_2D_3$ ($P < 0.05$)

$(OH)_2D_3$, infusion of neither human PTH(1-34) nor cAMP induced significant changes in plasma levels of respective ions at any dose levels.

DISCUSSION

It is well established that PTH and $1,25(OH)_2D_3$ are two major physio-logical factors in regulating $1,25(OH)_2D_3$ and $24,25(OH)_2D_3$ synthesis in mammals [2-4]. PTH stimulates $1,25(OH)_2D_3$ production through a mechanism involving cAMP. In contrast, $1,25(OH)_2D_3$ inhibits itself production and stimulates $24,25(OH)_2D_3$ production. $1,25(OH)_2D_3$ has been thought to be the sole physiological stimulator of $24,25(OH)_2D_3$ production. Thus, the pro-duction of $1,25(OH)_2D_3$ and $24,25(OH)_2D_3$ is considered to be tightly and reciprocally regulated in the balance of plasma concentrations of PTH and $1,25(OH)_2D_3$ [5]. Whether PTH inhibits $24,25(OH)_2D_3$ synthesis as an independent action besides its well known stimulatory effect on 1,25-$(OH)_2D_3$ synthesis has been obscure for a long time.

The present study clearly indicates that low doses (100pmol/h) of human PTH(1-34) infused into TPTX rats treated with 125ng $1,25(OH)_2D_3$ inhibit $24,25(OH)_2D_3$ production without any appreciable stimulation of $1,25(OH)_2D_3$ production. This suggests that besides its stimulatory effect on $1,25(OH)_2D_3$ production, PTH inhibits $24,25(OH)_2D_3$ production as an independent action by the much lower concentration than that stimulate $1,25(OH)_2D_3$ synthesis. Using the same rat infusion system as that used in this study, Takahashi et al reported that normal rats maintained on laboratory chow secrete PTH at a rate of 0.8-1.0 U/h [6]. This is com-parable to 50-60 pmol/h of the hormone. On the other hand, rats fed for 6-7 weeks the same synthetic vitamin D-deficient diet as that used in this study serete PTH at 6-8 U/h [6]. This is comparable to 360-480 pmol/h of the hormone. Thus, the inhibitory effect of PTH on $24,25(OH)_2D_3$ synthesis appears to be important physiologically. It is likely that $24,25(OH)_2D_3$ synthesis is more sensitive to PTH than $1,25(OH)_2D_3$ synthesis. It is apparent that the inhibitory action of PTH on $24,25(OH)_2D_3$ synthesis is independent of changes in plasma calcium and phosphorus.

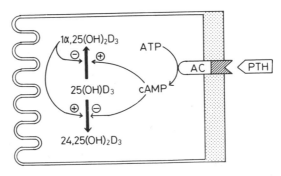

Figure 6

Schematic presentation of the main control mechanism of $25(OH)_2D_3$ metabolism in renal tubules.

Horiuch et al reported that PTH stimulates $1,25(OH)_2D_3$ synthesis in vivo through a mechanism involving cAMP [7]. Similarly, the inhibitory effect of PTH on $24,25(OH)_2D_3$ production appears to be mediated by cAMP. Recently, Armbrecht et al [8], Henry [9] and Matsumoto et al [10] reported that the inhibitory effect of PTH on $24,25(OH)_2D_3$ production were suggested in vitro studies. Our present study provides additional in vivo evidence for the previous studies. Low doses (<100 nmol/h) of cAMP constantly infused into TPTX rats treated with $1,25(OH)_2D_3$ dose-dependently inhibited $24,25(OH)_2D_3$ production without any appreciable stimulation of $1,25(OH)_2D_3$ production. Similarly, $24,25(OH)_2D_3$ production was markedly inhibited without stimulating $1,25(OH)_2D_3$ production when $1.0 \mu mol$ theophylline was constantly infused concomitantly with a submaximal dose (25 pmol/h) of human PTH(1-34) into the in vitro and the in vivo assays. These results indicate that cAMP is a common intracellular mediator of PTH action in regulating both stimulation of $1,25(OH)_2D_3$ production and inhibition of $24,25(OH)_2D_3$ synthesis. However, it is obscure how the difference of intracellular cAMP concentration may affect the process to stimulate $1,25(OH)_2D_3$ production or to inhibit $24,25(OH)_2D_3$ synthesis.

In conclusion, PTH inhibits $24,25(OH)_2D_3$ synthesis through a mechanism involving cAMP, besides its well known action to stimulate $1,25-(OH)_2D_3$ synthesis (Fig.6). cAMP functions as a common intracellular mediator in both PTH actions. Since physiological levels of PTH and cAMP inhibit $24,25(OH)_2D_3$ synthesis, this inhibitory effect appears to be important physiologically.

REFERENCES

1. Bligh,E.G., Dyer,W.J., 1959, A rapid method of total lipid extraction and purification, Can J Biochem Physiol., 37 : 97.
2. DeLuca,H.F., Schnoes,H.K., 1976, Metabolism and mechanism of action of vitamin D, Annu Rev Bio chem., 45 : 631.
3. Norman,A.W., Henry,H., 1974, 1,25-Dihydroxycholecalciferol — a hormonally active form of vitamin D_3, Recent Prog Horm Res., 30 : 431.
4. Fraser,D.R., 1980, Regulation of the metabolism of vitamin D, Phsiol Rev., 60 : 551.

5. Omdahl, J.L., 1978, Interaction of the parathyroid and 1,25-dihydroxy-vitamin D_3 in the control of renal 25-hydroxyvitamin D_3 metabolism, J Biol Chem., 253 : 8474.

6. Takahashi, H., Shimazawa, E., Horiuchi, N., Suda, T., Yamashita, K., Ogata, E., 1978, An estimation of the parathyroid hormone secretion rate in vitamin D deficient rats, Horm Metab Res., 10 : 161.

7. Horiuchi, N., Suda, T., Takahashi, H., Shimazawa, E., Ogata, E., 1977, In vivo evidence for the intermediary role of 3',5'-cyclic AMP in parathyroid hormone induced stimulation of 1α,25-dihydroxyvitamin D_3 synthesis in rats, Endocrinology, 101 : 969.

8. Armbrecht, H.J., Forte, L.R., Wongsurawat, N., Zenser, T.V., Davis, B.B 1984, Forskolin increases 1,25-dihydroxyvitamin D_3 production by rat renal slices in vitro, Endocrinology, 114 : 644.

9. Henry, H., 1985, Prathyroid hormone modulation of 25-hydroxyvitamin D_3 metabolism by cultured chick kidney cells is mimicked and enhanced by forskolin, Endocrinology, 116 : 503.

10 Matsumoto, T., Kawanobe, Y., Ogata, E., 1985, Regulation of 24,25-dihydroxyvitamin D-3 production by 1,25-dihydroxyvitamin D-3 and synthetic human parathyroid hormone fragment 1-34 in a cloned monkey kidney cell line (JTC-12), Biochim Biophys Acta, 845 : 358.

PARATHYROID HORMONE AND THE NERVOUS SYSTEM

DERANGEMENTS IN BRAIN SYNAPTOSOMES FUNCTION IN CHRONIC RENAL FAILURE: ROLE OF PARATHYROID HORMONE

Shaul G. Massry, Miroslaw Smogorzewski
and Anisul Islam

Division of Nephrology, The University of
Southern California, School of Medicine
Los Angeles, California

The neurotoxicity of excess blood levels of PTH in uremic state is well documented (1-4). This deleterious effect of the hormone is, at least in part, due to its ability to increase calcium content in brain (5-8). This is not surprisingly since the hormone enhances entry of calcium into many cells (9-11).

The mechanisms through which an increase in brain calcium adversely affects its function is not known. However, it is theoretically possible that alterations in the metabolism of neurotransmitters occur as a consequence of the increased calcium burden of the brain.

This study examined the effects of chronic renal failure (CRF) with and without secondary hyperparathyroidism and of excess PTH in the presence of normal renal function on norepinephrine (NE) metabolism and phospholipid contents of brain synaptosomes.

METHODS

Male Sprague-Dawley rats weighing 275-320 g were studied. The animals were fed normal rat chow (ICN Nutritional Biochemical, Cleveland, OH) throughout the study. One group of rats received intraperitoneal injection of 150 U/day of 1-84 PTH (Sigma Chemical Co., St. Louis, MO) for 21 days. The hormone was dissolved in normal saline and half of the daily dose was given in the morning and the other half in the late afternoon hours. The control animals received sham injections of vehicle (saline) only.

Studies were also performed after 21 days of chronic renal failure in the presence and absence of the parathyroid glands. Parathyroidectomy (PTX) was done by electrocautery, and the success of the procedure was ascertained by a decrease in plasma levels of calcium of at least 2 mg/dl. The mean value of plasma calcium for the 6 PTX rats that were included in the study fell from 9.95±0.08 to 7.60±0.11 mg/dl after parathyroidectomy. The PTX rats were allowed to freely drink water containing 50 g/l of calcium gluconate. This procedure is adequate to normalize plasma calcium in PTX rats. Seven days after PTX, the animals underwent right partial nephrectomy through a flank incision; a week later, a left nephrectomy was performed. The nephrectomy procedures were also performed in rats with intact parathyroid glands. Thus, this protocol provided 2 groups of animals with chronic renal failure (CRF): one with intact parathyroid glands (CRF-control) and the other without parathyroid glands (CRF-PTX).

All rats were sacrified at day 22 of the study by decapitation. Blood was collected in heparinized tubes for the measurements of creatinine, calcium and phosphorus. The forebrains of the animals were immediately removed, placed in ice-cold (4 °C) isolation media (320 mM sucrose, 0.2 mM K-EDTA, 5 mM Tris-HCl, pH 7.4) and chopped into small pieces with scissors. The chopped tissues were washed 3 times with isolation media. Synaptosomes were prepared according to the method of Booth and Clark (12) with minor modifications reported previously from our laboratory (13). Each forebrain yielded synaptosomes containing 12-16 mg of protein. The synaptosomal suspension was divided in 5 test tubes, frozen with liquid nitrogen and stored at -70 °C. At a later date the synaptosomes we thawed for the study of NE content, uptake and release, calcium content Na-K ATPase activity and phospholipid contents.

We have previously reported the various approaches to evaluate the intactness of the synaptosomes, their viability and the degree of contamination with mitochondria and endoplasmic reticulum (13,14). The anatomical intactness of the synaptosomes was ascertained by electron microscopic study of a section of the synaptosomal pellet and by measurements of lactic dehydrogenase (LDH) activity with and without 0.5% Triton (15). The values of LDH with Triton were four times those observed without Triton. The metabolic activity of the synaptosomes was assessed by measuring oxygen consumption with Clark oxygen electrode (Gilson Medical Electronics, Middelton, WI) using α - ketoglutarate and pyruvate as substrates (16); the values were similar to those obtained previously by others (12) and by us (13,14). The degree of contamination of the synpatosomes by extrasynaptosomal mitochondria and endoplasmic reticulum was evaluated by measurements of rotenone-insensitive NADH and NADPH cytochrome C reductase (17). The calculated mitochondrial contamination of our synaptosomal preparation was 7.2±0.61%.

NE content of brain synaptosomes was determined by radioenzymatic method described by DaPrada and Zurcher (18). The uptake and release of ^{3}H-NE was measured by a modification of the method of Pastuszko et al (19) which was detailed in a previous report from our laboratory (13). The activity of synaptosomal Na-K ATPase was estimated by measuring the hydrolysis of ATP (4 mM) in two buffered media, one without potassium (considered blank) since Na-K ATPase is inactive in it and the other contained 10 mM KCl (20). The details of the method was provided in a previous report from our laboratory (13). The estimation of calcium in synaptosomes was made by the method of Goldfarb and Rodnight (21) for the measurement of calcium in membrane fragments of cerebral cortex.

Synaptosomes (2-3 mg protein) phospholipids were extracted twice as described by Bligh and Dyer (23). The extract was evaporated and redissolved in methylene chloride and methanol 2:1 (v:v). The measurement of total and various phospholipid compounds were done by a modification of the method of a combined system of high performance liquid chromatography (HPLC) and automatic phosphorus analayzer described by Kaitaranta and Bessman (23). The HPLC was comprised of a 6000 A pump, a U6K injector (Waters Associates, Milford, MA) and an ultrasphere silica column of 4.6X250 mm packed with 5 u particles (Beckman Instrument, San Ramos, CA). An isocratic elution system with the mobile phase consisting of acetonitrile, methanol and sulfuric acid, 100:2.1:0.05 (v:v:v) was used. The eluate was directly channeled to an automated phosphorus analyzer (Alsab Scientific Products, Inc., Los Angeles, CA). A 20 nmol phosphorus standard was used in the autoanalyzer to allow quantification of the phospholipid peaks. The HPLC solvents were purchased from Burdick and Jackson through American Scientific Products (McGraw Park, IL), phosphatidylserine (PS), phosphatidylethanolamine (PE) and phosphatidylcholine (PC) standards were obtained from Sigma Chemical Company, St. Louis, MO), and phosphatidylinositol (PI) from Avanti Polar Lipids (Birmingham, ALA). Recoveries of the standard compounds were (%), PI, 78-80, PS 75-77, PE 71-73 and PC 75-78. The recovery of phospholipid phosphorus injected into the column was 66%.

Cholesterol in brain synaptosomes was determined using an assay based on enzymatic oxidation of cholesterol to cholest-4-en-3-one (Sigma Kit 352, Sigma Chemical Co., St. Louis, MO), and the results are expressed as nmoles/mg protein. Calcium content of synaptosomes and calcium concentration in plasma were determined by Perkin Elmer spectrophotometer, model 505 (Perkin Elmer Corporation, Norwalk, CN). Inorganic phosphorus and creatinine were measured with an autoanalyzer (Technicon Corp, Tarrytown, NY). The protein concentration of the synaptosomal pellet was determined by a modification of the method of Lowry et al (24).

Changes in parameters with time multiple measurements over time were evaluated by calculating area under the curve for each experiment. Data are expressed as mean $\pm$ SE and statistical significance was evaluated by parametric t-test.

RESULTS

The results are shown in Table 1 through 3 and figures 1 through 6. The treatment of rats for 21 days with 1-84 PTH did not cause a significant rise in the plasma levels of calcium but was associated with a significant ($p<0.01$) reduction in plasma levels of inorganic phosphorus; there were no significant changes in the blood levels of creatinine after PTH injection and the values were not different from control rats (Table 1).

The administration of 1-84 PTH was associated with a significant ($p<0.01$) reduction in NE content of synaptosomes as compared to control values, Figure 1. PTH treatment also caused a significant reduction in NE uptake (Figure 2) by and NE release from brain synaptosomes. The initial rate of NE uptake (1-15 min) was not affected by PTH treatment but the steady state NE uptake was significantly reduced.

The activity of Na-K ATPase in the synaptosomes obtained from PTH-treated rats was significantly lower than that of control animals, Figure 4. The calcium content of the synaptosomes in rats treated by PTH was significantly ($p<0.01$) higher than the values in control animals, Figure 5.

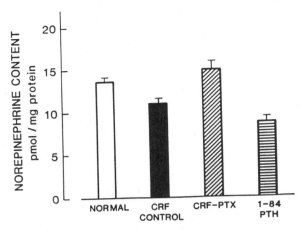

FIGURE 1. Norepinephrine content of brain synaptosomes in the various groups of animals studied. Each column represents the mean values and the bracket denotes 1 SE. There were 12 studies in normal and CRF-control and 6 studies in CRF-PTX and 1-84 PTH treated animals. Reproduced by permission from Smogorzewski et al (13).

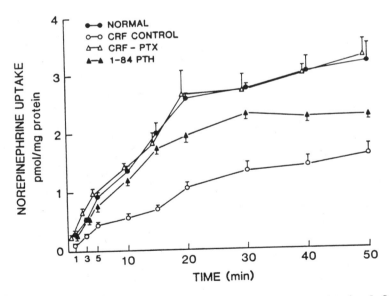

FIGURE 2. Norepinephrine uptake by brain synaptosomes obtained from 6 normal, 8 CRF-control, 6 CRF-PTX, and six 1-84 PTH treated animals. Each data point represents the mean value the bracket denotes 1 SE. Reproduced by permission from Smogorzewski et al (13).

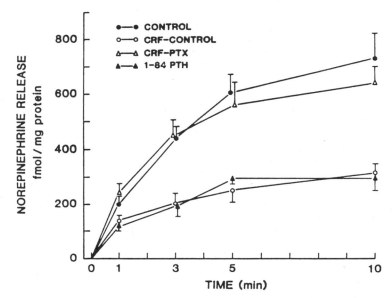

FIGURE 3. Norepinephrine release from brain synaptosomes obtained from 6 normal, 8 CRF-control, 6 CRF-PTX, and six 1-84 PTH treated animals. Each data point represents the mean values and the bracket denotes 1 SE. Reproduced by permission from Smogorzewski et al (13).

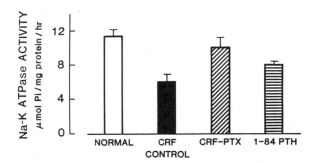

FIGURE 4. Na-K ATPase activity of brain synaptosomes in various groups of animals studied. Each column represents the mean value and the bracket denotes 1 SE. There were 9 studies in normal and 6 studies in the other groups of rats. Reproduced by permission from Smogorzewski et al (13).

Table 1 Blood Chemistry of Various Groups of Animals Studied

	Weight g	Plasma (mg/dl)		
		creatinine	calcium	phosphorus
Normal n=11	295±3	0.53±0.02	10.2±0.10	6.8±0.20
CRF-Control n=7	291±4	1.97±0.26*	9.8±0.25	8.6±0.77
CRF-PTX n=6	296±4	1.76±0.10*	10.3±0.19	6.2±0.30
1-84 PTH	276±2*	0.60±0.04	10.2±0.13	5.4±0.27*

Data are presented as mean ± SE
* $p < 0.01$ from control and/or 1-84 PTH

The nephrectomy procedure resulted in a significant ($p < 0.01$) rise in the plasma levels of creatinine with the values being three times higher than normal (Table 1). There were no significant differences between the plasma levels of calcium and phosphorus in CRF-control and CRF-PTX rats and the values were not different from those in normal animals except for a lower plasma phosphorus in CRF-PTX rats. NE content in synaptosome for CRF-control rats was significantly lower ($p < 0.01$) than in control animals or in CRF-PTX rats, figure 1. However, the decrease in NE content in CRF-control rats was significantly less than in PTH-treated animals. There was no significant difference between NE content of synaptosomes from CRF-PTX and normal rats. NE uptake by brain synaptosomes from CRF-control rats was significantly ($p < 0.01$) lower than that in control Figure 2. In contrast to PTH-treated rats, both the initial and the steady state NE uptake in CRF-control rats was significantly reduced. The NE uptake by synaptosomes from CRF-PTX animals was not different from that in normal rats. NE release from brain synaptosomes obtained from CRF-control rats was significantly ($p < 0.01$) lower than that in normal animals or CRF-PTX Figure 3. There was no significant difference in NE release between control and CRF-PTX rats.

The Na-K ATPase activity in the synaptosomes from CRF-control animals was significantly ($p < 0.01$) lower than in control rats, Figure 4. There was no significant difference between the Na-K ATPase activity of the synaptosomes from normal rats and CRF-PTX animals.

The calcium content of synaptosomes from CRF-control animals was significantly higher than that in normal rats or in CRF-PTX animals Figure 5, and there was no significant difference in the calcium content between the latter two groups.

The administration of 1-84 PTH to normal rats was associated with significant ($p < 0.01$) reduction in the brain synpatosomes content of PI, PS and PE as compared to values obtained from normal control animals (Table 2). There was no significant difference in the values of PC in synpatosomes from 1-84 PTH treated rats and control animals.

Similarly the PI, PS and PE content of brain synapsomes from CRF-control rats were significantly ($p < 0.01$) lower than values in control normal rats. The values of PI, PS and PE

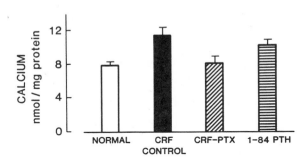

FIGURE 5. Calcium content of brain synaptosomes in the various groups of animals studied. Each column represents the mean of 6 studies and the bracket denotes 1 SE. Reproduced by permission from Smogorzewski et al (13).

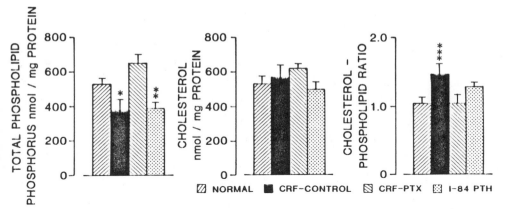

FIGURE 6. Total phospholipid phosphorus content, cholesterol content and cholesterol-phospholipid ratio of brain synaptosomes. Each column represents mean value of data obtained from 4 animals in each group. Each column represents mean value and brackets denotes 1 SE. * denotes p<0.05, ** indicates p<0.01, and *** represents p<0.025 from normal and CRF-PTX rats. Reproduced by permission from Islam et al (14).

Table 2. Synaptosomes Norepinephrine, Na-K ATPase, Phospholipids and Calcium in the Various Groups of Animals Studies

	Norepinephrine			Na-K ATPase	Calcium Content	Phospholipids			
	Content	Uptake	Release			PI	PS	PE	PC
Normal	13.6+0.55	110+5.9	5.1+0.47	11.4+0.74	7.1+0.50	4.9+0.31	45+2.7	76+3.9	195+10.5
CRF-Control	11.0+0.60	46+4.5	2.0+0.20	6.5+0.81	11.4+0.92	3.3+0.46*	35+2.0#	63+3.4**	176+7.9
CRF-PTX	14.8+1.02	107+2.9	4.3+0.57	10.8+0.62	8.0+0.62	5.5+0.47	47+4.2	88+8.5	219+18.0
1-84 PTH	8.6+0.55	87+4.0	2.3+0.2	8.3+0.58	10.0+0.80	2.4+0.14#	29+1.2#	62+3.8**	183+8.5

Data are presented as mean $\pm$ SE

Units for NE content are pmol/mg protein

Data for NE uptake are presented as area under the curve with the units for NE uptake are pmol/mg protein times 50 min and for NE release are pmol/mg protein times 10 min

Units for Na-K ATPase are µmol Pi/mg protein/hr

Units for calcium content are nmol/mg protein

PI = phosphatidylinositol, PS = phosphatidylserine, PE = phosphatidylethanolamine, and PC = phosphatidylcholine

Units for phospholipids are nmol phospholipid phosphorus/mg protein

Table 3. The Percent Molar Composition of Various Phospholipid Components of Brain Synaptosomes

	Total Phospholipid nmol Phospholipid Phosphorus/mg protein	PI	PS	PE	PC
			%		
Normal	528±25	0.96±0.04	8.5±0.45	15.0±0.90	40.2±1.32
CRF-Control	381±43*	0.72±0.05**	8.6±0.91	15.4±3.81	42.0±4.46
CRF-PTX	630±46	0.89±0.06	9.6±0.58	13.9±0.70	40.1±0.28
1-84 PTH	397±28*	0.72±0.02**	9.5±0.46	14.6±1.66	41.6±1.88

Reproduced by permission from Islam et al (19)

PI = Phosphatidylinositol; PS = Phosphatidylserine; PE = phosphatidylethanolamine; PC = phosphatidylcholine

Data are presented a mean ± SE

*$p < 0.01$ from normal and CRF-PTX

**$p < 0.05$ from normal and CRF-PTX

in the synaptosomes from CRF-control rats were not different from those obtained from 1-84 PTH treated animals (Table 2). There was no significant difference in the synaptosome content of PC among CRF-control, 1-84 PTH treated and normal rats.

Despite the presence of renal failure in the CRF-PTX rats, the PI, PS and PE contents of their brain synaptosomes were significantly (p<0.02) higher than those in CRF-control animals or 1-84 treated rats and were not different from values in normal control rats (Table 2).

In a separate study we examined the percent molar composition of the various phospholipid components of brain synaptosomes. These data are shown in Table 3. There were no significant difference between the percent of PS, PE and PC among the various groups of animals studied. However, there was a modest but significant (p<0.05) decrease in the percent PI in the CRF-control and PTH-treated rats.

Figure 6 depicts the total phospholipid phosphorus, cholesterol and cholesterol-phospholipid ratio in brain synaptosomes in the four groups of rats. Total phospholipid phosphorus contents were significantly (p<0.01) lower in CRF-control and 1-84 PTH treated rats than in normal control or CRF-PTX animals. Cholesterol contents of brain synaptosomes were not different among the various groups. Therefore, the cholesterol-phospholipid ratio was higher in CRF-control (p<0.025) and 1-84 PTH treated rats (did not reach significance) than in normal control and CRF-PTX rats.

DISCUSSION

CRF is associated with secondary hyperparathyroidism in man (25, 26), and dogs (27) and increased activity of the parathyroid glands is observed within few hours of induction of renal failure in rats (28). Although the blood levels of PTH were not measured in our animals, it is reasonable to assume that a state of secondary hyperparathyroidism did develop in the rats with CRF and intact parathyroid glands.

The results of the present study demonstrate that CRF exerts a variety of effects on norepinephrine metabolism of brain synaptosomes. CRF inhibits NE uptake and release by these structures and is associated with a decrease in their content of NE, total phospholipids, PI, PS and PE.

Two lines of evidence in our data indicate that these effects are related to the state of secondary hyperparathyroidism and not to other consequences of CRF. First, parathyroidectomy in CRF rats prevented these derangements in NE and phospholipid metabolism in brain synaptosomes. Indeed, the values of NE uptake and release by brain synaptosomes and their content of NE and phospholipids in CRF-PTX rats were not different from those in normal animals. Second, treatment of rats with normal renal function with 1-84 PTH produced abnormalities in NE and phospholipid metabolism of brain synaptosomes similar to those observed in CRF rats. Thus, it is apparent that the changes in NE and phospholipid metabolism of brain synaptosomes occur in animals with excess PTH whether renal failure is present or not.

Our observations that the calcium content of brain synaptosomes in CRF-control rats and in 1-84 PTH treated animals is elevated but is normal in CRF-PTX rats indicate that chronic exposure to excess PTH is associated with accumulation of calcium in brain synaptosomes. These data are in agreement with the reports of Fraser et al (29) that PTH enhances uptake of calcium by brain synaptosomes and that this effect is responsible for the augmented calcium influx in synaptosomes of rats with acute uremia (30). This accumulation of calcium in brain synaptosomes may contribute to the derangements in metabolism of NE and phospholipids of these structures.

Our data on NE release and uptake in all group of animals are made of an initial phase which most likely represents undirectional fluxes followed by a sustained phase which denotes net influx (uptake) or efflux (release). The evaluation of the slopes of the initial phases of NE uptake and release requires frequent measurements during the first 2 minutes. Such measurements were not made in our studies. Therefore, the results of NE uptake and release and presented as area under the curve which provides in large part the net influx or efflux, respectively, during the period of time of the study.

NE release by brain synaptosomes is regulated in part by calcium (31-34). An increase in calcium influx in brain synaptosomes is associated with an increase in NE release (34). Theoretically, one would expect that PTH, a hormone able to enhance calcium entry into cells, should stimulate rather than inhibit NE release. However, it is possible that chronic exposure to PTH and the associated chronic accumulation of calcium exert an inhibitory effect on NE release. Indeed, NE release was normal in CRF-PTX rats when calcium content of synaptosomes was also normal. A corollary to this phenomenon is found in the effects PTH on other systems. A stimulatory effect of acute exposure to the hormone have been noted in the heart (35-37) and leukocytes (38).

PS is important for the aggregation of synaptosomal vesicles, a step critical for the fusion of these vesicles with synaptosomal membrane and for the subsequent release of their content (39,40). A reduction in synaptosomal PS may, therefore, affect NE release. It is plausible that the decrease in PS content of the synaptosmes in CRF rats and PTH-treated animals plays an important role in the reduction of NE release from the brain synaptosomes of these animals. Acute renal failure is associated with decreased activity of Na-K ATPase of brain and brain synaptosomes (41-42). Our data demonstrate that chronic renal failure is also associated with reduced activity of Na-K ATPase. Since parathyroidectomy prevented the reduction in Na-K ATPase activity of brain synaptosomes from CRF rats and since treatment of rats with normal renal function with PTH produced a significant decrease in Na-K ATPase of brain synaptosomes, one can suggest that the changes in Na-K ATPase activity is related to the state of secondary hyperparathyroidism of CRF. It is possible that the effect of Na-K ATPase is due either to a direct effect of the chronic state of hyperparathyroidism or to the accumulation of calcium in brain synaptosomes induced by the chronic exposure to excess PTH or both. Further, the changes in synaptosomes phospholipids may also affect the activity of this enzyme.

The uptake of NE by brain synaptosomes is dependent on sodium gradient (43), requires energy and is dependent, directly or indirectly, on Na-K ATPase activity (44-45).

Indeed, NE uptake is inhibited by Ouabain (47,48). It is reasonable, therefore, to suggest that the decrease in NE uptake by brain synaptosomes in CRF-control rats and in 1-84 PTH treated animals may be due to the reduced Na-K ATPase activity (48).

It should be mentioned that the effect of PTH-treatment of normal animals and that of CRF in animals with intact parathyroid glands on NE uptake by brain synaptosomes were different. The former group of animals displayed a reduction in the steady state NE uptake only while the latter animals had a reduction in both the initial and the steady state rate of NE uptake. This difference occurred in the face of significantly lower activity of Na-K ATPase in the synaptosomes of CRF-control animals than in PTH-treated rats but with not significant difference in calcium content. These observations suggest that other factors in CRF besides excess PTH and/or calcium accumulation in synaptosomes may also cause inhibition of Na-K ATPase.

Our finding of reduced NE content in brain synaptosomes is in agreement with a previous data showing a decrease in NE content in brain of rats with chronic renal failure (49). A reduction in NE content of brain synaptosomes may be explained by alterations in NE uptake and release. Such an explanation would require the assumption that the inhibition in NE uptake is more marked than the inhibition of NE release. However, one cannot delineate the mechanisms responsible for alterations in NE content of synaptosomes without knowledge of their NE production. The processes regulating NE production are complex and may be coupled with NE release and be affected by calcium (50). It is possible that excess PTH and/or calcium accumulation in brain synaptosomes affect NE production either directly and/or through their influence on NE release. A reduction in the activity of tyrosine hydroxylase, a rats limiting step in NE production, may also produce a decrease in NE content. Data on the effect of PTH on the activity of this enzyme are not available. It should be mentioned, however, that Hennemann et al (51) reported that the activity of tyrosine hydroxylase is reduced in brain slices of rats with acute uremia. This change could have been due to the state of secondary hyperparathyroidism of acute uremia.

Several issues should be considered regarding the changes in synaptosomal content of phospholipids in CRF and PTH-treated rats. It is possible that alterations in synaptosomes phospholipids are affected by changes in plasma levels of phosphorus. However, the changes in phospholipids in synaptosomes from CRF rats and from those treated with PTH were not different despite lower plasma levels of phosphorus in the latter group. One can, therefore, suggest that plasma levels of phosphorus may not have played a major role in the genesis of the alterations in synaptosomes phospholipids in our studies.

The contents of total phospholipids, PI, PS and PE of the synaptosomes are determined by the rate of their synthesis and degradation. Our data cannot differentiate between changes in these two processes. However, chronic exposure to excess PTH have been shown to inhibit the activity of many cellular enzymes such as mitochondrial and myofibrillar creatinine phosphokinase of myocardium (37) and skeletal muscle (52) and carnitine palmitoyl transferase of skeletal muscle (53) and heart (54). It is possible, therefore, that chronic exposure to excess PTH may also inhibit the activity of enzymes involved in the synthesis of phospholipids in brain synaptosomes. It is of interest that two of the pathways responsible for the synthesis of PE involve the synthesis of PS (40); indeed, the predominant pathway of PS synthesis in animals is the base exchange reaction with PE. It is not surprising, therefore, to find that the synaptosomes contents of both PS and PE are decreased during chronic exposure to PTH, if the hormone reduces the synthesis of either compound.

The effects of chronic exposure to PTH on cellular enzymes activity of the myocardium and skeletal muscle have been attributed to PTH-induced accumulation of calcium in these organs (37,52,54) and a similar mechanism of action may be operative in brain synaptosomes as well.

Phosphatidylinositol metabolism is stimulated by binding of agonists to membrane receptor (55). Many reports indicate that acute exposure to PTH affects the turnover of PI causing a more rapid breakdown and resynthesis of this compound (56-58). It is possible that the balance between these two processes is disturbed with continued and chronic exposure to PTH resulting in reduced contents of PI.

The changes in the various phospholipids contents of brain synaptosomes may affect their function in many ways. We have already discussed the effects of these changes on NE release and Na-K ATPase. Since PI metabolism is critical for the response induced by agonist-receptor interaction (55), a reduction in synaptosomal PI may render them less responsive to many agonists and as such affect their function.

Membrane viscosity of mammalian cells is determined in large part by the cholesterol-phospholipid ratio in the plasma membrane (59). North and Fleischer examined the effect of changes in the cholesterol-phospholipid ratio of brain synaptosomes by manipulating the cholesterol content utilizing non-specific lipid transfer protein (60). They found that the reduction of the cholesterol-phospholipid ratio caused a significant decrease in sodium-dependent - aminobutyric acid (GABA) uptake by the synaptosomes while increasing the ratio did not affect GABA uptake. Our results showed that CRF in rats with intact parathyroid glands or 1-84 PTH treatment did not affect cholesterol content of brain synaptosomes; however, the cholesterol-phospholipid ratio in CRF-control rats was significant higher than in normal control or CRF-PTX animals due to the reduction in total phospholipid content.

REFERENCES

1. MASSRY, SG: The toxic effects of parathyroid hormone in uremia. Seminars Nephrol., 3:306-328, 1983.
2. ALLEN, EM, SINGER FR, MELAMED D: Electroencephalographic abnormalities in hypercalcemia. Clin. Sci., 20:15-20, 1970.
3. COOPER JD, LAZAROWITZ VC, ARIEFF AI: Neurodiagnostic abnormalities in patient with acute renal failure: Evidence for neurotoxicity of parathyroid hormone. J. Clin. Invest., 61:1448-1455, 1978.
4. COGAN MG, COVEY CM, ARIEFF AI: Central nervous system manifestations of hyperparathyroidism. Am. J. Med. 65:963-971, 1978.
5. ARIEFF AI, MASSRY SG: Calcium metabolism of brain in acute renal failure. J. Clin. Invest., 53:387-392, 1974.

6. ALFREY AC, MISHELL JM, BURKE J: Syndrome of dyspraxia and multifocal seizures with chronic hemodialysis. Trans. Am. Soc. Artif. Intern. Organs, 18:257-261, 1972.

7. GOLDSTEIN DA, MASSRY SG: Effect of parathyroid hormone administration and its withdrawl on brain calcium and electroencephalogram. Miner. Elect. Metab., 1:84-92, 1978.

8. AKMAL M, GOLDSTEIN DA, MULTANI S, MASSRY SG: Role of uremia, brain calcium and parthyroid hormone on changes in electroencephalogram in chronic renal failure. Am. J. Physiol., 246:F575-579, 1984.

9. WALLACH S, BELLAVIA JV, SHORR J, SCHAFFER J: Tissue distribution of electrolyte Ca^{47} and Mg^{28} in experimental hyper and hypoparathyroidism. Endocrinology, 78:16-28, 1966.

10. BORLE AB: Kinetic analysis of calcium movement in cell culture. II. Effect of calcium and parathyroid hormone in kidney cells. J. Gen. Physiol., 55:163-186, 1970.

11. CHAUSMER AB, SHERMAN BS, WALLACH S: The effect of parathyroid hormone on hepatic cell transport of calcium. Endocrinology. 90:663-672, 1972.

12. BOOTH RFG, CLARK JB: A rapid method for the preparation of relatively pure metabolically competent synaptosomes from rat brain. Biochem. J. 176:365-370, 1978.

13. SMOGORZEWSKI M, CAMPESE VM, MASSRY SG: Abnormal norepinephrine uptake and release in brain synaptosomes in chronic renal failure. Kidney Int. In press.

14. ISLAM A, SMOGORZEWSKI M, MASSRY SG: Effect of chronic renal failure and parathyroid hormone on phospholipid content of brain synaptosomes. Am. J. Physiol. 256:F705-F710, 1989.

15. Scandinavian Society for Clinical Chemistry and Clinical Physiology: Recommended method for the determination of four enzymes in blood. Scan. J. Clin. Lab. Invest., 33:291-306, 1974.

16. CHANCE B, WILLIAMS GR: Respiratory enzymes in oxidative phosphorylation. I. Kinetics of oxygen utilization. J. Biol. Chem. 217:383-393, 1955.

17. DUNCAN HM, MACKLER B: Electron transport systems of yeast. J. Biol. Chem. 24:1694-1697, 1966.

18. DaPRADA M, ZURCHER G: Simultaneous radioenzymatic determination of plasma and tissue adrenaline, noradrenaline and dopamine within the femtomole range. Life Sci., 19:1161-1174, 1976.

19. PASTUSZKO A, WILSON DF, ERECINSKA M: A role for transglutaminase in neurotransmitter release by rat brain synaptosomes. J. Neurochem., 46:499-508, 1986.

20. SAWAS AH, GILBERT JC: The effects of dopamine agonists and antagonists on Na^+-K^+ ATPase activities of synaptosomes. Biochem. Pharmacol., 31:1531-1533, 1982.

21. GOLDFARB PSG, RODNIGHT R: The role of bound potassium ions in the hydrolysis of low concentrations of Adenosine triphosphate by preparations of membrane fragments from ox brain cerebral cortex. Biochem. J. 120:15-24, 1970.

22. BLIGH EG, DYER WJ: A rapid method for total lipid extraction and purification. Can. J. Biochem. Physiol. 37:911-917, 1959.

23. KAITARANTA JK, BESSMAN SP: Determination of phospholipids by a combined liquid chromatograph-automated phosphorus analyzer. Anal. Chem. 53:1232-1235, 1981.

24. LOWREY OH, ROSENBROUGH NJ, FARR AL, RANDALL RT: Protein measurement with the Folin phenol reagent. J. Biol. Chem. 193:267-275, 1954.

25. BERSON SA, YALOW RS: Parathyroid hormone in plasma in

adenomatous hyperparathyroidism, uremia, and bronchogenic carcinoma. Science, 154:907-909, 1966.

26. MASSRY SG, COBURN JW, PEACOCK M, KLEEMAN CR: Turnover of endogenous parathyroid hormone in uremic patients and those undergoing hemodialysis. Trans. Am. Soc. Artif. Intern. Organs, 8:410-421, 1972.

27. AKMAL M, GODLSTEIN DA, MULTANI S, MASSRY SG: Role of uremia, brain calcium and parathyroid hormone on changes in electroencephalogram in chronic renal failure. Amer. J. Physiol. 246:F575-579, 1984.

28. JASTAK JT, MORRISON AB, RAISZ GL: Effect of renal insufficiency on parathyroid glands and calcium homeostasis. Amer. J. Physiol. 215:84-89, 1968.

29. FRASER CL, SARNACKI P: Parathyroid hormone-mediated changes in calcium transport. Amer. J. Physiol. 254:F837-F844, 1988.

30. FRASER CL, SARNACKI P, ARIEFF AI: Calcium transport abnormality in uremic rat brain synaptosomes. J. Clin. Invest. 76:1789-1795, 1985.

31. RUBIN RH: The role of calcium in the release of neurotransmitter substances and hormones. Pharmacol. Rev., 22:389-428, 1970.

32. RAITERI M, CERRITO F, CERVONI AM, LEVI G: Dopamine can be released by two mechanisms differentially affected by the dopamine transport inhibitor nomifensine. J. Pharmocol. Exp. Therap., 208:195-202, 1979.

33. ELGHOZI JL, LeQUAN-BUI KH, DEVYNK MA, MEYER P: Nomifensine antagonizes the ouabian-induced increase in dopamine metabolites in cerebrospinal fluid of the rat. Eur. J. Pharmacol, 90:279-282, 1983.

34. ASHLEY RH: External calcium, intrasynaptosomal free calcium and neurotransmitter release. Biochem. Biophys. Acta., 854:213-218, 1986.

35. BOGIN E, MASSRY SG, HARARY I: Effects of parathyroid hormone on rat cells. J. Clin. Invest., 67:1215-1227, 1981.

36. KAHOT Y, KLEIN KL, KAPLAN RA, SANDBORN WG, KUROKAWA K: Parathyroid hormone has a positive inotropic action in the rat. Endocrinology, 109:2252-2254, 1980.

37. BACZYNSKI R, MASSRY SG, KAHAN R, MAGOTT M, SAGLIKES Y, BRAUTBAR N: Effects of parthyroid hormone on myocardial energy metabolism in the rat. Kidney Int. 27:718-725, 1985.

38. DOHERTY CC, LaBELLE P, COLLINS JF, BRAUTBAR N, MASSRY SG: Effect of parathyroid hormone on random migration of human polymorphonuclear leukocytes. Am. J. Nephrol. 8:212-219, 1988.

39. WILSCHUT J, DUZGUNES N, HOEKSTRA D, PAPAHADJOPOULOS D: Modulation of membrane fusion by membrane fluidity: Temperature dependence of divalent cation induced fusion of phosphatidylserine vesicles. Biochem. 24:8-14, 1985.

40. YEALE P: The membranes of cells. Academic Press Inc., Orlando, Florida, 1987.

41. MINKOFF L, GAERTNER G, DARAB M, MERCIER C, LEVIN ML: Inhibition of brain sodium-potassium ATPase in uremic rats. J. Lab. Clin. Med. 80:71-78, 1972.

42. FRASER CL, SARNACKI P, ARIEFF AI: Abnormal sodium transport in synaptosomes from brain in uremic rats. J. Clin. Invest. 75:2014-2023, 1985.

43. PATON MD: Neuronal transport of noradrenaline and dopamine. Pharmacology, 21:85-95, 1980.

44: HOKIN LE: Purification and properties of the (sodium and potassium) activated adenosinetriphosphatase and

315

reconstitution of sodium transport. Ann. N.Y. Acad. Sci., 242:12-23, 1974.

45. BOGDANSKI DF: Mechanisms of transport for the uptake and release of biogenic amines in nerve endings. Adv. Exp. Med. Biol., 69:291-305, 1976.

46. VIZI ES: Na^+-K^+ activated adenosinetriphosphate as a trigger in transmitter release. Neuroscience, 3:367-384, 1978.

47. BOGDANSKI DF, TISARI AH, BRODI BB: Role of sodium, potassium, ouabain and reserpine in uptake, storage and metabolism of biogenic amines in synaptosomes. Life Sci. 7:419-428, 1968.

48. COLBURN RW, GOODWIN FK, MURPHY DL, BUNNEY WE, DAVIS JM: Quantitative studies of norepinephrine uptake by synaptosomes. Biochem. Pharmacol. 17:957-964, 1968.

49. ALI F, TAYEH O, ATTALLAH A: II. Plasma and brain catecholamines in experimental uremia: Acute and chronic studies. Life Sci. 37:1757-1764, 1985.

50. The Biochemical Basis of Neuropharmacology. Eds. COOPER JR, BLOOM FE, ROTH RH: Fifth Editon, Oxford Univerity Press, New York, 1986.

51. HENNENMANN H, HEVENDEHL G, HORLER E, HEIDLAND A: Toxic sympathicopathy in uremia. Proc. Eur. Dial. Transplant. Assoc. 10:166-170, 1973.

52. BACZYNSKI R, MASSRY SG, MAGOTT M, EL-BELBESSI S, KOHAN R, BRAUTBAR N: Effect of parathyroid hormone on energy metabolism of skeletal muscle. Kidney Int. 28:722-727, 1985.

53. SMOGORZEWSKI M, PISKORSKA G, BORUM PR, MASSRY SG: Chronic renal failure, parthyroid hormone and fatty acid oxidation in skeletal muscle. Kidney Int. 33555-560, 1988.

54. SMOGORZEWSKI M, PERNA AF, BORUM PR, MASSRY SG: Fatty acid oxidation in the myocardium. Effects of parathyroid hormone and CRF. Kidney Int. 34:794-803, 1988.

55. BERRIDGE MJ: Cell signaling through phospholipid metabolism. J. Cell. Sci. Suppl. 4:137-153, 1986.

56. LO H, LEHOTAY DC, KATZ D, MASSRY SG: Parathyroid hormone-mediated incorporation of ^{32}p orthophosphate into phosphatidic acid and phosphatidyl-inositol in renal cortical slices. Endocr. Res. Commun. 3:377-385, 1976.

57. MOLITORIS BA, HRUSKA KA, FISHMAN N, DAUGHADAY WH: Effect of glucose and parathyroid hormone on renal handling of myoinositol by isolated perfused dog kidney. J. Clin. Invest. 63:1110-1118, 1979.

58. FARESE RB, BIDOT-LOPEZ P, SABIR A, SMITH JS, SCHINBRECKLER B, LARSON R: Parathyroid hormone acutely increases phosphoinositides of the rabbit kidney cortex by a cycloheximide-sensitive process. J. Clin. Invest. 65:1523-1526, 1980.

59. SHINITZKY M, INBAR M: Microviscosity parameters and protein mobility in biological membrances. Biochem. Biophys. Acta 433:133-149, 1976.

60. NORTH P, FLEISCHER S: Alteration of synaptic membrane cholesterol-phospholipid ratio using a lipid transfer protein. Effect on γ-aminobutyric acid uptake. J. Biol. Chem. 258:1242-1253, 1983.

PTH INCREASES CA++ TRANSPORT IN RAT BRAIN SYNAPTOSOMES IN UREMIA

Cosmo L. Fraser and Allen I. Arieff

Divisions of Nephrology and Geriatrics, Department of Medicine
Veterans Administration Medical Center and University of California, San
Francisco
San Francisco, California

INTRODUCTION

Central nervous system (CNS) dysfunction is a major complication of patients with endstage renal failure. The clinical manifestations of this disorder are well described in several recent reviews (1). The biochemical basis for the CNS dysfunction of uremia is not well understood and is not completely corrected by dialysis. Studies of the CNS in humans and animals with renal failure have revealed no consistent pathologic changes (2) and biochemical studies in the brain of animal models of renal failure have also been generally unrevealing. The brain content of several ions (Na, K, Mg, C1, bicarbonate) and water are normal (2,3), and so is brain intracellular pH (pH_i) (3). Brain content of high-energy phosphate compounds (ATP, phosphocreatine) is also normal, although their turnover rate appears to be decreased (4). It appears that there may be altered permeability of the uremic brain to certain molecules, such as sodium, potassium, and inulin (5).

Among the few pathological findings in uremic brain which have been described is increased brain content of calcium, which appears to be parathyroid hormone (PTH) dependent (6). There are also associated abnormalities of the electroencephalogram, which are also felt to be dependent on PTH (7,8). Additionally, it is also felt that increased levels of aluminum in the brain may be responsible for some forms of uremic encephalopathy (9). However, removal of some of the potential "uremic neurotoxins", such as aluminum or PTH, does not necessarily reverse the encephalopathy, although parathyroidectomy in uremic subjects does result in improvement of both physiologic testing and the electroencephalographic abnormalities (10). Thus, it appears that other biochemical alterations are most likely present in uremia, and these alterations may play a significant role in the development of uremic encephalopathy. Further elucidation of these abnormalities in *in vivo* whole animal models appears to be rather difficult.

With studies in *in vitro* systems, other investigators have found abnormalities in both enzyme activity and certain transport phenomena. In erythrocytes from uremic subjects, it has been shown (11-13) that there may be abnormalities of sodium transport. In extracts from uremic rat brain, the Na-K ATPase enzyme activity was reported to be normal to low (14,15).

Because of the difficulty of directly measuring calcium transport in the brain of mammalian species, recent workers have performed calcium transport studies in an *in vivo* system called synaptosomes. These are membrane vesicles that are formed from presynaptic nerve terminals in the brain (16) by homogenization and differential centrifugation of the cerebral cortex. Under these conditions the presynaptic nerve terminals are sheared off and reseal to form intact vesicles called synaptosomes (17-19). Many enzymatic and metabolic properties which are identical to the intact nerve cell have been demonstrated in synaptosomes, and transport studies with sodium and neurotransmitter substances have also been evaluated (16,20-22). Under these conditions, the synaptosomes have proven to be a reliable and highly reproducible model with which to study alterations in CNS function.

There are five major pathways by which calcium can either enter or leave synaptosomes. These include voltage dependent Na^+ channel, voltage dependent Ca^{++} channel, Na-Ca exchanger and Ca-ATPase pump. The Na-Ca exchanger and the Ca-ATPase pump are the two major calcium efflux pathways, while the Na^+-Ca^{++} exchange participates in both calcium influx and calcium efflux (23-25). In nonexcitable cells, these transport mechanisms serve to actively extrude calcium against a high calcium concentration gradient of 10,000:1 (outside to inside cell). Calcium transport by the Na^+-Ca^{++} exchanger is dependent on the sodium concentration gradient such that calcium is transported in a direction opposite to that of the sodium movement (26). The larger the sodium gradient, the greater the amount of calcium which will be exchanged for sodium (27). The stoichiometry for this process is such that three sodiums are exchanged for each calcium transported (28).

In the present studies, experiments were carried out to determine the effect of uremia on calcium transport in synaptosomes. However, based on the results of the studies, additional experiments were performed to determine if PTH was responsible for the calcium transport abnormalities that were observed.

METHODS

Experiments were performed on 200 gm male Sprague Dawley rats (29) and were carried out in normal (BUN = 20 ± 3 mg/dl), uremic (BUN = 250 ± 25 mg/dl), uremic parathyroidectomized (PTX-U) (BUN = 230 ± 18 mg/dl) and PTX-U rats which received 2.8 μg/day PTH x 7 days. Rats were made acutely uremic by performing bilateral ureteral ligation under general anesthesia (16). Depending on the experimental protocol, at between 30-45 hours of uremia, they were decapitated and their forebrains removed and placed in ice cold isolation media (320 mM sucrose, 0.2 mM K-EDTA, 5 mM TRIS-HCl, pH 7.4 at 0-4°C). In the PTX-U rats that were treated with parathyroid extract, decapitation was performed at approximately 30 hours of uremia (BUN = 180 mg/dl) vs. 45 hours in the uremic group. This modification was necessary because PTX-U rats which received PTH did not generally survive beyond 35 hours of acute uremia. In these instances all groups that were simultaneously studied were sacrificed at the same time.

Isolation of Synaptosomes

After the forebrain was removed and placed in ice cold isolation media, it was minced finely with scissors and washed thoroughly with the same media to remove all trace of blood. The brain extract was homogenized slowly, and centrifuged with a Beckman centrifuge at graded spins of 1300 G and 18000 G to obtain the crude synaptosomal-mitochondrial pellet (16). The purified synaptosomal fraction was then obtained by differential centrifugation on a discontinuous Ficoll gradient. At the end of the spin, the synaptosomal fraction was resuspended in isolation media and kept on ice until transport studies were performed.

Assessment of Metabolic Properties of Synaptosomes

Protein concentration of the synaptosomal preparations were determined as described by Lowry et al. (30). Internal synaptosomal volume prior to performing uptake studies was measured using ^{14}C-methoxy inulin and tritiated water as described by Padan and associates (31). During experimental conditions, internal volumes were followed using tritiated mannitol as a marker for intracellular water (16). Tritiated mannitol was used to follow vesicular volume during the experiments instead of ^{14}C-methoxy inulin because of the convenience of counting both $^{45}Ca^{++}$ and $^{3}H^{+}$ simultaneously. Oxygen consumption studies were carried out as previously described (16). The degree of contamination of the synaptosomal preparations by extrasynaptosomal mitochondria and endoplasmic reticulum was assessed using a Gilford recording spectrophotometer Model 240. Activities of both rotenone insensitive NADH and NADPH cytochrome c reductase were used as surface markers for both mitochondria and endoplasmic reticulum (16). The intactness of the synaptosomal membrane was evaluated by measuring lactate dehydrogenase (LDH) activity during NADH oxidation in the absence and presence of the detergent Triton X100 (16,29,32).

Na$^+$-Ca^{++} Exchange Assay

One-half ml synaptosomal suspension (approximately 5 mg protein) was incubated for 10 minutes in 2 ml of pre-equilibrium media at 37°C (29). The pre-equilibrium media consisted of 140 mM NaCl, 1 mM $MgSO_4$, 10 mM glucose, 5 mM HEPES-TRIS at pH 7.4. The suspension was centrifuged at 20000 G for 5 minutes, and the final pellet was resuspended in 400 μl of the same pre-equilibrium media and stored at 0-4°C until transport studies were started (29). In studies which involved the sodium ionophore monensin, the sodium loaded vesicles were incubated for 5 minutes in 20 μM monensin prior to the initiation of the calcium transport.

Transport was initiated by adding approximately 50 μg protein to 95 μl of external media which contained 140 mM KCl, 1 mM $MgSO_4$, 10 mM glucose, 10 μM $CaCl_2$, 0.1 μCi $^{45}Ca^{++}$ and 5 mM HEPES-TRIS, pH 7.4 at 25°C. After the desired periods of incubation, uptake was terminated by adding to the reaction mixture 2 ml of ice cold 150 mM KCl solution. This mixture was immediately vacuum filtered through a 0.45 μm pore size cellulose-acetate membrane and washed with 2 ml of the ice cold KCl solution. The filters were then dissolved in PCS and counted by a Packard counter. The zero time points were obtained by adding 2 ml of stop solution to 95 μl of the external media, and to this mixture was added 5 μl of synaptic vesicles. The mixture was filtered and counted as described above.

ATP-Dependent Calcium Transport Assay

In this assay, synaptosomes were loaded with pre-equilibrium media containing 140 mM KCl, 1 mM $MgSO_4$, 10 mM glucose and 5 mM HEPES-TRIS, pH 7.4, at 25°C (29). Five μl of synaptosomes (approximately 50 μg protein) were then added to 95 μl of external media and allowed to incubate at 25°C for the desired time period. The external media contained 140 mM KCl, 1 mM $MgSO_4$, 10 mM glucose, ±1 mM TRIS-ATP, 10 μM $CaCl_2$, 0.5 μCi $^{45}Ca^{++}$, 5 mM HEPES-TRIS, pH 7.4. Calcium uptake was terminated at the appropriate time of incubation as discussed above.

Assessment of Parathyroid Status in Parathyroidectomized Rats

Parathyroidectomized rats (Ca = 9.8 ± 0.2 mg/dl) on calcium gluconate supplement were obtained from Harlan (Indianapolis, IN). Prior to study, calcium supplementation was discontinued and only animals in which serum calcium fell to <7.0 mg/dl after 48 hours were chosen for the study (33). Dietary calcium was then resumed in the chosen animals, and was maintained throughout the duration of the study. Normal nonparathyroidectomized rats maintained serum calcium at approximately 10.2 ± 0.3 mg/dl. Uremic parathyroidectomized rats treated with PTH, were injected intraperitoneally once daily with 2.8 μg PTH in cysteine hydrochloride vehicle (33). Some parathyroidectomized normal rats were treated in a similar manner with 100 μg PTH. Injections were started one week prior to uremia and maintained throughout the 35 hours of ureteral ligation. Serum calcium in this group was maintained at approximately 10.2 ± 0.3 mg/dl.

RESULTS

The internal volume of both normal and uremic synaptosomes were measured and no difference was found between the two groups. The value of 3.5 ± 0.6 µl/mg protein and 3.4 ± 0.4 µl/mg protein were similar to those obtained by other investigators (34). The results of the degree of contamination of the synaptosomal fraction by free mitochondria and endoplasmic reticulum (ER) were also evaluated with both rotenone-insensitive NADH and NADPH cytochrome c reductase as markers. The NADH-cytochrome c reductase is a marker for both the outer mitochondrial membrane and the ER (35,36), whereas the NADPH-cytochrome c reductase is a specific marker only for the ER (35). It was found that there were only ~6.4 and 5.7% contamination of the normal and uremic synaptosomes, respectively, with free mitochondria. Additionally, we evaluated contamination by ER in normal and uremic synaptosomes and found that the degree of contamination by ER and uremic synaptosomes were quite small and not significantly different from each other (5% vs. 7%, respectively).

The integrity of the synaptosomal plasma membrane was evaluated by measuring LDH activity in the absence and presence of the detergent Triton X-100 (37). As shown previously (16), specific activities of LDH in the absence of Triton X-100 were found to be 136 ± 15.0 nmol/min per mg protein and 150 ± 15 nmol/min per mg protein in normal and uremic synaptosomal fractions, respectively. These values increased to 995 ± 35 nmol/min per mg protein and 920 ± 40 nmol/min per mg protein, respectively, in the presence of 0.5% Triton X-100. The six-fold increase of LDH activity after lysis of the synaptosomes demonstrates an intactness of both groups of synaptosomes before lysing with detergent. In both normal and uremic synaptosomes, the respiratory rates are not significantly different from each other (4.3 ± 0.12 nmol/min per mg protein vs. 4.6 ± 0.2 nmol/min per mg protein, respectively). This similarity in rate of respiration was also observed in the presence of other substrates, such as glucose, ADP, and succinate, a substrate for both mitochondrial and synaptosomal respiration (18,36).

To evaluate the effect of parathyroidectomy on calcium transport by Na-Ca exchanger, studies were carried out in vesicles prepared from rats which were either normal, uremic or uremic parathyroidectomized (PTXU). In the uremic group, uptake was significantly greater ($p < 0.005$) than in normal, while in the PTXU group uptake was not increased above normal control (Figure 1). Uptake in uremia was approximately 25% greater than in normal, and approximately 70% greater than in synaptosomes from PTXU rats. Since except for their parathyroid status, the rats were otherwise biochemically similar to each other, it appears that parathyroidectomy alone prevented the increase in calcium uptake in uremia.

Studies were then performed to evaluate the effect of parathyroidectomy on ATP dependent calcium uptake in inverted vesicles. Figure 2 shows ATP dependent calcium uptake in vesicles from rats that were either normal, uremic or uremic parathyroidectomized. Calcium uptake in the uremic group was significantly ($p < 0.005$) greater than normal between 15 and 60 seconds. However, in vesicles prepared from PTX-U rats, calcium uptake was not increased as in the nonparathyroidectomized uremic group. Uptake in the PTX-U group remained similar to that observed in vesicles from normal rats. In either the absence of ATP or in the presence of the calcium ionophore, no uptake was observed (Figure 2).

We next investigated the effect which PTH may have on calcium transport in synaptosomes. Figure 3 shows calcium uptake by the Na-Ca exchanger in synaptosomes obtained from either normal, uremic, PTX-U or PTX-U rats that were treated with 2.8 µg PTH. As described above uptake in uremic vesicles was significantly ($p < 0.005$) greater than in normal by approximately 26%, while uptake in PTX-U rats treated with vehicle alone showed a 58% reduction in uptake from that observed in uremia (Figure 3). However, in synaptosomes from PTX-U rats treated with PTH, calcium uptake was increased by approximately 80% above that in PTX-U rats. Thus, based on these data it does appear that

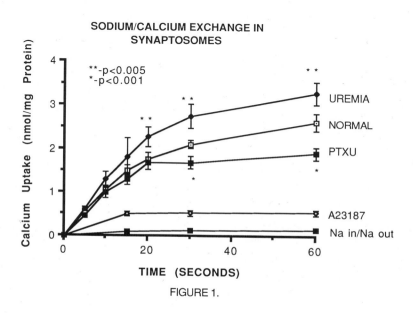

FIGURE 1.

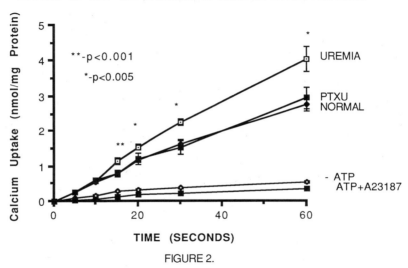

EFFECT OF ATP ON CALCIUM UPTAKE IN SYNAPTOSOMES

FIGURE 2.

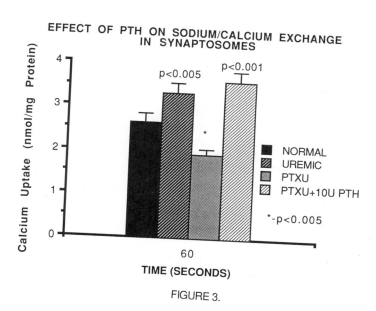

FIGURE 3.

in uremia, the parathyroid status of the rats has a direct effect on synaptosomal calcium transport.

To determine the possible relationship between the uremic environment and PTH on calcium transport, the uremic environment was eliminated by performing transport studies in synaptosomes from normal (nonuremic) rats. Studies were performed in vesicles from rats that were either normal, parathyroidectomized (PTX) or parathyroidectomized but in addition treated with either 2.8 µg or 110 µg of parathyroid hormone. Figure 4 shows calcium uptake by the Na-Ca exchanger which was decreased by 27% in the PTX group as compared to normal (nonparathyroidectomized) control. Additionally, uptake was increased by 23% and 43% above PTX value with either 2.8 µg or 110 µg of parathyroid hormone, respectively. Similarly, by ATP dependent calcium transport uptake in the PTX group was reduced by 27% from normal control (Figure 5). Contrary to what we observed with Na$^+$ gradient stimulation, 2.8 µg PTH did not result in any increase in uptake above PTX values. However, with a higher dose of PTH (110 µg), uptake was increased by approximately 32% above the value seen in parathyroidectomized rats. The final amount of calcium accumulated in synaptosomes in the presence of 110 µg PTH was not significantly different from normal in either of the two transport mechanisms studied (Figures 4 and 5). At the lower concentration of PTH (2.8 µg), calcium uptake by the Na-Ca exchanger was 31% greater than uptake due to ATP stimulation (Figures 4 and 5). From these data, it is also evident that whereas in uremia parathyroidectomy resulted in no significant decrease in ATP stimulated uptake below normal control value (Figure 2), in nonuremic rats, parathyroidectomy leads to a significant decrease in uptake of approximately 27% below normal control (Figure 5). This suggests that in uremia, additional factors other than PTH may be responsible for the increased calcium uptake with ATP stimulation. This is different from what was observed with Na$^+$ gradient stimulation of calcium uptake, where parathyroidectomy of either the normal or the uremic group resulted in a 27% decrease in uptake below the values of normal control (Figures 1 and 3). It thus appears that the Na-Ca exchanger and the ATP dependent calcium transport mechanism in synaptosomes have different sensitivities to PTH. It also appears that PTH dependent calcium uptake due to ATP stimulation is enhanced by uremia (PTX group in Figure 2 vs. Figure 5), while uptake due to N$^+$ gradient stimulation is not (PTX group in Figure 1 vs. Figure 4).

SUMMARY

The results of these studies suggest that calcium transport in synaptosomes isolated from uremic rat brain synaptosomes is increased in uremia. It also appears that the increase in calcium transport by both the Na-Ca exchanger and the ATP dependent calcium transport mechanisms in synaptosomes is dependent on PTH. The effect of PTH on the Na-Ca exchanger appears to be independent of the uremic environment, while the PTH action on the Ca-ATPase pump is enhanced by the uremic environment. PTH dependent calcium transport has also been described in other membranes (38-40). Scoble and associates recently showed that there are sodium dependent and sodium independent calcium transport pathways in canine renal proximal tubular basolateral membrane vesicles that were PTH dependent (40). It was also shown that the binding of calcium to canine brush-border membrane vesicles was enhanced by PTH (39). In other laboratories, it was also shown that calcium uptake by the Na-Ca exchanger into rat renal cortex basolateral membrane vesicles is decreased by 40% after parathyroidectomy and returned to normal after infusion of PTH into parathyroidectomized animals (38). Recently, Hruska and associates also showed that PTH produces a rise in cytosolic calcium in cultured canine renal proximal tubular cells that was not mimicked by cAMP (40). Thus, the results of all these studies from different laboratories suggest that a relationship does exist between parathyroid hormone and calcium transport in various tissues. These findings are consistent with our observation that PTH regulates calcium transport in synaptosomes.

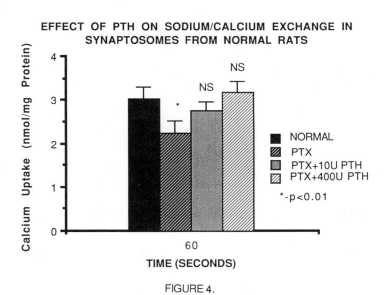

EFFECT OF PTH ON SODIUM/CALCIUM EXCHANGE IN SYNAPTOSOMES FROM NORMAL RATS

FIGURE 4.

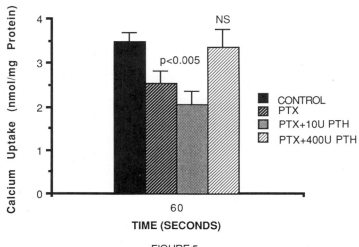

FIGURE 5.

REFERENCES

1.	P. E. Teschan and A. I. Arieff, Uremic and dialysis encephalopathies, in: "Cerebral Energy Metabolism and Metabolic Encephalopathy", D. W. McCandless, ed., Plenum Publishing Corp. New York (1985).

2.	A. I. Arieff, Effects of water, electrolyte and acid base disorders on the central nervous system, in: "Fluid, Electrolyte and Acid-Base Disorders", A. I. Arieff and R. A. DeFronzo, ed., Churchill Livingstone. New York (1985).

3.	C. A. Mahoney and A. I. Arieff, Central and peripheral nervous system effects of chronic renal failue, Kidney Int. 24: 170-177 (1983).

4.	C. A. Mahoney, P. Sarnacki and A. I. Arieff, Uremic encephalopathy: Role of brain energy metabolism, Am. J. Physiol. 247(Renal Fluid Electrolyte Physiol. 16): F527-F532 (1984).

5.	R. A. Fishman, Permeability changes in experimental uremic encephalopathy, Arch. Int. Med. 126: 835 (1970).

6.	A. I. Arieff and S. G. Massry, Calcium metabolism of brain in acute renal failure: effects of uremia, hemodialysis and parathyroid hormone, J. Clin. Invest. 53: 387-392 (1974).

7.	R. Guisado, A. I. Arieff and S. G. Massry, Changes in the electroencephalogram in acute uremia: Effects of parathyroid hormone and brain electrolytes, J. Clin. Invest. 55: 738-745 (1975).

8.	J. D. Cooper, V. C. Lazarowitz and A. I. Arieff, Neurodiagnostic abnormalities in patients with acute renal failure. Evidence for neurotoxicity of parathyroid hormone, J. Clin. Invest. 61: 1448-1455 (1978).

9.	A. C. Alfrey, G. R. LeGrande and W. D. Kaehny, The dialysis encephalopathy syndrome. Possible aluminum intoxication, N. Engl. J. Med. 294: 184-188 (1976).

10.	M. G. Cogan, C. Covey, A. I. Arieff, A. Wisnieski, O. Clark, V. C. Lazarowitz and W. Leach, Central nervous system manifestations of hyperparathyroidism, Amer. J. Med. 65: 963 (1978).

11.	L. G. Welt, J. R. Sachs and T. J. McManus, An ion transport defect in erythrocytes from uremic patients, Trans. Assoc. Am. Phys. 77: 169-181 (1964).

12.	C. H. Cole, J. W. Balfe and L. G. Welt, Induction of an ouabain-sensitive ATPase defect by uremic plasma, Trans. Assoc. Am. Phys. 81: 213-220 (1968).

13.	J. W. Woods, J. C. Parker and B. S. Watson, Perturbation of sodium-lithium countertransport in red cells, N. Engl. J. Med. 308: 1258-1261 (1983).

14.	S. Van den Noort, R. E. Eckel, K. Brine and J. T. Hrdlicka, Brain metabolism in uremic and adenosine-infused rates, J. Clin. Invest. 47: 2133-2142 (1968).

15.	L. Minkoff, M. Gaertner, C. Darah, C. Mercier and M. L. Levin, Inhibition of brain sodium-potassium ATPase in uremic rats, J. Lab. Clin. Med. 80: 71-78 (1972).

16.	C. L. Fraser, P. Sarnacki and A. I. Arieff, Abnormal sodium transport in synaptosomes from brain of uremic rats, J. Clin. Invest. 75: 2014-2023 (1985).

17.	V. P. Whittaker, I. A. Michaelson, R. Jeanette and A. Kirkland, The separation of synaptic vesicles from nerve ending particles (synaptosomes), Biochem. J. 90: 293-303 (1964).

18.	E. G. Gray and V. P. Whittaker, The isolation of nerve endings from brain, J. Anat. 96: 79-87 (1962).

19.	E. De Robertis, Ultrastructure and cytochemistry of the synaptic region, Science. 156: 907-914 (1967).

20.	V. P. Whittaker, The synaptosome, in: "Handbook of Neurochemistry", A. Lajtha, ed., Plenum Press. New York (1969).

21.	L. D. Lewis, U. Ponten and B. K. Siesjo, Arterial acid-base changes in unanesthetized rats in acute hypoxia, Respir. Physiol. 19: 312-321 (1973).

22.	A. Pastuszko, D. F. Wilson, M. Erecinska and I. A. Silver, Effects of in vitro and lowered pH on potassium fluxes and energy metabolism in rat brain synaptosomes, J. Neurochem. 36: 116-123 (1981).

23.	M. P. Blaustein and C. J. Oborn, The influence of sodium and calcium fluxes in pinched-off nerve terminals in vitro, J. Physiol. 247: 657-686 (1975).

24.	P. Kalix, Uptake and release of calcium in rabbit vagus nerve, Pflugers Arch. ges. Physiol. 326: 1-14 (1971).

25.   H. Reuter and N. Seitz, The dependence of calcium efflux from cardiac muscle on temperature and external ion composition, J. Physiol. 195: 451-470 (1968).

26.   M. P. Blaustein and A. L. Hodgkin, The effect of cynamine on the efflux of calcium from squid axon, J. Physiol. (Lond.). 200: 497-527 (1969).

27.   M. L. Michaelis and E. K. Michaelis, Ca++ fluxes in resealed synaptic plasma membrane vesicles, Life Sci. 28: 37-45 (1981).

28.   E. Carafoli and S. Longoni, The plasma membrane in the control of the signalling function of calcium, in: "Cell Calcium and the Control of Membrane Transport", L. J. Mandel and D. C. Eaton, ed., The Rockefeller University Press. New York (1987).

29.   C. L. Fraser, P. Sarnacki and A. I. Arieff, Calcium transport abnormality in uremic rat brain synaptosomes, J. Clin. Invest. 76: 1789-1795 (1985).

30.   O. H. Lowery, N. J. Rosenberg, A. L. Farr and R. J. Randall, Protein measurements with Folin-phenol reagent, J. Biol. Chem. 193: 265-275 (1951).

31.   E. Padan, D. Zilberstein and H. Rottenberg, The proton electrochemical gradient in escherichia coli cells, Eur. J. Biochem. 63: 533-541 (1976).

32.   H. U. Bergmeyer, H. Klotzsch, H. Mollering, M. Nelbock-Hochstetter and K. Beauchamp, Biochemical reagents (Section D), in: "Methods of Enzymatic Analysis", H. U. Bergmeyer, ed., Academic Press. New York (1965).

33.   A. Causton, B. Chorlton and G. A. Rose, An improved assay for parathyroid hormone, observing the rise of serum calcium in thyroparathyroidectomized rats, J. Endocrinol. 33: 1-12 (1965).

34.   C. Deutch, C. Drown, U. Rafalowska and I. A. Silver, Synaptosomes from rat brain: morphology, compartmentation, and transmembrane pH and electrical gradients, J. Neurochem. 36: 2062-2072 (1981).

35.   J. W. Gurd, L. R. Jones, H. R. Mahler and W. J. Moore, Isolation and partial characterization of rat brain synaptic plasma membranes, J. Neurochem. 22: 281-290 (1974).

36.   D. S. Beattie, Enzyme localization in the inner and outer membranes of rat liver mitochondria, Biochem. Biophys Res Commun. 31: 901-907 (1968).

37.   M. K. Johnson and V. P. Whittaker, Lactate dehydrogenase as a cytosolic marker in brain, Biochem. J. 88: 404-409 (1963).

38.   A. Jayakumar, L. Cheng, C. T. Liang and B. Sacktor, Sodium gradient-dependent calcium uptake in renal basolateral membrane vesicles, J. Biol. Chem. 259(17): 10827-10833 (1984).

39.   S. Khalifa, S. Mills and K. A. Hruska, Stimulation of calcium uptake by parathyroid hormone in renal brush-border membrane vesicles, J. Biol. Chem. 258(23): 14400-14406 (1983).

40.   K. A. Hruska, M. Goligorsky, J. Scoble, M. Tsutsumi, S. Westbrook and D. Moskowitz, Effects of parathyroid hormone on cytosolic calcium in proximal tubular primary cultures, Am. J. Physiol. 251(20): F188-F198 (1986).

41.   J. E. Scoble, S. Mills and K. A. Hruska, Calcium transport in canine renal basolateral membrane vesicles; effects of parathyroid hormone, J. Clin. Invest. 75: 1096-1105 (1985).

RELATION OF SERUM PARATHYROID HORMONE TO

COGNITIVE FUNCTION IN ELDERLY FEMALES

S. Morimoto, F. Masugi, T. Hironaka, T. Shiraishi, K. Itoh,
H. Yamamoto, E. Koh, T. Onishi, T. Ogihara and Y. Kumahara

Department of Medicine and Geriatrics
Osaka University Medical School, Osaka, Japan

INTRODUCTION

Senile dementia is one of the serious diseases of the aged. The cause(s) of this disease is unknown, but the role of calcium (Ca) in regulation of the mental state of elderly subjects is receiving increasing attention.[1] Chronic nutritional deficiency of Ca has been suggested to induce aberrations in mineral metabolism resulting in the abnormal accumulation of Ca and non-essential trace metals in neurons.[2] Possible associations of the well-known Ca-regulating hormones parathyroid hormone (PTH),[3-7] calcitonin (CT)[8,9] and 1,25-dihydroxyvitamin D [1,25-$(OH)_2$D][10,11] with senile dementia have been reported. However, there have been few precise measurements of Ca and Ca-regulating hormones in elderly subjects with senile dementia. In this study, we measured Ca-related factors in elderly females with and without dementia. Cases of dementia were classified into Alzheimer- and vascular-types on the bases of cognitive function and ischemic score. We found that the circulating level of PTH was significantly elevated in cases of dementia especially of the Alzheimer-type.

MATERIALS AND METHODS

Sixty "healthy" elderly female subjects with a mean ($\pm$ SD) age of 79 $\pm$ 7 years (range 63 - 94 years), who did not have a major cerebrovascular accident, renal failure, or diabetes mellitus were studied. None of them were receiving any drug that might alter Ca metabolism. All these subjects were hospitalized, and received about 600 mg of Ca/day. Their cognitive function was examined by the Dementia Screening Scale of Hasegawa,[12] (Table 1), and on the basis of their score for cognitive functions, they were classified as predementia-dementia (score 0 - 21.5, n = 42) and normal-borderline (score 22 - 32.5, n = 18). The subjects in the predementia-dementia group were further classified into Alzheimer-type (n = 22) and vascular-type (n = 20) dementia according to the ischemic score of Rosen et al..[13] Blood samples of these subjects were obtained in the early morning after an overnight fast. The serum and urinary levels of Ca, inorganic phosphate (Pi) and creatinine (Cr), were determined in a Technicon autoanalyzer. Corrected serum levels of Ca (cCa) were calculated by the formula of Payne et al..[14] The serum PTH level was measured with a commercially available RIA kit (Eiken Immunochemical Lab., Tokyo,

Table 1. Dementia Screening Scale of Hasegawa.[12]

Questions	Score
1. What is the date?	0, 3
2. Where are you? (name of place)	0, 2.5
3. What is your age?	0, 2
4. How long have you been here?	0, 2.5
5. Where were you born?	0, 2
6. When was the second world war?	0, 3.5
7. How many days are there in a year?	0, 2.5
8. Who is the prime minister?	0, 3
9. Subtract 7 from 100, then 7 from 93, and so on.	0, 2, 4.
10. Name of numbers in reverse order. (e.g., 6.8.2; 3.5.2.9)	0, 2, 4.
11. Indicate five things and recall them.	0, 0.5, 1.5, 2.5, 3.5

The elderly female subjects were classified according to cognitive function as normal (score 31–32.5), borderline (22–30.5), predementia (10.5–21.5) and dementia (0–10).

Japan) using antiserum directed towards the carboxy-terminal portion of the peptide.[15] Plasma CT was measured by RIA as described previously with antiserum directed towards the mid-portion of the peptide.[15] The serum levels of 25-hydroxyvitamin D (25–OHD) was determined by protein binding assay[16] and that of 1,25-$(OH)_2$D by radioreceptor assay,[17] after separation of these compounds by HPLC, as described previously. All samples from the subjects were examined in the same assay to reduce the between assay variation. Values are expressed as means $\pm$ SD. Statistical analyses were performed by Student's t test, and Spearman's rank correlation analysis.

Table 2. Serum and Urinary Levels of Various Parameters in Elderly Female Subjects in Predementia-dementia and Normal-borderline Groups.

Serum and urinary parameters	Normal range in young subjects	Elderly female subjects		Significance of difference between groups of elderly females
		Predementia-dementia group (n=42)	Normal-borderline group (n=18)	
Age (years)		80.2 $\pm$ 7.2	77.8 $\pm$ 5.5	NS
Hasegawa score		11.5 $\pm$ 5.7	26.5 $\pm$ 3.2	p<0.01
Serum level				
Ca (mg/dl)	8.4 – 10.2	8.75 $\pm$ 0.51	9.06 $\pm$ 0.66	p<0.05
cCa (mg/dl)	8.4 – 10.2	9.28 $\pm$ 0.48	9.31 $\pm$ 0.61	NS
Pi (mg/dl)	3.0 – 4.5	3.10 $\pm$ 0.41	3.25 $\pm$ 0.52	NS
Cr (mg/dl)	0.3 – 1.5	0.92 $\pm$ 0.21	0.98 $\pm$ 0.17	NS
PTH (ng/ml)	0.18 – 0.46	0.42 $\pm$ 0.16	0.30 $\pm$ 0.16	p<0.05
CT (pg/ml)	<150	36.8 $\pm$ 24.0	47.0 $\pm$ 24.4	NS
25–OHD (ng/ml)	7 – 35	7.32 $\pm$ 3.22	8.33 $\pm$ 4.25	NS
1,25-$(OH)_2$D (pg/ml)	20 – 60	26.1 $\pm$ 14.0	37.6 $\pm$ 17.3	NS
Urinary level				
Ca (mg/gCr)	30 – 300	199 $\pm$ 132	128 $\pm$ 72	p<0.02
Pi (mg/gCr)	300 – 800	578 $\pm$ 252	606 $\pm$ 365	NS

NS: not significant.

RESULTS

Table 2 summarizes the serum and urinary levels of Ca-related factors in the predementia-dementia and normal-borderline groups. Compared with the normal-borderline group the predementia-dementia group showed significant decrease in the serum level of Ca ($p<0.05$), and significant increases in the serum level of PTH ($p<0.05$) and urinary level of Ca (in mg of Ca per g of Cr; $p<0.02$).

Table 3 summarizes the mean levels of serum and urinary Ca-related parameters in subjects with Alzheimer-type and vascular-type dementia and those in the normal-borderline group. There was no significant difference in the mean ages of the three groups. The mean values for the scores for cognitive function in the groups with Alzheimer-type and vascular-type dementia were not significantly different. The group with Alzheimer-type dementia showed more marked abnormalities in serum and urinary parameters than the group with vascular-type dementia: unlike the latter, this group showed a significant decrease in the serum Ca level, and significant increases in the serum PTH level and urinary Ca level. However, the group with vascular-type dementia showed a tendency of decrease in the serum level of CT. The serum levels of $1,25-(OH)_2D$ tended to be lower in the groups with Alzheimer-type and vascular-type dementia than in the normal-borderline group, although the differences were not significant.

Table 4 summarizes the correlation between the score for cognitive function and the values of serum and urinary parameters in all the subjects studied, and in combined groups of normal-borderline and Alzheimer-type dementia, and normal-borderline and vascular-type dementia, and the significance of differences among these three groups. The results show that subjects with severe dementia had higher levels of serum PTH and

Table 3. Serum and Urinary Levels of Parameters in Elderly Female Subjects in the Alzheimer-type Dementia, Vascular-type Dementia, and Normal-borderline Broups.

Serum and urinary parameters	Normal range in young subjects	Predementia-Dementia group		Normal-Borderline group (n = 18)
		Alzheimer-type (n = 22)	Vascular-type (n = 20)	
Age (year)		80.7 ± 6.9	79.6 ± 7.7	77.8 ± 5.5
Hasegawa score		$10.8 \pm 5.1^{**}$	$12.2 \pm 6.3^{**}$	26.5 ± 3.2
Serum level				
Ca (mg/dl)	8.4 – 10.2	$8.60 \pm 0.44^{*}$	8.80 ± 0.56	9.06 ± 0.66
cCa (mg/dl)	8.4 – 10.2	9.22 ± 0.50	9.35 ± 0.45	9.31 ± 0.46
Pi (mg/dl)	3.0 – 4.5	3.15 ± 0.33	3.04 ± 0.48	3.25 ± 0.52
Cr (mg/dl)	0.3 – 1.5	0.94 ± 0.22	0.89 ± 0.21	0.98 ± 0.17
PTH (ng/ml)	0.18 – 0.46	$0.46 \pm 0.19^{*\alpha}$	0.38 ± 0.11	0.30 ± 0.16
CT (pg/ml)	<150	40.2 ± 29.6	$33.6 \pm 17.1^{\dagger}$	47.0 ± 24.4
25-OHD (ng/ml)	7 – 35	7.05 ± 3.45	8.33 ± 4.25	8.33 ± 4.25
$1,25-(OH)_2D$ (pg/ml)	20 – 60	25.0 ± 12.7	27.6 ± 16.0	37.6 ± 17.3
Urinary level				
Ca (mg/gCr)	30 – 300	$239 \pm 157^{**\alpha}$	161 ± 92	128 ± 72
Pi (mg/gCr)	300 – 800	605 ± 268	550 ± 228	606 ± 265

Significant differences between values in the normal-borderline group and Alzheimer-type or vascular-type dementia group ($^{\dagger}p<0.1$, $^{*}p<0.05$, $^{**}p<0.01$), and between the Alzheimer-type and vascular-type dementia groups ($^{\alpha}p<0.1$) are shown.

Table 4. Correlation between the Score for Cognitive Function and
the Serum and Urinary Parameters, in All Elderly Female Subjects,
and in Combinations of Groups of Normal-borderline with
Alzheimer-type Dementia, and with Vascular-type Dementia.

Serum and urinary parameters	Normal-Borderline & Alzheimer & Vascular (n = 60)		Normal-Borderline & Alzheimer-type (n = 40)		Normal-Borderline & Vascular-type (n = 38)	
	r	p	r	p	r	p
Age	−0.199	NS	−0.176	NS	−0.200	NS
Serum level						
Ca	0.162	NS	0.258	NS	0.070	NS
cCa	−0.048	NS	0.014	NS	−0.128	NS
Pi	0.122	NS	0.095	NS	0.193	NS
Cr	0.041	NS	0.117	NS	0.049	NS
PTH	−0.331	p<0.05	−0.485	p<0.01	−0.164	NS
CT	0.141	NS	0.080	NS	0.397	p<0.05
25-OHD	0.039	NS	0.008	NS	−0.034	NS
$1,25-(OH)_2D$	0.257	NS	0.309	p<0.1	0.216	NS
Urinary level						
Ca	−0.286	p<0.05	−0.378	p<0.05	−0.116	NS
Pi	0.005	NS	−0.210	NS	0.224	NS

Statistical significance was calculated by Spearman's rank correlation
analysis. NS: not significant.

urinary Ca, and the changes were more marked in the combined group of
normal-borderline and Alzheimer-type dementia. Moreover, in the latter
group, the serum level of $1,25-(OH)_2D$ tended to be lower in subjects with
more severe dementia. On the other hand, the combine group of normal-
borderline and vascular-type dementia did not show these features, but
instead showed a significant decrease in serum CT level in subjects with
more severe dementia.

DISCUSSION

In this study we examined the relation of the serum and urinary
levels of Ca-related factors to senile dementia in 60 "healthy" elderly
female subjects. Compared with the normal-borderline group, predementia-
dementia group, especially subjects with Alzheimer-type dementia, showed
significantly lower serum Ca, and significantly higher serum PTH and
urinary Ca levels, and tended to have a lower serum $1,25-(OH)_2D$ level.
These changes in Ca-related factors were more prominent in demented
subjects of the Alzheimer-type than in those of the vascular-type. These
results suggest that mild elevation of the serum PTH level due to excess
loss of Ca in the urine may be important in decrease in the cognitive state
of female subjects with senile dementia of the Alzheimer-type.
A possible association of PTH with dementia has also been suspected
in diseases other than senile dementia. Associations of primary and
secondary hyperparathyroidism with dementia have been reported.[3] PTH is
also suspected to be a causal factor of cerebral symptoms including
abnormality in the electroencephalogram of patients with renal failure who
have elevated circulating levels of this hormone due to secondary
hyperparathyroidism.[4-6] Moreover, in uremic dogs, normalization of the

electroencephalogram was observed after parathyroidectomy, and increased abnormality of the electroencephalogram was observed after infusion of PTH.[7] However, the significance of PTH in pathogenesis and its clinical meaning are still controversial.[18]

In this study we found that subjects with vascular-type dementia showed a decreased level of serum CT. CT is reported to prevent immune-arteriosclerosis in animals,[8] and to improve chronic cerebral obliterance arteriopathies clinically.[9] Since vascular-type dementia is thought to be due to arteriosclerosis of brain arteries, a decreased level of CT may contribute to the development of this type of senile dementia.

In our series of patients, the serum level of $1,25-(OH)_2D$ tended to be decreased in dementia of both the Alzheimer-and vascular-type, although the decreases were not statistically significant. Recently a receptor for 1,25-dihydroxyvitamin D_3 [$1,25-(OH)_2D_3$], an active form of vitamin D, was found in the brain and $1,25-(OH)_2D_3$ was suggested to have roles in the brain.[10-11] $1,25-(OH)_2 D_3$ was also shown to elevate the choline acetyl-transferase activity in brain nuclei of rats, suggesting that $1,25-(OH)_2D_3$ affects cholinergic activity in several discrete regions of the brain and may play a role in neuroendocrine regulation.[11] Since a specific relationship between cholinergic transmitter pathology and Alzheimer's disease has been reported,[19] $1,25-(OH)_2D$ may have a direct role in development of dementia.

Further studies are required on the precise significance of the changes in Ca-related factors seen in this study, and especially the roles of PTH, CT and $1,25-(OH)_2D$ in the development of senile dementia, including the time courses of development of dementia in subjects with different changes in Ca-related factors.

REFERENCES

1. T. Fujita, Aging and calcium, Miner. Electrolyte Metab. 12:149 (1986).
2. Y. Yase, Calcium, metals and nervous system in the elderly, J. Nutr. Sci. Vitaminol. 31:S37 (1985).
3. J. Luxenberg, L. Z. Feigenbaum, and J. M. Aron, Reversible long-standing dementia with normocalcemic hyperparathyroidism, J. Am. Geriatr. Soc. 32:546 (1984).
4. J. D. Cooper, V. C. Lazarowitz, and A. I. Arieff, Neurodiagnostic abnormalities in patients with acute renal failure, J. Clin. Invest. 61:1448 (1978).
5. D. A. Goldstein, E. I. Feinstein, L. A. Chui, R. Pattabhiraman, and S. G. Massry, The relationship between the abnormalities in electroencephalogram and blood levels of parathyroid hormone in dialysis patients, J. Clin. Endocrinol. Metab. 51:130 (1980).
6. M. G. Cogan, C. M. Covey, A. I. Arieff, A. Wisniewski, and O. H. Clark, Central nervous system manifestations of hyperparathyroidism, Am. J. Med. 65:963 (1978).
7. R. Guisado, A. I. Arieff, and S. G. Massry, Changes in the electro-encephalogram in acute uremia, J. Clin. Invest. 55:738 (1975).
8. L. Robert, D. Brechemier, G. Godeau, M. L. Labat, and G. Milhaud, Prevention of experimental immunarteriosclerosis by calcitonin, Biochem. Pharmacol. 26:2129 (1977).
9. F. Insinna, and P. Sarcone, Clinical research on effects of calcitonin in the treatment of chronic cerebral and peripheral obliterans arteriopathies, Int. Angiol. 4:39 (1985).
10. W. E. Stumpf, M. Sar, and S. A. Clark, Brain target sites for 1,25-dihydroxyvitamin D_3, Science 215:1403 (1982)
11. J. Sonnenberg, V. N. Luine, L. C. Krey, and S. Christakos, 1,25-Dihydroxyvitamin D_3 treatment results in increased choline acetyltransferase activity in specific brain nuclei, Endocrinology 118:1433 (1986).

12. K. Hasegawa, Dementia screening scale, in "Score Book of Geriatric Assessment," L. Israel, D. Kozarevic, and N. Sartrius, eds., S Kager, Basel (1984).
13. W. G. Rosen, R. D. Terry, P. A. Fuld, R. Katzman, and A. Peck, Pathological verification of ischemic score in differentiation of dementias, Ann. Neurol. 7:486 (1980).
14. R. B. Payne, A. J. Little, R. B. William, and J. R. Milner, Interpretation of calcium in patients with abnormal serum protein, Br. Med. J. 4:643 (1973).
15. S. Morimoto, M. Tsuji, Y. Okada, T. Onishi, and Y. Kumahara, The effect of oestrogen on human calcitonin secretion after calcium infusion in elderly female subjects, Clin. Endocrinol. 13:135 (1980).
16. Y. Shimotsuji, and Y. Seino, Competitive protein binding assay for 25-hydroxycholecalciferol. Methods Enzymol. 67:466 (1980).
17. Y. Seino, T. Shimotsuji, K. Yamaoka, M. Ishida, T. Ishii, S. Matsuda, C. Ikehara, H. Yabuuchi, and S. Dokoh, Plasma 1,25-dihydroxyvitamin D concentrations in cords, newborns, infants and children. Calcif. Tissue Int. 30:1 (1980).
18. D. Shore, M. R. Wills, J. Savory, and R. J. Wyat, Serum parathyroid hormone concentrations in senile dementia, J. Gerontol. 35:656 (1980).
19. P. Davis, and A. J. F. Malony, Selective loss of central cholinergic neurons in Alzheimer's disease, Lancet 2:1403 (1976).

PARATHYROID HORMONE AND PAIN

Carlo Gennari

Institute of Medical Semeiotics
University of Siena
Siena, Italy

INTRODUCTION

In recent years, it has been suggested that calcitonin (CT), in addition to well known action on calcium and phosphate metabolism, may also exert effects as a neuromodulator. In fact, evidence has been given
that CT potentiates haloperidol-induced catalepsy in rats (1), decreases glutammic acid decarboxylase (GAD) activity in the substantia nigra
(2), decreases plasma prolactin level in rats and in healthy subjects
(3,4), induces analgesia in animals and man (5,6), and inhibits gastric
acid secretion and feeding in rats (7,8).

Recently, it has been observed that parathyroid hormone (PTh), the
physiological antagonist of CT, determines some behavioral and neurochemical effects opposite to those found after CT administration. These
effects include a reduction of haloperidol-induced catalepsy and an
increase in GAD activity in the substantia nigra (9), and an increase
in plasma prolactin level in rats (10). Furthermore, intracerebroventricular (ICV) injection of PTH induces hyperalgesia in the rat (11).

The responses of the two peptides administered centrally address the
attention to the presence of CT and PTH receptors in the central nervous
system. In fact, salmon calcitonin receptors have been identified in
rat and man with the highest binding in the midbrain and brainstem (12,
13). In addition, messenger RNA encoding the precursors of CT has been
detected in the rat nervous system (14). and CT has been identified in
human brain and cerebrospinal fluid (15,16).

Surprisingly, little is known regarding the presence of PTH and PTH-
binding sites in the central nervous system. Like CT, PTH was found to
elevate the intracellular concentration of cyclic AMP in primary cultures
of rat brain cells (17). In these studies it has been shown that a competitive antagonist of PTH inhibits the PTH-induced accumulation of
cyclic AMP in cultured brain cells (17). In this system the potency of
PTH is at least three times higher than that of CT and is comparable to
the potency of PTH in stimulating adenylate cyclase in kidney cells.
The responsiveness of cultured brain cells to PTH constitutes a conside-

New Actions of Parathyroid Hormone
Edited by S. G. Massry and T. Fujita
Plenum Press, New York

rable, albeit indirect, evidence for the presence of PTH receptors. In
analogy to the situation with CT, it appears worthwhile to look for PTH
in the brain and for physiological and behavioral effects of the hormone
in the central nervous system.

HYPERALGESIC ACTIVITY OF PTH

The first study suggesting a possible central hyperalgesic activity
of PTH has been conducted in rats (11). The interest of this study was
centered on the effect of ICV injection of bovine PTH (1-84) or its fragments 1-34, 44-68 or 65-84 on pain threshold. The effects on pain
threshold were evaluated using the tail-flick or hot-plate tests, and
results were expressed as percent change in reaction times. The whole
molecule (1-84) or the fragments 1-34 and 44-68 of PTH significantly decreased the reaction time in both tail-flick and hot-plate test. In contrast, the fragment 65-84 failed to affect pain threshold.

It is well known that about one-half of patients with primary hyperparathyroidism is symptomatic for abdominal, joint or bone pain. Recently,
in five patients with hypercalcemia and probable primary hyperparathyroidism, all symptomatic with bone and joint pain, we have selectively
investigated the effects of parathyroid surgery on pain, as measured by
a visual analogue scale (Fig. 1). In four of five patients single parathyroid adenomas were removed; to the rapid improvement in hypercalcemia
and in parathyroid hyperactivity, as evaluated by the measurement of nephrogenous cyclic AMP (NcAMP) corresponded a progressive improvement in
pain. In the fifth patient the adenoma was not found at surgery, so that
no significant postoperative improvement was observed not only in serum
calcium level and NcAMP, but also in pain score. This clinical observation
suggests that in patients with primary hyperparathyroidism pain may be
dependent on parathyroid hyperactivity.

The question arises if the hyperalgesic activity of PTH is related
to a direct effect on brain or is indirectly related to the PTH-induced
increase in calcium levels in body fluids. An increased sensitivity to
pain is common to hypercalcemia of different origin (18) and calcium ion
is certainly involved in some mechanism or system of pain modulation.
In fact, evidence has been given that calcium antagonizes the analgesic
action of morphine and that this effect can be enhanced by manipulations
that increase brain membrane permeability to calcium and can be reversed
by decreasing calcium availability (19). It is also unclear whether pe-
ripherally produced PTH may penetrate the blood-brain barrier (BBB).

PTH AND CALCIUM IN CEREBROSPINAL FLUID

The cerebrospinal fluid (CSF) and brain compositions are strictly
protected by the BBB selectivity and integrity. Available data indicate
that the concentrations of calcium and phosphorus in CSF are not affected
in conditions associated with excess or deficiency of PTH (20,21). On
the other side, contrasting data exist on the possibility that the hormone may cross the BBB. Some authors have shown that an increase in the
blood levels of PTH produced by PTH infusion or by stimulation of endogenous release of the hormone is not associated with a rise in the concentration of PTH in CSF (22). More recently, in sheep and human subjects
evidence has been given that PTH readily cross the BBB (23).

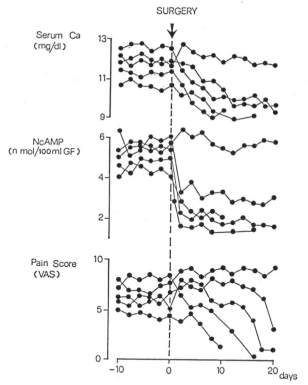

Fig. 1. Effects of parathyroid surgery on serum calcium,
nephrogenous cyclic AMP (NcAMP) and pain, as
measured by a visual analogue scale, in 5 patients
with primary hyperparathyroidism, symptomatic with
bone and joint pain.

To evaluate the possibility that PTH crosses the BBB, the concentrations of immunoreactive PTH (N-terminal and middle-molecule antibodies)
and of total calcium were measured in serum and CSF of 17 human subjects,
all symptomatic for bone or joint pain. Seven patients were suspected
of having pain due to vertebral disk disease and were scheduled for
myelography; 7 patients had hypercalcemia due to metastatic bone involvement from solid tumors; 3 patients had primary hyperparathyroidism.
In all cases immunoreactive PTH was present in CSF and its concentration
was lower in CSF that in the peripheral circulation. We have found a
direct and significant relationship between the CSF and blood levels of
both the amino-terminal and the middle-molecule fragment of PTH (Figs. 2,
3). On the contrary, no significant relationship was found between the
CSF and the blood levels of total calcium (Fig. 4). These results provide evidence that PTH crosses the BBB in man and that the concentration
of PTH in CSF is a function of the concentration of the hormone in the
peripheral circulation.

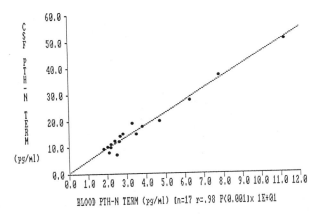

Fig. 2. Relationship between the concentration of PTH-N terminal in blood and cerebrospinal fluid (CSF) in normo- and hypercalcemic patients.

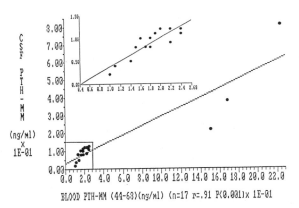

Fig. 3. Relationship between the concentration of PTH middle molecule (44-68) in blood and cerebrospinal fluid (CSF) in normo- and hypercalcemic patients.

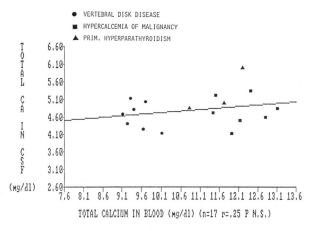

Fig. 4. Relationship between total concentration of calcium in blood
and CSF in normo- and hypercalcemic patients.

PTH AND CENTRAL NERVOUS SYSTEM FUNCTION

Recent work in animals and man has suggested that abnormal central
nervous system function in acute or advanced renal failure is correlated
with the presence of elevated serum PTH levels. Electroencephalographic
abnormalities have been frequently observed in patients with primary or
secondary hyperparathyroidism (24,25). A direct and significant relationship between the abnormalities in electroencephalogram and the blood
levels of the amino-terminal fragment of PTH has been found in dialysis
patients (24). In addition, it has been shown that parathyroidectomy in
uremic patients and the removal of the parathyroid adenoma in patients
with primary hyperparathyroidism is associated with improvement or normalization of electroencephalogram (24,25). Finally, it has been observed
that in parathyroidectomized animals rendered hypercalcemic, electroencephalographic abnormalities do not occur (26). These results suggest that
PTH, but not the calcium ion, may have a detrimental effect on the central
nervous system (27,28).

The mechanism by which PTH disturbs central nervous system function
is unclear, although the occurrence of psychosis or abnormalities in
learning and memory processes in patients with hypercalcemia and hyperparathyroidism has been described (29,30). At this regard, learning and memory processes appear to be increased by a rise in extracellular calcium
(31) and decreased by a block of transmembrane calcium flux (32). Recently,
the acquisition of active avoidance response has been studied in rats
injected intracerebroventricularly with CT, PTH or PTH-related fragments
(33). Animals were trained to avoid the inconditioned stimulus of an
electrical footshock delivered through the grid floor of a shuttle-box

task. PTH 1-84 and its fragment 65-84 facilitated the acquisition of active avoidance behavior, and increased the percentage of animals reaching the learning criterion (33). On the contrary, the fragments 1-34 and 44-68 of PTH inhibited the acquisition of active avoidance behavior (33). This would imply that the behavioral effects of the various PTH fragments do not parallel the hyperalgesic effects. In fact, PTH 65-84 that is most effective in facilitating avoidance acquisition, is totally devoid of any hyperalgesic activity (11). These data seem to indicate that PTH may mediate its action on the central nervous system by different mechanisms.

PTH AND INTRACELLULAR CALCIUM

The mechanism through which PTH may act directly on brain cells, inducing behavioral and neurochemical effects, is still being investigated. PTH is known to augment entry of calcium into a variety of mammalian cells (34) and excess hormone increased the calcium content of various tissues, including peripheral nerves (35) and brain (20). An increase in intracellular calcium level may affect cell function directly, since intracellular calcium is a critical cell messenger, or by inducing changes in cell membrane permeability and integrity. Apart from this speculative interpretation, it is remarkable that PTH induces some biochemical effects on cells opposite to those observed with CT.

In animals and man it has been shown that the characteristic PTH hypercalcemia, that takes hours to develop, is preceded by an initial hypocalcemic phase (36-38). On the contrary, the classic CT hypocalcemia is preceded by a transient increase in serum calcium (38,39). The rapid PTH- and CT-induced changes in target cell calcium content may account for the early changes observed in serum calcium. These data fit in line with the hypothesis that the primary event in initiating the action of PTH is to cause a calcium inflow into the cell, and that the primary event of CT action on calcium cellular fluxes is to cause a decrease in intracellular concentration of calcium (38,39).

The red blood cell (RBC) is a target organ for PTH and CT. PTH has been shown to cause a significant influx of calcium into RBC (40), to stimulate the membranal Ca-ATPase activity (40), to decrease the deformability by increasing membrane rigidity (41), and to elevate the osmotic fragility of normal human RBC in vitro in a dose-dependent manner (40). CT has been shown to cause a significant calcium efflux from RBC by acting on Ca-ATPase system (42), and to increase the deformability of human RBC both in vitro and in vivo studies (43).

Finally, the possibility exists that PTH and CT may affect inositol phospholipids of cell membrane, thus producing alterations in agonist-receptor interaction (44). Recently, evidence has been given that PTH produces a dose-dependent immediate stimulation of inositol triphosphate (IP_3) production by kidney cell lines in culture (45). On the other hand, CT has been shown to inhibit the phospholipid hydrolysis and the production of IP_3 stimulated by norepinephrine in rat hippocampal slices (46).

In conclusion, activation of multiple mechanisms of cell signaling by PTH and CT may be important in regulating the cellular response to any one signal, not only in the classical target cells of the two hormones (kidney and bone cells), but also in brain cells.

CALCIOTROPIC HORMONES AND PAIN SENSITIVITY

A final point should be addressed. It is possible that the effects
of calciotropic hormones on behavior and on pain sensitivity may be due
to different and more complex mechanisms. In fact, CT-induced analgesia
and PTH-induced hyperalgesia can be the result of changes in the neurotransmitter and opioid systems regulating pain.

The mechanism through which CT induces analgesia is still debated.
At this regard, three theoretical pathways have been proposed. These include: a) increasing endogenous opioid release; b) altering the release
of neurotransmitters, such as catecholamines or serotonin; c) binding
directly to specific pain regulating sites in the central nervous system.
Evidence has been obtained for and against each of these hypotheses. In
animal and man the intravenous infusion of CT determines a sudden and
dose-dependent increase in circulating B-endorphin (47,48). Nevertheless,
the role of endogenous opiates as mediators for the analgesic effect of
CT remains controversial, since there are conflicting reports of the
ability of opiate antagonists, such as naloxone and levallorphan, to
antagonize this effect (49,50). Concerning the second hypothesis, a series
of recent studies suggest that the integrity of the serotonergic system
is required for CT-induced analgesia. In fact, it has been shown that
serotonin blocking and depleting agents antagonize the analgesic activity
of the hormone (10). Regarding the hypothesis of a direct analgesic effect of CT on the central nervous system, recent studies indicate that
there is a dense clustering of calcitonin binding sites in the areas of
the brain that regulate and modulate pain (51). The binding assay using
rat brain has shown that salmon calcitonin has a greater affinity than
mammalian calcitonins, i.e. porcine and human (52). These experimental
data suggest that the central effect of the hormone is probably different
with calcitonin of different species. The hypothesis that calcitonins
exert different potencies in producing analgesia has been recently tested
in patients with osteolytic metastases and bone pain. In this study it
has been demonstrated that salmon calcitonin is more effective in reducing
bone pain than human calcitonin (53). Thus, further studies are needed
to better clarify the mode of action of calcitonin as analgesic agent.

As it concerns the hyperalgesic activity of PTH, it is possible that
the hormone may influence the release of some neurotransmitters, such as
norepinephrine and acetylcholine, that exert a central action (33).
Furthermore, we cannot exclude that PTH-induced hyperalgesia may be dependent on an opioid mechanism. Studies are in progress in our laboratory
to establish whether opiate system is involved in the hyperalgesic effect
of PTH.

REFERENCES

1. G. Clementi, A. Prato, R. Bernardini, F. Nicoletti, F. Patti, D. De
   Simone, and U. Scapagnini, Effects of calcitonin on the brain of
   aged rats, Neurobiol. Aging 4:229-232 (1983).
2. F. Nicoletti, G. Clementi, F. Patti, P.L. Canonico, R.M. Di Giorgio,
   M. Matera, G. Pennisi, L. Angelucci, and U. Scapagnini, Effects of
   calcitonin on rat extrapyramidal motor system: behavioral and
   biochemical data, Brain Res.250:381-385 (1982).

3. G. Clementi, F. Nicoletti, F. Patacchioli, A. Prato, F. Patti, M. Matera, and U. Scapagnini, Hypoprolactinemic action of calcitonin and the tuberoinfundibular dopaminergic system, _J. Neurochem._ 40:885-886 (1983).

4. R. Isaac, R. Merceron, G. Coillens, J.P. Raymond, and R. Ardaillou, Effects of calcitonin on basal and thyrotropin releasing hormone stimulated prolactin secretion in man, _J. Clin. Endocrinol. Metab._ 50:1011-1015 (1980).

5. A. Pecile, S. Ferri, P.C. Braga, and V.R. Olgiati, Effects of intracerebroventricular calcitonin in the conscious rabbit, _Experientia_ 31:332-333 (1975).

6. C. Gennari, Clinical aspects of calcitonin in pain, _Triangle_ 22:157-163 (1983).

7. J. E. Morley, A. S. Levine, and S. E. Silvis, Intraventricular calcitonin inhibits gastric acid secretion, _Science_ 214:671-673 (1981).

8. W. J. Freed, M. J. Perlow, and R. J. Wyatt, Calcitonin: inhibitory effect on eating in rats, _Science_ 206:850-852 (1979).

9. F. Nicoletti, G. Clementi, F. Patti, A. Prato, R. M. Di Giorgio, and U. Scapagnini, Effects of parathyroid hormone on haloperidol induced catalepsy and nigral GAD activity, _Eur. J. Pharmacol._ 88: 135-136 (1983).

10. G. Clementi, F. Drago, M. Amico-Rowas, A. Prato, E. Rapisarda, F. Nicoletti, G. Rodolico, and U. Scapagnini, Central actions of calcitonin and parathyroid hormone, _in_: "Calcitonin 1984: Chemistry, Physiology, Pharmacology, and Clinical Aspects", A. Pecile ed., Excerpta Medica, Amsterdam, pp. 279-286 (1985).

11. G. Clementi, M. Amico-Roxas, F. Nicoletti, E.C. Fiore, A. Prato, and U. Scapagnini, Hyperalgesic activity of parathyroid hormone and its fragments in male rats, _Brain Res._ 295:376-377 (1984).

12. J. A. Fischer, S. M. Sagar, and J. B. Martin, Characterization and regional distribution of calcitonin binding sites in the rat brain, _Life Sci._ 29:663-671 (1981).

13. F. A. Tschopp, H. Henke, J. B. Petermann, P. H. Tobler, R. Janzer, T. Hökfelt, J. M. Lundberg, C. Cuello, and J. A. Fischer, Calcitonin gene-related peptide and its binding sites in the human central nervous system and pituitary, _Proc. Natl. Acad. Sci. USA_ 82:248-252 (1985).

14. M. G. Rosenfeld, S. G. Amara, and R. M. Evans, Alternative RNA processing: determining neuronal phenotype, _Science_ 225:1315-1320 (1984).

15. J. A. Fischer, P. H. Tobler, M. Kaufmann, W. Born, H. Henke, P.E. Cooper, S. M. Sagar, and J.B. Martin, Calcitonin: regional distribution of the hormone and its binding sites in the human brain and pituitary, _Proc. Natl. Acad. Sci. USA_ 78:7801-7805 (1981).

16. D. M. Pavlinac, L. W. Lenhard, J. G. Parthemore, and L. J. Deftos, Immunoreactive calcitonin in human cerebrospinal fluid, _J. Clin. Endocrinol._ 50:717-720 (1980).

17. F. Loffler, D. Van Calker, and B. Hamprecht, parathyrin and calcitonin stimulate cyclic AMP accumulation in cultured murine brain cells, _The EMBO J._ 1:297-302 (1982).

18. G. R. Mundy, and T. J. Martin, The hypercalcemia of malignancy: pathogenesis and management, _Metabolism_ 31:1247-1277 (1983).

19. F. Guerrero-Munoz, M. De Lourdes Guerrero, E. Leong Way, and C. Haoli, Effect of B-endorphin on calcium uptake in the brain, Science 206:89-91 (1979).

20. A. I. Arieff, and S. G. Massry, Calcium metabolism of brain in acute renal failure, J. Clin. Invest. 53:387-392 (1974).

21. D. A. Goldstein, M. Romoff, E. Bogin, and S. G. Massry, Relationship between the concentrations of calcium and phosphorus in blood and cerebrospinal fluid, J. Clin. Endocrinol. Metab. 49:58-62 (1979).

22. M. Akmal, D. A. Goldstein, S. A. Tuma, P. Fanti, R. Pattabhiraman, and S. G. Massry, The effect of parathyroid hormone (PTH) on the blood-brain barrier, Clin. Res. 31:52A (1983).

23. A. D. Care, and N. H. Bell, Evidence that parathyroid hormone crosses the blood brain barrier, in: "IXth International Conference on Calcium Regulating Hormones and Bone Metabolism", Nice oct. 25-nov. 1, 1986, Volume of Abstracts, Abstract 122, p. 181 (1986).

24. D. A. Goldstein, E. I. Feinstein, L. A. Chui, R. Pattabhiraman, and S. G. Massry, The relationship between the abnormalities in electroencephalogram and blood levels of PTH in dyalisis patients, J. Clin. Endocrinol. Metab. 51:130-134 (1980).

25. E. M. Allen, F. R. Singer, and D. Melamed, Electroencephalographic abnormalities in hypercalcemia, Neurology 20:15-23, 1970.

26. R. Guisado, A. I. Arieff, and S. G. Massry, Changes in the electroencephalogram in acute uremia. Effects of parathyroid hormone and brain electrolytes, J. Clin. Invest. 55:738-745 (1975).

27. S. G. Massry, Neurotoxicity of parathyroid hormone in uremia. Kidney Int. 28(suppl. 17):S5-S11 (1985).

28. M. G. Cogan, C. M. Covey, A. I. Arieff, A. Wisniesky, O. H. Clark, V. Lazarowitz, and W. Leach, Central nervous system manifestations of hyperparathyroidism, Am. J. Med. 65:963-971 (1978).

29. J. W. Gatewood, C. H. Organ, and B. T. Mead, Mental changes associated with hyperparathyroidism, Am. J. Psychiatry 132:129-132 (1975).

30. J. L. Crammer, Calcium metabolism and mental disorder, Psychol. Med. 7:557-560 (1977).

31. M. E. Gibbs, C. L. Gibbs, and K. T. Ng, A possible physiological mechanism for short-term memory, Physiol. Behav. 20:619-627 (1978).

32. M. E. Gibbs, C. L. Gibbs, and K. T. Ng, The influence of calcium on short-term memory, Neurosci. Lett. 14:255-360 (1979).

33. G. Clementi, F. Drago, A. Prato, S. Cavaliere, A. Di Benedetto, F. Leone, U. Scapagnini, and G. Rodolico, Effects of calcitonin, parathyroid hormone and its related fragments on acquisition of active avoidance behavior, Physiol. Behav. 33:913-916 (1984).

34. A. B. Borle, Calcium metabolism at the cellular level, Fed. Proc. 30:1944-1950 (1973).

35. D. A. Goldstein, L. A. Chui, and S. G. Massry, Effect of parathyroid hormone and uremia on peripheral nerve calcium and motor nerve conduction velocity, J. Clin. Invest. 62:88-93 (1978).

36. J. A. Parsons, R. M. Neer, and J. T. Potts Jr., Initial fall of plasma calcium after intravenous injection of parathyroid hormone, Endocrinology 89:735-740 (1971).

37. W. G. Robertson, M. Peacock, D. Atkins, and L. A. Webster, The ef-

fect of parathyroid hormone on the uptake and release of calcium by bone in tissue culture, Clin. Sci. 43:715-718 (1972).

38. A. Caniggia, and C. Gennari, Early effects of calcitonin in man: comparison with the early effects of parathyroid hormone, in: "Calcium Regulating Hormones", R. V. Talmage, M. Owen, J. A. Parsons, eds., Excerpta Medica, Amsterdam, pp. 154-156 (1975).

39. A. Caniggia, C. Gennari, F. Piantelli, and A. Vattimo, Initial increase of plasma radioactive calcium after intravenous injection of calcitonin in man, Clin. Sci. 43:171-180 (1972).

40. E. Bogin, S. G. Massry, J. Levi, M. Djaldeti, G. Bristol, and J. Smith, Effect of parathyroid hormone on osmotic fragility of human erythrocytes, J. Clin. Invest. 69:1017-1025 (1982).

41. C. Gennari, M. Montagnani, R. Civitelli, D. Agnusdei, R. Nami, and S. Bigazzi, Calcitonina, ormone paratiroideo, ione calcio, 3,5-adenosinmonofosfato ciclico (AMPc) e deformabilità eritrocitaria, La Ricerca Clin. Lab. 15(suppl. 1):465-473 (1985).

42. D. K. Parkinson, and I. C. Radde, Calcitonin action on membrane ATPase - a hypothesis, in: "Calcitonin 1969. Proceedings of the Second International Symposium", Heinemann Medical Books, London, pp. 466-471 (1970).

43. C. Gennari, M. Montagnani, R. Nami, R. Civitelli, P. Bartalini, C. Bianchini, and E. Maioli, The effects of calcitonins on erythrocyte filtration and calmodulin content in man, in: "VIII International Conference on Calcium Regulating Hormones", Kobe, Japan october 16-24, 1983, abstracts book p. 33 (1983).

44. H. Lo, D. C. Lehotay, D. Katz, and G. S. Levey, Parathyroid hormone-mediated incorporation of ^{32}P orthophosphate into phosphatidic acid and phosphatidylinositol in renal cortical slices, Endocr. Res. Commun. 3:377-385 (1976).

45. K. A. Hruska, D. Moskowitz, P. Esbrit, R. Civitelli, S. Westbrook, and M. Huskey, Stimulation of inositol triphosphate and diacylglycerol production in renal tubular cells by parathyroid hormone, J. Clin. Invest. 79:230-239 (1987).

46. G. Clementi, and U. Scapagnini, Personal communication, (1987).

47. J. J. Rohner, D. Planche, and F. Boudouresque, Calcitonin induced analgesia: experimental study suggesting both a morphine-like and a cortisone-like effect, Calcif. Tissue Int. 36(suppl.):S78 (1984).

48. C. Gennari, Calcitonin and bone metastases of cancer, in: "Calcitonin 1980. Chemistry, Physiology, Pharmacology, and Clinical Aspects", A. Pecile ed., Excerpta Medica, Amsterdam, pp. 277-287 (1981).

49. M. Yamamoto, S. Kumagai, S. Tachikawa, and M. Maeno, Lack of effect of levallorphan on analgesia induced by intracerebroventricular application of porcine calcitonin in mice, Europ. J. Pharmacol. 55:211-213 (1979).

50. P. C. Braga, S. Ferri, A. Santagostino, V. R. Olgiati, and A. Pecile, Lack of opiate receptor involvement in centrally induced calcitonin analgesia, Life Sci. 22:971-978 (1978).

51. H. Henke, F. A. Tschopp, and J. A. Fischer, Distinct binding sites for calcitonin gene-related peptide and salmon calcitonin in rat central nervous system, Brain Res. 360:165-171 (1985).

52. H. Nakamuta, S. Furukawa, M. Koida, H. Yajima, R. C. Orlowski, and R. Schlueter, Specific binding of ^{125}I-salmon calcitonin to rat brain: regional variation and calcitonin specificity, Japan J. Pharmacol. 31:53-60 (19817.

53. C. Gennari, S. M. Chierichetti, M. Piolini, C. Vibelli, D. Agnusdei, R. Civitelli, and S. Gonnelli, Analgesic activity of salmon and human calcitonin against cancer pain: a double-blind, placebo-controlled clinical study, Curr. Ther. Res. 38:298-308 (1985).

AGING AND PARATHYROID HORMONE

AGING AND PARATHYROID HORMONE

Takuo Fujita

Third Division, Department of Medicine
Kobe University School of Medicine

INTRODUCTION

Aging is always associated with abnormalities of calcium metabolism as shown by the universal phenomenon of age-dependent bone loss. Parathyroid hormone, the longest known calcium regulating hormone, is also involved in aging. Since 99 % of calcium in human body is found in the bone, bone loss is almost synonymous with calcium loss. Looking back the history of evolution,it is likely that life developed for the first time in the sea. On analyzing the human body, we find an unmistakable piece of evidence that we also came from the sea, rather than from the earth, the resemblance in the elements composing human body with components of seawater, but not those of the earth. Nine of the 10 most commonly occurring elements including calcium are the same between seawater and human body H, O, C, N, Na, Ca, S, K and Cl, whereas the soil contains only 5 of these, along with unfamiliar elements such as Al, Ti, Si and Fe. The most important difference between the environment of fishes living in seawater and that of land-abiding creatures including human beings in the abundance of calcium in the seawater, in contrast to the lack of calcium in the air. Land-abiding creatures including human beings are more deficient in calcium than fishes living in seawater, since food is the only source of calcium supply in the former, whereas as much calcium as necessary may be taken from seawater by fish through the gill (Fig 1). Absence of parathyroid glands in fish and their constant presence in land-abiding creatures may indicate the need for parathyroid glands in calcium-deficient environment.

As shown in Fig. 2,total body calcium decreases and bone calcium as we age, reflecting the progression of calcium deficiency. Prompted by such continued negative calcium balance, possibly through repeated, mild and transient hypocalcemia, PTH secretion rises, producing secondary hyperparathyroidism. Serum PTH measurement in normal subjects indicated an age-bound rise as shown in Fig. 3. Osteoporosis and secondary hyperparathyroidism therefore always accompanies aging. PTH brings calcium out of the bone and some of the calcium coming out of the bone deposits in the soft tissue.

New Actions of Parathyroid Hormone
Edited by S. G. Massry and T. Fujita
Plenum Press, New York

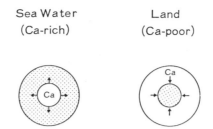

Sea Water
(Ca-rich)

Land
(Ca-poor)

Fig 1. Creatures living in seawater containing abundant calcium such as fish are in the state of calcium excess. Land-
abiding creatures breathing air are more deficient in calcium
than fishes. Parathyroid glands, always found in land-
abiding animals, are never found in fishes. The need for the
parathyroid glands has probably appeared in calcium deficient
environment.

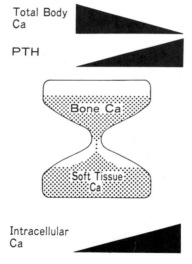

Total Body
Ca

PTH

Bone Ca

Soft Tissue
Ca

Intracellular
Ca

Fig 2. Sandclock of aging
In a calcium-deficient environment in which all land-abiding
creatures are placed, total body calcium decreases along
with aging, with concomitant rise in PTH. Bone loses calcium
and soft tissues like blood vessels and brain gain calcium
at the same time, PTH increases intracellular calcium
and blunt the extracellular/intracellular concentration
gradient.

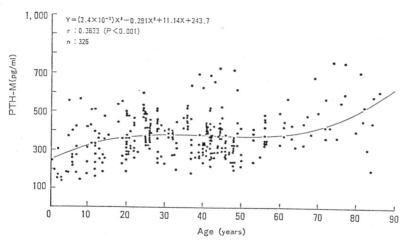

$Y = (2.4 \times 10^{-3})X^3 - 0.291X^2 + 11.14X + 243.7$
$r : 0.3633\ (P < 0.001)$
$n : 326$

Fig 3. Serum PTH in normal subjects measured by the use of antibody recognizing mid-and C-terminal portion. The best fit is obtained by three component curve consisting of a rise in growth. Constant values in adulthood and a final rise in old age.

EPIDEMIOLOGICAL STUDY

Towards the tip of the Kii Peninsula, the southern tip of the Japan mainland, two contrasting communities were selected for epidemiological studies. The mountain community of Kozagawa mainly engaged in forestry, with low calcium intake and less exposure to sunshine was also known because of a high incidence of amyotrophic lateral sclerosis. The seacoast community of Oshima mainly engaged in fishery, on the other hand, has taken enough calcium from seafood and bathed in abundant sunshine all the year round. The pertinent results in the epidemiological comparison between these two communities are summarized in Table 1. Death due to cardiovascular and cerebrovascular disease was more frequent in the mountain community despite low serum cholesterol.

Table 1. Comparison between mountain (Kozagawa) and seacoast (Oshima) communities

	Mountain	Seacoast
Body Height	Short	Normal
Lumbago	Frequent	Less Frequent
Bone Mass	Low	Normal
Serum P	Low	Normal
Serum Cholesterol	Low	Normal
Serum Protein	Low	Normal
Aortic Calcification	Frequent	Less Frequent

The mountain people were shorter, complained of more lumbago, with lower bone mass as suggested by narrower clavicular cortical thickness, and more frequent aortic calcification in chest X-ray picture. Serum phosphorus, cholesterol and total protein were lower, suggesting general malnutrition. The fact that lower calcium and vitamin D intake was associated with lower bone mass and more pronounced aortic calcification may support the concept of calcium shift from the bone to soft tissue in the process of aging.[2][3]

In another study on elderly hospitalized patients[4], serum calcium was found to be an important determinant of the prognosis. In a multi-factorial analysis to determine factors contributing to death due to any cause during hospitalization or survival until high serum creatinine was found to contribute to death and high serum calcium quite significantly to survival. Since hypocalcemia is usually accompanied by secondary hyperparathyroidism, tendency to hypocalcemia may indicate more advanced changes of calcium metabolism towards aging (Fig 4).

CALCIUM PARADOX OF AGING

The abnormalities of calcium metabolism associated with aging may be called calcium paradox of aging. [5] When insufficient calcium is available in food, absorption is incomplete due to vitamin D deficiency or other causes, or calcitonin action is insufficient, the bone loses so much calcium that a large amount of calcium is deposited in soft tissues such as blood vessels and brain to cause hypertension, arteriosclerosis and senile dementia. On the contrary, when sufficient calcium is ingested,

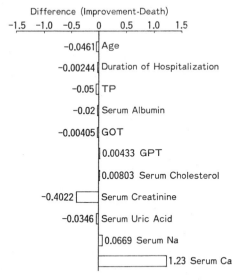

Fig 4. Multifactorial analysis of the factors contributing to death or survival of elderly hospitalized patients. Scale to the left contributes to death, whereas the scale to the right, to survival. Negative contribution of serum creatinine and positive contribution of serum calcium to survival is most conspicuous.

absorbed and held in the bone by the action of calcitonin, little calcium is deposited in the soft tissue. Thus the amount of calcium available from the digestive tract and the amount deposited in the soft tissue is by no means parallel, but is rather in opposite directions each other, or paradoxical (Fig 5).

In addition to aging, calcium paradox is also found in chronic renal failure. Since aging is characterized by progressive loss of renal function, it may not be surprising that aging and chronic renal failure have many things in common (Table 2). Since the kidney is the only site of 1,25(OH)$_2$ vitamin D synthesis under normal situation, decrease of serum 1,25(OH)$_2$ vitamin D$_3$ in both of these conditions with consequent decrease of intestinal calcium absorption is expected. Secondary

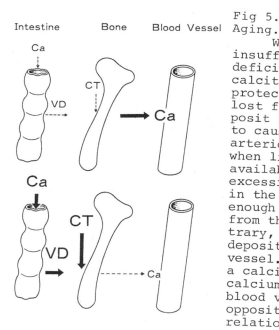

Intestine   Bone   Blood Vessel

Fig 5. Calcium Paradox of Aging.

When calcium intake is insufficient, vitamin D is deficient or not enough calcitonin is available to protect bone, calcium is lost from the bone to deposit in the blood vessel to cause hypertension or arteriosclerosis. Thus when little calcium is available from the the gut, excessive calcium is found in the blood vessel. When enough calcium is absorbed from the gut, on the contrary, little calcium is deposited in the blood vessel. Thus the amout a calcium absorbed and calcium deposited in the blood vessel are found in opposite or paradoxical relationship.

hyperparathyroidism, bone loss and increased calcium deposition in the soft tissue is also seen in both of these conditions. Decrease of immune function and increase of malignancy in renal failure and secondary hyperparathyroidism may be explained by blunting of extracellular/intracellular calcium concentration gradient through the action of PTH. In case calcium deficiency represents one of the factors causing many of the age-associated diseases related to calcium maldistribution throughout the body, such as osteoporosis[6], hypertension[7], arteriosclerosis[8] and possibly senile dementia[9], it follows that calcium supplementation along with agents to facilitate intestinal absorption of calcium may open a way to prevent these disease.

Table 2

Aging and Chronic Renal Failure

	Aging	Chronic Renal Failure
Renal Function	Decrease	Decrease
Serum 1,25(OH)-vitamin D_3	Decrease	Decrease
Intestinal Calcium Absorption	Decrease	Decrease
Serum PTH	Increase	Increase
Bone Mass	Decrease	Decrease
Calcium in Blood Vessel	Increase	Increase
Calcium in Brain	Increase	Increase
Immune Function	Decrease	Decrease
Malignancy	Increase	Increase

SUMMARY

1. Human, like all other land-abiding creatures, are calcium-deficient compared to fish. Such calcium deficiency becomes more pronounced in advancing age.
2. Insufficient Ca intake, decreased intestinal Ca absorption, and insufficient renal synthesis of 1,25(OH) vitamin D all contributes to Ca deficiency in aging.
3. Secondary hyperparathyroidism characterizes Ca metabolism in aging with Ca shift from bone to soft tissue causing osteoporosis on one hand, and hypertension, arteriosclerosis and senile dementia on the other. Action of PTH to increase intracellular Ca also tends to blunt extra/intracellular Ca concentration gradient, leading to generalized cell hypofunction in aging.

CONCLUSION

There is need for a unified concept to explain age-associated change of calcium distribution both on a whole body and individual cell basis. Calcium deficiency with secondary hyperparathyroidism may be the key to understand aging.

REFERENCES

1. T. Fujita, Aging and Calcium, Mineral & Electrolyte Metabolism 12: 149 (1986).
2. T. Fujita, Y. Okamoto, T. Tomita, Y. Sakagami, K. Ota and M. Ohata, Calcium metabolism in aging inhabitants of mountain versus seacoast communities in the Kii Peninsula, J. Amer. Geriat. Soc. 25:254 (1977).
3. T. Fujita, Y. Okamoto, Y. Sakagami, K. Ota and M. Ohata, Bone changes and aortic calcification in aging inhabitants of mountain versus seacoast communities in the Kii Peninsula, J. Amer. Geriat. Soc. 32:124 (1984).
4. T. Fujita, Serum Calcium an important determinant of the survival of elderly patients, Kobe J. Med. Sci. 30:1 (1984).
5. T. Fujita, Calcium and your health, Japan Publications (1987)
6. B.E.C. Nordin, Calcium balance and calcium requirement in osteoporosis, Amer. J. Clin. Nutrition 1: 384 (1962).
7. D.A. McCarron, C.D. Morris and C. Cole, Dietary calcium in human hypertension, Science 217:267 (1987).
8. N.D. Crawford, Hardness of drinking water and cardiovascular disease Proc. Nutr. Soc. 31:347 (1972).
9. A.I. Arieff and S.G. Massry, Calcium metabolism of the brain in acute renal failure, J. Clin. Invest. 53:387 (1974).

PARATHYROID HORMONE IN AGING RAT

Dike N. Kalu

Department of Physiology
The University of Texas Health Science Center
San Antonio, Texas 78284-7756, USA

INTRODUCTION

One of the first clear documentations that the physiological system undergoes aging was made over twenty-five years ago by Nathan Shock (1). He measured the indices of the physiological functions of many organ systems and demonstrated that their functional efficiency declined progressively with advancing age. Although this finding has acquired the status of a logo in the field of gerontological research on account of the frequency of its presentation at scientific meetings, the data on which it is based have been criticized especially because they are cross-sectional and, therefore, subject to interpretational problems. Also, some of the data such as the decline with aging in basal metabolic rate have been contested, and some physiological indices such as blood cholesterol and blood pressure actually go up rather than down with advancing age. In addition, there is increasing concern regarding the difficulties in determining whether an age-related physiological decline is a manifestation of primary aging processes or is secondary to extrinsic factors such as disease or lifestyle (2, 3).

Another way to illustrate the impact of aging is by examining the survival curves of different populations. A survival curve is simply a graphical representation of what proportion of people of the same age, or animals of the same species born at the same time, are alive at any point in time with advancing age. About 50 years ago, McCay (4) demonstrated that restricting the food intake of rats prolongs their life span. This observation has been repeatedly confirmed by other investigators in mice, rats, and hamsters (5, 6). In a study by Yu et al (6), Group A rats were fed ad libitum and Group R rats were fed 60% of the mean ad libitum food intake from 6 weeks of age until they died. In the protected environment of the laboratory the ad libitum fed rats had an almost rectangular survival curve with a mean length of life of 701 days, a median length of life of 714 days and a maximum length of life of 963 days. The food restricted animals lived much longer. Their survival curve was shifted to the right, and they had a mean length of life of 986 days, a median length of life of 1047 days and a maximum length of life of 1435 days. It has also been shown that in rodents, life-prolonging food restriction, in addition, retards age-related physiological deteriorations and age-related disease processes such as chronic nephropathy (7). This decade is witnessing a resurgence of interest in these fascinating actions of food restriction partly because food restriction is the only manipulation known to increase the life span of mammals. As such, it is a powerful tool for probing the aging process. In rats (8-10) as well as in humans (11-13), aging is associated with a progressive increase in circulating parathyroid hormone (PTH) that may be involved in aging bone loss (9-12). Since the underlying reasons for the increase as well as its consequences are uncertain, several years ago we undertook to explore the influence of aging on serum PTH and bone and assess whether any age-related changes are modulated by life-prolonging food restriction (9, 10).

EXPERIMENT 1

Specific pathogen-free (SPF) rats, purchased from Charles River Laboratories at 28 days of age and housed in our barrier facility to maintain their SPF status, were used in these studies. In the first experiment, two groups of rats were studied. One group was fed ad libitum and the other was fed 60% of the mean ad libitum food intake throughout their lives. The compositions of the rat diets were such that ad libitum and food restricted animals consumed the same amount of dietary calcium per day. From 6 weeks of age until senescence, 10 rats were bled at periodic intervals from each dietary group following an overnight fast. We observed that with aging, serum immunoreactive PTH increased in the rats fed ad libitum, and that the rats experienced loss of bone towards the end of their life span (9, 10). The increase in PTH was biphasic; an initial progressive increase occurred from 6 months to 24 months of age and was followed by a marked increase at 27 months of age. Both the increase in PTH and the terminal loss of bone were prevented by the restriction of food intake. Serum total calcium was slightly lower in the food restricted rats and in both dietary groups, serum phosphate decreased with aging.

The findings from this study raised the following questions. (a) Was the rise in serum PTH with aging due to the accumulation of inactive PTH fragments? (b) Did PTH not rise in the food-restricted animals because of their relatively higher dietary calcium intake? (c) Did the age- and dietary-modulated changes in PTH relate to alterations in kidney and intestinal functions? (d) Do other calcium-regulating hormones display similar age-related and dietary-modulated changes as those that occurred in PTH levels? (e) Can the age-related rise in PTH be prevented by dietary means other than food restriction, and what will be the consequence to aging bone loss?

EXPERIMENT 2

To address the above questions, a second experiment was carried out with three groups of animals. Rats in Group A were fed ad libitum Diet A with casein as the protein source as in the first study. Group B rats were fed Diet B (with casein as the protein source) at 60% of the mean ad libitum food intake as in the first study. However, the calcium content of Diet B was the same as that of Diet A with the result that in this second experiment Group B rats consumed per day 60% of the dietary calcium intake of Group A rats. This is in contrast to the first study where the calcium content of Diet B was adjusted such that rats in Groups A and B ingested similar amounts of calcium per day. Group C rats were fed ad libitum Diet C in which soy protein replaced casein as the protein source. Seven or more rats from each dietary group were bled and sacrificed at periodic intervals with aging, and serum PTH was measured with Nichols Institute intact-N-terminal PTH radioimmunoassay (RIA). In addition, renal pathology, renal function, femur density, intestinal calcium absorption, urine calcium, serum total calcium, blood ionized calcium, serum phosphate and serum calcitonin and vitamin D metabolites were measured.

We observed that serum immunoreactive PTH and calcitonin increased progressively with aging in the Group A rats. The increase was markedly suppressed by food restriction, and in the case of PTH by soy protein diet as well. Serum creatinine increased with aging after 18 months of age and both dietary regimens of Groups B and C rats retarded the increase. Aging was associated with a progressive fall in serum 25(OH)vitamin D, and loss of bone occurred during the terminal part of life in the ad libitum fed animals. These were prevented by food restriction while soy protein diet delayed the onset and magnitude of the bone loss. Ad libitum (casein) and food-restricted rats absorbed similar fractions of ingested calcium. Serum total but not blood ionized calcium or urinary calcium excretion was lower in the food-restricted than in the ad libitum (casein) fed rats, except at 24 months of age when they were similar. Serum phosphate decreased progressively with aging, with no dietary modulated differences between the ad libitum (casein) and food restricted animals.

DISCUSSION

Our findings in the two experiments confirm previous observations that serum PTH increases with aging (8-13). Most of the earlier reports on age-related increase in serum PTH were based on antisera that recognized the biologically inactive, carboxyl-terminal part of PTH as well. It is for this reason that in our second study PTH was measured with the Nichols Institute intact-N-terminal specific RIA, which is believed to measure bioactive PTH (14). Consequently, the age-dependent increase we observed in the serum PTH levels of male Fischer 344 rats in the second experiment is likely due to an increase in biologically active PTH. The suppression of this increase in serum PTH levels by food restriction confirms the findings from our first experiment in which we used a PTH RIA based on antibody of uncertain antigenic specificity (9, 10). In that study, the dietary calcium intake of the restricted rats was adjusted such that they ingested similar amounts of calcium per day as the ad libitum fed rats. Since they weighed less than the ad libitum fed rats, it is possible that the suppression of PTH levels in the food restricted animals related to their higher dietary calcium intake per unit body weight. This possibility was ruled out by our second study because the calcium contents of the diets of the ad libitum fed and food restricted rats were the same and the food restricted animals ingested per day only 60% of the calcium intake of the ad libitum fed animals. It is noteworthy that soy protein diet fed ad libitum was just as effective as food restriction in suppressing the age-related increase in serum PTH especially since the casein diet and the soy protein diet differed only in their protein source, and the rats consumed similar amounts of the diets per day (15).

That the increase with age in serum PTH in our rats is related to renal disease is supported by the well documented occurrence of secondary hyperparathyroidism in renal disease (16), the increase in the incidence and severity of chronic nephropathy with aging in the male Fischer 344 rats (7), and by our finding that after 18 months of age serum creatinine increased progressively in the animals fed casein containing diet ad libitum. The finding that food restriction and soy protein diet inhibited the increase in both serum PTH and serum creatinine indicates that these dietary manipulations might act to lower PTH levels, in part, by preventing age-related decline in renal function. The mechanism by which age-related decrease in renal function increases PTH secretion is not clear but it may relate to phosphate retention resulting in hypocalcemic stimulation of the parathyroid glands (16). However, aging in rats is not associated with hyperphosphatemia (9, 17). On the contrary, the plasma phosphate of rats in these studies was found to decrease progressively with aging with no decrease in plasma calcium that could account for the age-related increase in circulating PTH. It is also noteworthy that the initial increase in serum PTH from 6 to 18 months in the second experiment occurred when renal function appeared not to be compromised as determined by serum creatinine concentration, and that in both studies the prevention of age-related hyperparathyroidism by food restriction was associated with the inhibition of senile bone loss. Although soy protein was just as effective as food restriction in preventing age-related hyperparathyroidism, it did not, as food restriction, totally prevent the loss of bone found in the aged rats, but only delayed the onset and magnitude of the bone loss. Consequently, age-related bone loss in Fischer 344 male rats and its modulation by diet appear not to be due solely to changes in parathyroid hormone levels.

Our finding that in rats aging resulted in a progressive decrease in serum 25(OH)vitamin D that was prevented by food restriction is of particular interest, especially since a similar decrease has been reported in humans (18, 19). Although the level of circulating 25-hydroxyvitamin D in humans is potentially subject to a variety of influences such as sunlight, seasons and diet, the rat, in the stringently controlled environment of the laboratory with respect to diet, lighting, temperature and humidity is less subject to such influences. Our observations on serum 25-hydroxyvitamin D may, therefore, reflect the well documented decline that occurs with aging in hepatic protein synthesis and its modulation by food restriction (20, 21) since vitamin D-25-hydroxylase that catalyzes the formation of 25(OH)vitamin D is a liver enzyme (22). Surely more investigations such as the effects of aging and the experimental manipulations of these studies on intestinal absorption of vitamin D, on plasma vitamin D levels and on the metabolic clearance of 25-hydroxyvitamin D from plasma are required to fully explain our findings. It is noteworthy that serum 1,25(OH)$_2$vitamin D, which is formed by renal hydroxylation of 25(OH)vitamin D, was mostly higher in the food restricted rats but did not show the same age-related and dietary modulated changes as 25(OH)vitamin D. The significance, if any, of the differences in the levels of the vitamin D metabolites to the protection of the food-restricted animals from age-related bone loss remains to be determined.

CONCLUSION

We conclude that in the male Fischer 344 rats: (a) age-related increase in serum PTH precedes age-related decline in renal function; (b) age-related decline in renal function likely contributes to age-related hyperparathyroidism which in turn contributes to senile bone loss; (c) food restriction inhibits age-related hyperparathyroidism and senile bone loss; (d) and on the basis of the data from rats fed soy protein containing diet a decline in renal function and progressive hyperparathyroidism are not inevitable consequences of aging in the ad libitum fed rats.

REFERENCES

1.   Shock NW. Discussion on mortality and measurement. In: Strehler BL, Ebert JD, Glass HB, Shock NW (eds.), The Biology of Aging: A

Symposium, American Institute of Biological Sciences, Washington DC, 1960, p.23.

2. Masoro EJ. Biology of aging: Current state of knowledge. Arch Intern Med 147:166, 1987.

3. Rowe JW, Andres R, Tobin JB, Norris AH, Shock NW. The effect of age on creatinine clearance in man: a cross-sectional and longitudinal study. J Gerontol 31:155, 1976.

4. McCay CM, Crowell MF, Maynard LM. The effect of retarded growth upon the length of life span and upon the ultimate body size. J Nutrition 10:63, 1935.

5. Barrows CH Jr, Kokkonen GC. Comparative nutrition during aging. Comp Anim Nutr 4:274, 1981.

6. Yu BP, Masoro EJ, Murata I, Bertrand HA, Lynd FT. Life span study of SPF Fischer 344 male rats fed ad libitum or restricted diets: longevity, growth, lean body mass and disease. J Gerontol 37:130, 1982.

7. Maeda H, Gleiser CA, Masoro EJ, Murata I, McMahan CA, Yu BP. Nutritional influences on aging of Fischer 344 rats: II. Pathology. J Gerontol 40:671, 1985.

8. Armbrecht HJ, Forte LR, Halloran BP. Effect of age and dietary calcium on renal 25-OH-D metabolism, serum 1,25(OH)$_2$D and PTH. Am J Physiol 246:E266, 1984.

9. Kalu DN, Hardin RR, Cockerham R, Yu BP, Norling BK, Egan JW. Lifelong food restriction prevents senile osteopenia and hyperparathyroidism in F344 rats. Mech of Ageing and Devt. 26:103, 1984.

10. Kalu DN, Hardin RR, Cockerham R, Yu BP. Aging and dietary modulation of rat skeleton and parathyroid hormone. Endocrinology 115:1239, 1984.

11. Berlyne GM, Ben-Ari J, Kushelevsky A, Idelman A, Galinsky D, Hirsch M, Shainkin R, Yagil R, Zlotnik M. The aetiology of senile osteoporosis: secondary hyperparathyroidism due to renal failure. Q J Med New Ser XLIV:505, 1975.

12. Wiske PS, Epstein S, Bell NH, Queener SF, Edmondson J, Johnston CC. Increases in immunoreactive parathyroid hormone with age. N Engl J Med 300:1419, 1979.

13. Gallagher JC, Riggs BL, Jerbak CM, Arnaud CD. The effect of age on serum immunoreactive parathyroid hormone in normal and osteoporotic women. J Lab Clin Med 95:373, 1980.

14. Toverud SW, Boass A, Garner SC, Endres DB. Circulating parathyroid hormone concentrations in normal and vitamin D-deprived rat pups determined with an N-terminal-specific radioimmunoassay. Bone and Mineral 1:145, 1986.

15. Iwasaki K, Gleiser CA, Masoro EJ, McMahan CA, Seo E-J, Yu BP. The influence of dietary protein source on longevity and age-related disease processes of Fischer rats. J Gerontol, in press.

16. Slatopolsky E, Caglar JP, Pennell JP, Taggart DD, Canterbury JM, Reiss E, Pricker NS. On the pathogenesis of hyperparathyroidism

17. Kiebzak GM, Sacktor B. Effect of age on renal conservation of phosphate in the rat. Am J Physiol 21:F399, 1986.

18. Peacock M, Francis RM, Selby PL, Vitamin D and osteoporosis. In: Dixon A St. J, Russell RGG, Stamp TCB (eds). Osteoporosis: a multidisciplinary problem. Academic Press Inc., London, 1983, p.245.

19. Tsai K-S, Wahner HW, Offord KP, Melton LJ III, Kumar R, Riggs BL. Effect of aging on vitamin stores and bone density in women. Calcif Tissue Int 40:241, 1987.

20. Birchenall-Spark MC, Roberts MS, Staecker J, Hardwick JP, Richardson A. Effect of dietary restriction on liver protein synthesis in rats. J Nutrition 115:944, 1985.

21. Ward WF. Nutritional modulation of liver protein turnover in the aging Fischer 344 rat. Federation Proceedings 46:567 (Abstract), 1987.

22. Ponchon G, Kennan AL, DeLuca HF. Activation of vitamin D by the liver. J Clin Invest 48:2032, 1969.

CLINICAL TOPICS

THE NEUROMUSCULAR MANIFESTATIONS OF PRIMARY HYPERPARATHYROIDISM IN HUMANS

Dean T. Yamaguchi* and Charles R. Kleeman*

*Medical and Research Services, Veterans Administration Medical Center, West Los Angeles, +The Research Institute, Cedars-Sinai Medical Center, Division of Nephrology, Cedars-Sinai Medical Center, and UCLA School of Medicine, Los Angeles, CA

INTRODUCTION

The clinical manifestations of primary hyperparathyroidism can be of an immense spectrum from no symptomatology to the severest expression of the disease with renal stones, bone pain and fractures, gastrointestinal complaints, and neuropsychiatric manifestations. It is the purpose of this discussion to focus on the neuromuscular manifestations of hyperparathyroidism and to see whether parathyroid hormone (PTH) by itself or the other biochemical alterations induced by increased circulating levels of PTH, such as hypercalcemia or hypophosphatemia, can be implicated in the neuromuscular aberrations attributed to hyperparathyroidism.

A review of standard and well-known endocrine texts in the USA and in Europe was done to determine if there was any correlations between the frequency and nature of the reference to neuromuscular symptoms or signs and the year of publication of the book or its later editions. No such correlation was found. It became clear that most texts with more than one edition simply stated that the symptoms, when present, were related to the degree of hypercalcemia.

The incidence of neuromuscular disease in primary hyperparathyroidism has been reported to be approximately four percent (49 of 1205 patients summarized from 1954-1971) [1]. Weakness was the main neuromuscular symptom in these patients. Other smaller series prior to 1970 report incidences of weakness and/or fatigability as 64% (21 of 33 patients) [2] and 7% (6 of 91 patients) [3]. Review of the literature from the early 1970s to the present revealed that there are 88 more patients reported as having neuromuscular complaints [4-20]. Most of the reported patients were individual cases. However, of four series of patients with surgically proven primary hyperparathyroidism, the incidence of neuromuscular signs and symptoms ranged from a high of 61.5% [20] down to 37.5% [18] and 24-25% [8,17].

New Actions of Parathyroid Hormone
Edited by S. G. Massry and T. Fujita
Plenum Press, New York

CLINICAL MANIFESTATIONS

Generalized weakness and easy fatigability seemed to be the most common neuromuscular symptoms. More specifically, weakness was mostly localized to the lower extremities with proximal musculature mainly affected. Rarely, pain in affected muscle groups was reported (13). Physical examination of the neuromuscular system in those patients with specific neuromuscular complaints yielded a gamut of findings from only slightly decreased muscle strength or normal strength of the lower extremity proximal muscles and normal deep tendon reflexes to proximal muscle wasting, atrophy, and severely diminished strength and muscle tone and absent or hyperactive deep tendon reflexes. An example of the most extreme degree of hypotonia was described in a case reported by Barr and Bulger. al. (Fig. 1) (21). Seven of the above 88 patients were described as having gait abnormalities (4,5,8,14) characterized by a "waddling" or "ataxic" type of gait. Two of the 88 patients were reported as having a tremor (6,9). One patient's neuromuscular syndrome was severe enough to result in respiratory depression (10).

In addition to neuromuscular complaints related to the peripheral nervous system and muscles of the extremities, lesions perhaps involving more central neural or muscular structures were also evident in a number of patients. Abnormal tongue movements were reported in 12 patients (8). Glossal atrophy, hoarseness, dysphagia, dysarthria, mastication difficulties, and diplopia were found in a smaller number of patients (5,7-9). The above symptoms and physical findings suggest cranial nerve involvement or primary muscular involvement of the head and neck.

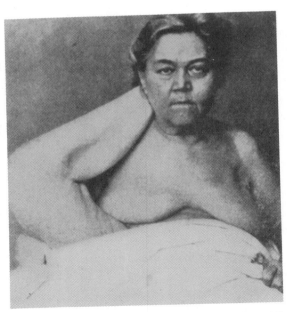

Fig. 1. Patient with severe hyperparathyroidism and marked hypotonicity (from Barr
and Bulger (21).)

Less commonly reported are abnormalities of the sensory system. Twelve of the 88 patients with neuromuscular symptoms had sensory disturbances. Most commonly, paresthesias and dysesthesias were related symptoms. Decreased vibratory sensation appeared to be the most common physical finding demonstrated in one series -- 8 of 16 patients with neuromuscular complaints had decreased vibratory sensation (8)

Neurological workup of patients with both motor and sensory deficits and primary hyperparathyroidism has been mainly that of nerve conduction studies, electromyography (EMG), and muscle biopsy. A hyperparathyroidism-associated myopathy was concluded on the basis of EMGs showing, in general, short duration (millisecond range), polyphasic potentials, usually with low amplitude (microvolt range) (3,22-25). These EMGs were felt to be consistent with a primary myopathy since such EMGs were also noted in other myositis-type of disease. Muscle biopsies revealed scattered atrophic fibers with some areas of muscle fiber degeneration. Rarely neutrophilic infiltration of muscle fibers was observed (24). Other histologic data showed loss of transverse striations, granular-vacuolar degeneration of fibers with enlarged sarcolemmal nuclei or clumping of nuclei. Where specified, type 1 muscle fibers (white or quick contraction fibers) appeared to be involved to a greater extent than type 2 fibers (red or prolonged contraction fibers) (25). Conclusion from these biopsies was that these specimens were representative of primary myopathy, at times suggestive of a myositis. Interestingly, a role for vascular insufficiency in the establishment of the myopathy was suggested due to findings of thickened basement membranes of endomysial blood vessels (25). Virtually all series or isolated reports have found normal nerve conduction velocities and distal sensory latencies in upper and lower extremity nerves sampled (3,8,9,14-16). Only three patients could be identified where nerve conduction velocities were abnormal, these three patients had neuromuscular symptoms. One patient had motor conduction impairment, another had sensory conduction impairment (18), while in a third patient, details were not given and the nerve conduction velocities were "abnormal" suggesting either a myopathy or neuropathy (19).

However, later descriptions (i.e. after 1971 in general) of the neuromuscular syndrome of hyperparathyroidism arrive at different conclusions of the type of neuromuscular disease based on EMG and muscle biopsy. A detailed study of 16 patients with primary hyperparathyroidism and evidence of neuromuscular disease (weakness, muscle atrophy, etc.) was done at the NIH in 1972 (12). In 12 of the patients, nerve conduction studies and EMGs were done. Nerve conduction velocities and distal sensory latencies were normal in all 12 patients. Ten of the 12 patients had abnormal EMGs. These EMG abnormalities ranged from high-amplitude, long duration, often polyphasic potentials, to short-duration, small amplitude, short polyphasic potentials. Others had decreased numbers of motor units under voluntary control on maximal effort. High amplitude, long duration potentials are suggestive of denervation. These investigators further believe that the low amplitude, short duration potentials are not due to previously described primary myopathy but that this type of potential can be seen in neuropathic disease "in which there is non-function or death of some but not all axonal twigs of many motor units and in which collateral reinervation is not prominent" (12).

The EMG data suggesting a neuropathic origin of these abnormal potentials is supported by the muscle biopsy specimens from 15 or 16 patients. Patten et. al (12) could not find evidence of a pure myopathy from the biopsies. Thus, myopathic evidence of necrosis, phagocytosed or regenerating muscle fibers, inflammatory cells, or increased fibrosis was not seen. Atrophy of muscles fibers was the most prevalent finding. The vast majority of atrophic fibers occurred in type 2 muscle fibers rather than type 1 fibers. The atrophic fibers also stained prominently with a NADPH-tetrazolium reductase reaction, a feature of muscle denervation. Since denervation of muscles causes greater atrophy of type 2 rather than type 1 fibers, it was concluded that the muscle abnormalities were secondary to denervation-like nerve dysfunction. Similarly, single fiber EMG by others (15,16) also support the conclusion of a neurogenic origin of the muscular abnormalities seen in primary hyperparathyroidism; paired blocking and unresponsive to edrophonium was suggestive of a synchronous release of acetylcholine at the neuromuscular junction.

THE UCLA EXPERIENCE

Between the years 1955 and 1985, approximately 200 cases of primary hyperparathyroidism were operated on at UCLA Medical Center. One hundred five of these cases were retrospectively and randomly selected from the medical files as part of a review of primary hyperparathyroidism at UCLA from the time the institution opened through 1985 -- approximately 30 years. Special attention was not necessarily paid to the neuromuscular syndromes, however, the degree of muscle weakness was graded in severity from 1[+] to 4[+]. 1[+] -- definite subjective complaint of some weakness in walking and climbing stairs; 2[+] -- further weakness with some difficulty getting up from a sitting position; 3[+] -- objective evidence of muscle weakness on exam with increasing complaints; 4[+] -- could not rise from a sitting position or rise from bed without help with definite muscle weakness. In reviewing these cases, we did not record the actual neurologic exam or laboratory test of neurological or muscular dysfunction.

Demographic features of the 105 patients with primary hyperparathyroidism were as follows: 21 males, mean age 47 ± 15 years; 84 females, mean age 53 ± 15 years; 11 blacks and 94 whites. Forty-four patients had weakness (42%). Overt neurological abnormalities that seemed consistent with neuromuscular disease in primary hyperparathyroidism was rarely seen. There was no relationship of the degree of weakness to the serum calcium (Fig. 2) or serum phosphorous levels. Furthermore, there was no correlation between the severity of neuromuscular dysfunction and the half-decade in which the given case was discovered during the period mid-1950s to mid-1985 (Fig. 3). PTH assay was not done at UCLA before 1973. PTH assays were available in 69 patients. There was no correlation between the severity of the weakness and the magnitude of the increase in serum PTH as presented as multiples of the upper limit of normal of any given assay for PTH.

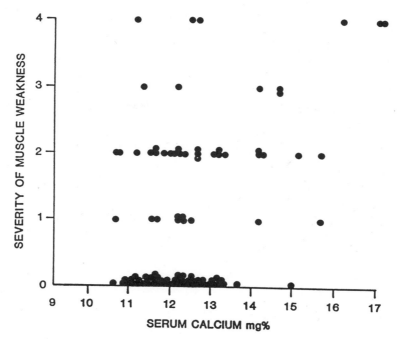

Fig. 2. The severity of muscle weakness related
to the level of hypercalcemia in primary
hyperparathyroidism.

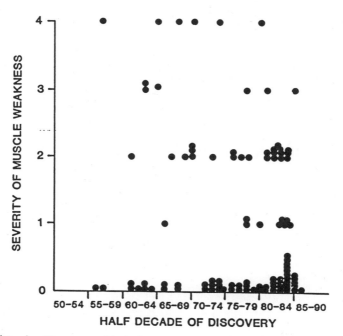

Fig. 3. The severity of muscle weakness in primary
hyperparathyroidism related to the half decade
when the disease was discovered.

NEUROMUSCULAR DISEASE AND BIOCHEMICAL ABNORMALITIES INDUCED BY PTH

The mechanism of how primary hyperparathyroidism can lead to neuromuscular manifestations is certainly unclear although there are numerous possibilities due to the biochemical abnormalities induced by high circulating levels of PTH. Hypercalcemia, hypophosphatemia, hypomagnesemia, or acid/base disturbances and associated hypokalemia may be hypothesized to contribute to the neuromuscular dysfunction.

Reports from the literature, however, tend to agree that the degree of hypercalcemia per se does not appear to correlate with the severity of the neuromuscular manifestations (9,12,19,22,24-26). In fact, neuromusucular manifestations in secondary hyperparathyroidism resulting from causes other than renal failure are similar to those reported in primary hyperparathyroidism (proximal muscle weakness, muscle atrophy, involuntary tongue movements, decreased vibratory sensation). These same clinical findings occur in patients with normocalcemia or hypocalcemia (3,22,27). Further, EMG studies and muscle biopsies from these patients appear similar to those from patients with primary hyperparathyroidism.

Similarly, the degree of hypophosphatemia does not seem to correlate with the severity of neuromuscular disease although it is well known that severe phosphate depletion with serum phosphate levels below 1 mg/100 ml can result in alterations in cardiac muscle (cardiomyopathy) as well as skeletal muscle (rhabdomyolysis) (28).

Other potential causes for neuromuscular disease in primary hyperparathyroidism may be due to an associated proximal renal tubular acidosis (29) and attendant hypokalemia and/or hypomagnesemia. Hypomagnesemia resulting from decreased proximal tubular reabsorption has been shown to enhance potassium excretion (30,31). However, when infrequently reported in those patients with primary hyperparathyroidism and neuromuscular disease, serum potassium and magnesium concentrations were normal. It should be noted that serum levels of ions such as phosphate, magnesium and potassium which are primarily intracellular ions may be misleading in determining a truly depleted or repleted state of tissue such as muscle. Thus, correlation between degree of clinical neuromuscular disease and intracellular ionic levels may yet exist.

The clinical syndrome of proximal muscle weakness and gait abnormalities (waddling gait) has been well-described in osteomalacia due to vitamin D deficiency (32,33), suggesting a potential link between abnormal vitamin D metabolism and neuromuscular disease in primary and secondary hyperparathyroidism (9,22). With secondary hyperparathyroidism, muscular weakness in general responds well to vitamin D replacement (3,22) although determination of vitamin D or its most potent metabolite, 1,25 dihydroxycholecalciferol (1,25D) was not done in those patients responding to vitamin D replacement. In primary hyperparathyroidism, it is expected that the increased levels of circulating PTH would stimulate 1a-hydroxylase in the proximal tubule of the kidney to enhance 1,25D production. In one patient with primary hyperparathyroidism and severe neuromuscular disease, serum 1,25D level was indeed found to be elevated (33). No such vitamin D determinations were made in any of the other reports or series describing neuromuscular disease in primary hyperparathyroidism. Thus it is difficult to reconcile what specific role vitamin D plays in the etiology of the neuromuscular manifestations. However, it is clear that there are remarkable subjective and objective similarities between those cases of primary hyperparathyroidism with neuromuscular disease and cases of secondary hyperparathyroidism due to vitamin D deficiency, excluding the cases of secondary hyperparathyroidism due to chronic renal failure. It is plausible that the increase in PTH levels results in an increased demand for 25-hydroxycholecalciferol (25D) and calcium in primary hyperparathyroidism (34). Individuals who develop primary hyperparathyroidism and who have marginal intakes of calcium and/or vitamin D over years would, therefore, have a relative deficiency of vitamin D and its metabolites. Therefore, the neuromuscular syndrome observed in primary hyperparathyroidism and the neuromuscular manifestations noted in secondary hyperparathyroidism may be a reflection of a disorder of vitamin D metabolism.

CELLULAR ASPECTS OF PTH AND VITAMIN D INTERACTIONS

PTH itself could directly affect muscle and/or neuronal tissues to account for the clinical syndrome of neuromuscular disease in hyperparathyroid states. At least in dogs, administering PTH to normal animals resulted in a decrease in motor nerve conduction velocities and an increase in nerve calcium content (35). Recently, Fraser and Sarnacki (36) have reported direct PTH action on nerve synaptosomes derived from rat brain cortex. PTH increased Ca^{2+} uptake by 19% in synaptosomes independent of cAMP levels in synaptosomes. It is well-established that upon depolarization of synaptosomes, an increased rate of Ca^{2+} uptake occurs that can be correlated to an increase in the rate of neurotransmitter release (37). Thus, an increase in free cytosolic calcium concentration $[Ca^{2+}]_i$ may be a trigger for neurosecretion at nerve terminals.

Studies by Nachshen (38) have shown that Na^+/Ca^{2+} exchange plays a role in the recovery of basal $[Ca^{2+}]_i$ after an increase in $[Ca^{2+}]_i$ in nerve terminals. PTH can directly stimulate Na^+/Ca^{2+} exchange at least in isolated renal cells (39); the stimulation of Na^+/Ca^{2+} exchange was correlated with an increase in cellular cAMP as Na^+-dependent Ca^{2+} transport and cAMP generation had similar concentration dependencies and time course of action. Interestingly, at least in bone, PTH has been shown to depolarize osteoblast-like cells from rabbit long bones (40). Thus, it is possible that PTH may cause increases in $[Ca^{2+}]_i$ in nerve terminals by the depolarization of nerve terminals. The increase in $[Ca^{2+}]_i$ would lead to a release of the neurotransmitter, acetylcholine at nerve terminals. Augmentation of Na^+/Ca^{2+} exchange activity may quickly decrease $[Ca^{2+}]_i$ toward resting levels, thus preparing the nerve terminals for further Ca^{2+} entry stimulated by PTH and further release of neurotransmitter. The constant repetitive cycling of depolarization, Ca^{2+} influx, and neurotransmitter release with subsequent hydrolysis of acetylcholine, may deplete nerve terminals of acetylcholine, thus accounting for defective neuromuscular transmission. It has been suggested that edrophonium chloride, an acetylcholinesterase inhibitor may be a useful drug in defining neuromuscular abnormalities in hyperparathyroidism. In fact Kaplan et al. (16,17) suggest that edrophonium-insensitive paired blocking by single-fiber EMG found in primary hyperparathyroidism could be explained by dysfunction of acetylcholine release.

PTH is known to directly affect muscle. Bogin et. al. (41) described positive inotropic and chonotropic effects of PTH on cardiac muscle. PTH has also been shown to stimulate cAMP production in cardiac muscle (42). However, little is known about the metabolic effects of PTH on skeletal muscle. In fact, in rat hemicorpus preparations, acute PTH infusion did not affect glucose uptake, protein synthesis or degradation, or release of amino acids from muscle (43). No data is available specifically concerned with the effect of PTH on calcium homeostasis or other ion fluxes in skeletal muscle. Furthermore, we are not aware of specific studies of the effect of PTH on calcium transport in nerve cell bodies in the spinal cord.

At the cellular level, evidence is accumulating that 1,25D is able to affect cytosolic calcium independent of a genomic action via calcium binding protein. In hepatocytes, 1,25D was shown to increase $[Ca^{2+}]_i$ gradually over 5 minutes after in vitro administration. Furthermore, an increase in $[Ca^{2+}]_i$ was also correlated with decreased production of 25D in hepatocytes (44). The early effect of 1,25D suggests plasma membrane interaction of a target cell with 1,25D. Indeed, 1,25D stimulates ^{47}Ca accumulation into duodenal tissue from rachitic chicks within 20-30 minutes (45). Furthermore, 1,25D hyperpolarizes rabbit chondrocytes but not muscle (46,47).

It is possible that 1,25D or other vitamin D metabolites may interact with PTH in such a way as to modify the effect of PTH on second messenger generation and ultimate physiologic function in nerve terminals (Fig.4). In a well-known target tissue of PTH, the osteoblast, PTH has been shown to increase $[Ca^{2+}]$ by both cAMP-independent and cAMP-dependent calcium channels (48). Furthermore, 1,25D attenuates cAMP generation in response to PTH. The mechanism of how 1,25D attenuates PTH mediated cAMP response is suggested to be at the PTH receptor-N (stimulatory guanine nucleotide binding regulatory protein) complex (49). Lieberherr et al. (50) reported that 1,25D inhibited basal accumulation of cAMP while 25D and 24,25 dihydroxycholecalciferol (24,25D) enhanced basal cAMP content in rat calvariae. However, these investigators did not find a suppressive action of 1,25D on PTH ability to stimulate cAMP production despite an apparent inhibition of PTH-stimulated cAMP accumulation by 1,25D (since cAMP levels were lower in calvariae stimulated with PTH and 1,25D compared to PTH alone). In addition, 25D and 24,25D have been shown to inhibit calcium uptake by bone cells in vitro (51).

In summary, if it can be shown that PTH and vitamin D metabolites, 1,25D, 24,25D, and 25D, can act directly at the

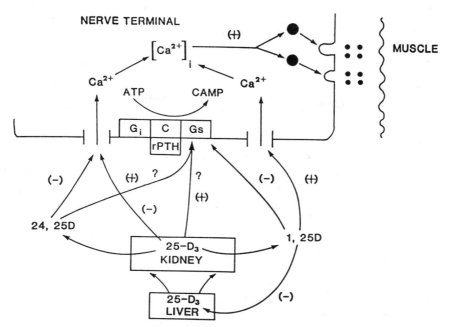

Fig. 4. Hypothesis to explain the neuromuscular abnormalities in PHP. The interrelationship between PTH
and vitamin D metabolites: normal conditions.

nerve terminal, one can speculate that for proper coordinated
release of acetylcholine at the nerve terminal, closely
regulated second messenger function of Ca^{2+} and cAMP must
occur. PTH can increase both $[Ca^{2+}]_i$ and cAMP. 1,25D can
perhaps suppress cAMP production while 24,25D and 25D can
enhance cAMP accumulation but also antagonize an increase in
$[Ca^{2+}]_i$. The modulating effect of 24,25D and 25D on PTH-
stimulated $[Ca^{2+}]_i$ may be a key in coordinating acetylcholine
release. In primary hyperparathyroidism, increased PTH
activity occurs. This activity stimulates renal la-hydroxylase
to increase 1,25D production. Together, PTH and 1,25D can
immensely augment Ca^{2+} entry into the nerve terminal to cause
acetylcholine depletion and/or dysfunctional release. Since an
increase in 1,25D can suppress 25D production and thus
indirectly suppress 24,25D production, relatively lower levels
of these latter two vitamin D metabolites may be present. The
ability of 24,25D to antagonize the PTH and 1,25D rise in
$[Ca^+]_i$ and their ability to establish an adequate level of
cAMP in the nerve terminals may then not occur. This imbalance
at the nerve terminal and the myoneural junction may lead to
the clinical syndrome of neuromuscular disease in primary
hyperparathyroidism (Fig. 5). In secondary
hyperparathyroidism, due to a deficiency of vitamin D and,
therefore, of 25D, 24,25D, and 1,25D metabolites, lack of an
inhibitory effect of 24,25D and of 25D on PTH-activated Ca^{2+}
channels may allow an augmented stimulation of Ca^{2+} entry into
the nerve terminal by PTH. Thus, the end result on Ca^{2+} and
subsequent neurotransmitter release may be the same in both
primary and secondary hyperparathyroidism.

1° HYPERPARATHYROIDISM

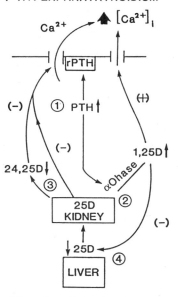

2° HYPERPARATHYROIDISM

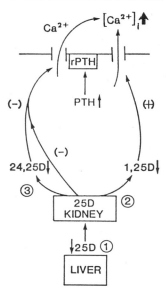

Fig. 5. Hypothesis to explain the neuromuscular abnormalities in PHP. The interrelationship between PTH and vitamin D metabolites: primary and secondary hyperparathyroidism.

Finally, review of the literature, and those patients with muscle weakness and primary hyperparathyroidism described from the UCLA Medical Center show no correlation with serum calcium levels (Fig. 2). However, it should be noted that a rise in extracellular calcium without a proportionate increase in $[Ca^{2+}]_i$ may effect neuromuscular transmission. The excitability of nervous tissue is determined by the difference between the resting membrane potential, Em, and the threshold potential, Et (52). Hypercalcemia, or a rise in extracellular ionized calcium raises the Et, thereby making the firing of an action potential much more difficult. This would translate into a decreased neuromuscular excitability. In this way, hypercalcemia, independent of the schema presented above, could contribute to weakness and reduced muscle tone.

FUTURE DIRECTIONS

In order to further investigate the potential role of vitamin D in the development of neuromuscular disease in primary hyperparathyroidism, the following suggestions are offered.

(1) Prior to and post-operatively in patients with hyperparathyroidism, serum levels of 1,25D, 24,25D, and 25D would be helpful in establishing the vitamin D status of the patient. (2) A careful dietary history should be obtained, specifically with respect to quantitating the amount of calcium intake in patients with primary hyperparathyroidism. (3) Careful and pointed history and physical examination of patients with neuromuscular complaints should be established. Specifically, a careful neurological examination should be done. If any positive historical and/or physical findings appear, EMG and/or muscle biopsy should be contemplated to try

to obtain more objective data pinpointing neuromuscular dysfunction. If available, single fiber EMG with edrophoniam provocation should be tried. (4) For in vitro investigative work on the potential mechanism of how vitamin D metabolites interact with PTH at nerve terminals, one must first examine the direct effect of PTH and vitamin D metabolites, spearately or in concert, in neurotransmitter release. (5) If direct effects of PTH and/or vitamin D metabolites can be shown to affect neutotransmitter release, then the involvement of potential second messengers such as $[Ca^{2+}]_i$ and cAMP on neutrotransmitter release can be studied. How vitamin D modifies the known PTH second messengers of $[Ca^{2+}]_i$ and cAMP · finally be determined to show if the models hypothesized to explain the neuromuscular abnormalities in primary hyperparathyroidism can be substantiated.

REFERENCES

1. Rabin, D. and T.J. McKenna, 1982, Clinical Endocrinology and Metabolism. 672p. Grune Publisher, New York.
2. Vicale, C.T., 1949. The diagnostic features of a muscular syndrome resulting from hyperparathyroidism, osteomalacia owing to renal tubular acidosis, and perhaps related disorders of calcium metabolism. Trans. Amer. Neurological Assoc. 74:143.
3. Smith, R. and G. Stern, 1967. Myopathy, osteomalacia and hyperparathyroidism. Brain 90:593.
4. Caughey, J.E., G. Parendeh, L.B. Cohen, and M. Vameghi, 1971. Multiple endocrine adenomatosis with metabolic myopathy. N.Z. Med. J. 74:18.
5. Cape, C.A., 1971. Increased phosphorylase activity in muscle in hyperparathyroid disease. Neurology 21:638.
6. Goodhue, W.W., J.N. Davis and R.S. Porro, 1972. Ischemic myopathy in uremic hyperparathyroidism. JAMA 221:911.
7. Hines, J.R. and J.R. Suker, 1973. Some unusual manifestations of parathyroid disease. Surg. Clinics of No. Am. 53:221.
8. Aurbach, G.D., L.E. Mallette, B.M. Patten, D.A. Heath, J.L. Doppman and J.P. Bilezikian, 1973. Hyperparathyroidism: recent studies. Ann.Int. Med. 79:566.
9. Caplan, R.H. and K.C. Bogart, 1974. Myopathy in primary hyperparathyroidism. Wisc. Med. J. 73:527.
10. Soucie, J., 1974. Letter: Hypercalcemia and neuromuscular disease. Ann. Int. Med. 81:128.
11. Tashima, C.K., 1974. Letter: Hypercalcemia and neuromuscular disease. Ann. Int. Med. 81:129.
12. Patten, B.M., J.P. Bilezikian, L.E. Mallette, A. Prince, W.K. Engle and G.D. Aurbach, 1974. Neuromuscular disease in primary hyperparathyroidism. Ann. Int. Med. 80:182.
13. Gerster, J.C., T.L. Vischer, A. Panchaud, P. Burchhardt, E. Courvoisier and G.H. Fallet, 1975. Myalgies dans l'hyperparathyroidie primaire: un diagnostic differentiel de la polymyalgia rheumatica. Schweiz. Med. Wschr. 105:623.
14. Rollinson, R.D. and B.S. Gilligan, 1977. Primary hyperparathyroidism presenting as a proximal myopathy. Aust. N.Z. J. Med. 7:420.
15. Kaplan, P.E., J.R. Hines, J.E. Leestma and H.J. Ruder, 1980. Neuromuscular junction transmission deficit in a patient with primary hyperparathyroidism. Electromyog. Clin Neurophysiol. 20:359.

16. Kaplan, P.E., H.J. Ruder and J.R. Hines, 1982. Neuromuscular junction dysfunction in primary hyperparathyroidism: A new hypothesis. Electromyog. Clin. Neurophysiol. 22:239.

17. Tibblin, S., N. Palsson and J. Rydberg, 1983. Hyperparathyroidism in the lederly. Ann. Surg. 197:135.

18. Ljunghall, S., G. Akerstrom, G. Johansson, Y. Olsson and E. Stalberg, 1984. Neuromuscular involvement in primary hyperparathyroidism. J. Neurology 231:263.

19. Yalowitz, D.L., A.S. Brett and J.M. Earll, 1984. Far-advanced primary hyperparathyroidism in an 18-year-old man. Am. J. Med. 77:545.

20. Wersall-Robertson, E., B. Hamberger, H. Ehren, E. Eriksson and P.O. Granberg, 1986. Increase in muscular strength following surgery for primary hyperparathyroidism. Acta. Med. Scan. 220:233.

21. Barr, D., P. Bulger, Amer. J. Med. Sc. 179:449, 1930.

22. Prineas, J.W., A.S. Mason and R.A. Hanson, 1965. Myopathy in metabolic bone disease. Br. Med. J. 1:1034.

23. Bischoff, A. and E. Esslen, 1965. Myopathy with primary hyperparathyroidism. Neurology 15:64.

24. Frame, B., E.G. Heinze, Jr., M.A. Block and G.A. Manson, 1968. Myopathy in primary hyperparathyroidism. Observations in three patients. Ann. Int. Med. 68:1022.

25. Cholod, E.J., M.D. Haust, A.J. Hudson and F.N. Lewis, 1970. Myopathy in primary familial hyperparathyroidism. Am. J. Med. 48:700.

26. Kendall-Taylor, P. and D.M. Turnbull, 1983. Endocrine myopathies. Br. Med. J. 287:705.

27. Mallette, L.E., B.M. Patten and W.K. Engel, 1975. Neuromuscular disease in secondary hyperparathyroidism. Ann. Int. Med. 82:474.

28. Brautbar, N. and C.R. Kleeman, 1987. Hypophosphatemia and hyperphosphatemia: clinical and pathophysiologic aspects. In Clinical Disorders of Fluid and Electrolyte Metabolism. Eds. M.H. Maxwell, C.R. Kleeman and R.g. Narins, 4th Ed. McGraw Hill Book Co., New York, pp. 789.

29. Pessah, M. and W. Frank, 1974. Letter: hyperparathyroidism and renal tubular acidosis. Ann. Int. Med. 80:116.

30. Ginn, H.E. and L.L. Shanbour, 1967. Phosphaturia in magnesium-deficient rats. Am. J. Physiol. 212:1347.

31. Shils, M.E., 1969. Experimental human magnesium depletion. Medicine (Baltimore) 48:61.

32. Ekbom, K., R. Hed, L. Kirstein and K.E. Astrom, 1965. Weakness of proximal limb muscles, probably due to myopathy after partial gastrectomy. Acta Medica Scan. 176:493.

33. Thage, O., 1970. Metabolic neuropathies and myopathies in adults. Clinical aspects. Acta Neuro. Scand. 46 (Suppl. 43):120.

34. Kleeman, C.R., K. Norris and J.W. Coburn, 1987. Is the clinical expression of primary hyperparathyroidism a function of the long-term vitamin D status of the patient? Min. Elec. Metab. 13:305.

35. Goldstein, D.A., L.A. Chui and S.G. Massry, 1978. Effect of parathyroid hormone and uremia on peripheral nerve calcium and motor nerve conduction velocity. J. Clin. Invest. 62:88.

36. Fraser, C.L. and p. Sarnacki, 1987. Parathyroid hormone facilitates calcium transport in rat brain synaptosomes by cAMP independent pathway. Kidney Int. 31:347A.

37. Blaustein, M.P., 1975. Effects of potassium, veratridine and scorpion venom on calcium accumulation and transmitter release by nerve terminals in vitro. J. Physiol.247:617.

38. Nachshen, D.A., 1985. Regulation of cytosolic calcium concentration in presynaptic nerve endings isolated from rat brain. J. Physiol. 363:87.

39. Sacktor, B., H. Hanai, M. Ishida and C.T. Liang, 1986. Action of PTH on Na^+-Ca^{2+} exchange in isolated renal cells. Kidney Int. 29:171A.

40. Chow, S.Y., Y.C. Chow, W.S.S. Jee and D.M. Woodbury, 1984. Electro-physiological properties of osteoblast-like cells from the cortical endosteal surface of rabbit long bones. Calcif. Tissue Int. 36:401.

41. Bogin, E., S.G. Massry and I. Harary, 1981. Effect of parathyroid hormone on rat heart cells. J. Clin. Invest. 67:1215.

42. Massry, S.G., D.A. Goldsteion, M. Akmal and E. Gogin. The role of parathyroid hormone as a uremic toxin. In: 12th Annual Contractors Conference, Artificial kidney -- Chronic Uremia Program, 1979, p. 49.

43. Wassner, S.J. and J.B. Li, 1987. Lack of acute effect of parathyroid hormone within skeletal muscle. Int. J. Ped. Neph. 8:15.

44. Baran, D.T. and M.L. Milne, 1986. 1,25 dihydroxyvitamin D increases hepatocyte cytosolic calcium levels,. A potential regulator of vitamin D-25-hydroxylase. J. Clin. Invest. 77:1622.

45. Fullmer, C.S., M.E. Brindak, S. Edelstein and R.H. Wasserman, 1984. Early and direct effect of 1,25-dihydroxycholecalciferol on calcium uptake by duodena of rachitic dhicks (41972). Proc. Soc. Exp. Biol. Med. 177:455.

46. Edelman, A., C.L. Thil, M. Garadedian, T. Anagnostopoulos and S. Balsan, 1983. Genome-independent effects of 1,25 dihydroxyvitamin D-3 on membrane potential. Biochem. Biophys. Acta 732:300.

47. Edelman, A., C.L. Thil, M. Garabedian, J.J. Plachot, H. Guillozo, J. Fritsch, S.R. Thomas and S. Balsan, 1985. Vitamin D metabolite effects on membrane potential and intracellular potassiuim activity in rabbit cartilage. Min. Elec. Metrab. 11:97.

48. Yamaguchi, D.T., T.J. Hahn, A. Iida-Klein, C.R. Kleeman and S. Muallem, 1987. Parathyroid hormone-activated calcium channels in an osteoblast-like osteosarcoma cell line: cAMP-dependent and cAMP-independent calcium channels. J. Biol. Chem. 262:7711.

49. Catherwood, B.D., 1985. 1,25-dihydroxycholecalciferol and glucocorticosteroid regulation of adenylate cyclase in an osteoblast-like cell line. J. Biol. Chem. 260:736-743.

50. Lieberherr, M. Garabedian, H. Guillozo, C.L. Thil and S. Balsan, 1980. In vitro effect of vitamin D_3 metabolites on rat calvaria cAMP content. Calcif. Tissue Int. 30:209.

51. Dziak, R., 1978. Effects of vitamin D_3 metabolites on bone cell calcium transport. Calcif. Tissue Int. 26:65.

52. Shanes, A.M., 1968. Electrochemical aspects of physiological and pharmacological action in excitable cells II the action potential and excitation. Pharmacol. Rev. 10:165.

HYPOPARATHYROIDISM: A CLINICAL REVIEW

A. McElduff and S. Posen

Department of Endocrinology, Royal North Shore
Hospital, Sydney, N.S.W., Australia. 2065

Introduction

The term "hypoparathyroidism" describes a variety of
conditions characterised by a decrease in some or all of the
action of parathyroid hormone (PTH), the net result of which in
the untreated state is hypocalcaemia.

Mechanism of Action of PTH

PTH, an 84 amino acid single chain peptide, is formed from
pre-pro-PTH in the parathyroid glands. PTH is released in
response to a fall in extra-cellular calcium concentration, it
enters the circulation and interacts with PTH receptors in various
target tissues. The 1-34 amino terminal fragment which retains
full biological activity, is present in the circulation with
intact 1-84 PTH and biologically inactive C-terminal fragments.

PTH has a number of physiological effects. In the kidney, it
causes an increase in phosphate clearance, a decrease in calcium
clearance and an increase in the production of 1,25 dihydroxyvitamin D_3 ($1,25(OH)_2D_3$) from 25 hydroxyvitamin D_3 ($25OHD_3$). PTH
also increases the tubular absorption of magnesium and the
clearance of bicarbonate, sodium and free water. In bone, PTH
produces two effects. It causes a rapid release of calcium
probably in part dependent on the availability of $1,25(OH)_2D_3$.
PTH also causes a more gradual increase in bone remodelling
possibly independent of vitamin D metabolites (1). In the
intestine PTH enhances calcium absorption via $1,25(OH)_2D_3$. A
direct effect may also exist (2).

At the cellular level PTH binds to its receptor, the PTH-PTH
receptor complex interacts with the guanine nucleotide binding (G)
regulatory subunit, which then activates adenylate cyclase so that
cyclic AMP (cAMP) is produced. cAMP, by mechanisms unknown, but
probably via a series of kinases, mediates the various PTH
effects. PTH may act via non-cAMP mediated response pathways (3).

The overall effect of PTH is an increase in the concentration
of calcium and a decrease in the concentration of phosphate in the
extracellular fluid (see 4 for reviews).

New Actions of Parathyroid Hormone
Edited by S. G. Massry and T. Fujita
Plenum Press, New York

Hypoparathyroidism (i) Due to PTH Deficiency

PTH deficient patients are classified as <u>post-surgical</u> (currently the largest group) and <u>idiopathic</u>. Within the idiopathic group several entities are recognized. In some patients PTH deficiency is associated with other endocrine or non-endocrine diseases such as Addison's disease or pernicious anaemia, and it is believed that these disorders have an "<u>autoimmune</u>" basis (5). Others have associated <u>branchial cleft dysembryogenesis</u> with thymic dysfunction such as Di George's syndrome. Subtle thymic abnormalities may be responsible for fungal infections and T cell abnormalities associated with idiopathic hypoparathyroidism (6). Furthermore it is possible that the thymic dysfunction is in some way responsible for the development of the "autoimmune" diseases. Some patients with idiopathic hypoparathyrodism have no demonstrable lymphocyte abnormality and no other endocrinopathies. Rare causes of PTH hyposecretion include iron-overload, ^{131}I therapy, metastatic disease and hypomagnesaemia. More subtle defects in PTH release and/or secretion probably exist, although they are not yet well described. For example, in patients with pancreatitis or other severe illnesses, hypocalcaemia may occur in the presence of relatively low PTH concentrations which may constitute a "secretory" defect (7).

Hypoparathyroidism (ii) Due to PTH Resistance

This syndrome or group of syndromes is characterised by the failure of PTH to elicit a normal response (8). This diagnosis cannot be made unless it has been demonstrated that some or all responses to administered PTH are abnormal. Unless these diagnostic criteria are met, patients with immunoreactive but biologically inactive PTH (see p.3) will be misdiagnosed as hormone resistant when they are in fact hormone deficient.

PTH resistance may be <u>temporary</u>, as in premature infants (9) or hypomagnesaemia (10), or <u>permanent</u> as in pseudohypoparathyroidism (8). Resistance may also be <u>selective</u> so that hyperparathyroid bone disease may coexist with hypocalcaemia and documented renal PTH resistance (11). The failure of specific target organs, e.g. the kidney, is a model for selective PTH resistance. The renal resistance to PTH in chronic renal failure (CRF) is associated with normal responses in the skeleton where PTH may cause significant histological changes. This model may help to explain some unusual subtypes of pseudohypoparathyroidism characterised by parathyroid bone disease in the presence of documented renal PTH resistance. The mechanisms for these discordant effects in different tissues are not understood.

Malabsorption may be associated with PTH-resistant "hypoparathyroidism" because in some malabsorptive states $1,25(OH)_2D_3$ cannot increase calcium absorption. As in patients with CRF, hyperparathyroid bone disease can coexist with hypocalcaemia. Osteomalacia may cause a degree of skeletal PTH resistance which may be reversed by appropriate treatment.

At the cellular level PTH resistance can result from any

dysfunction at any site in the PTH response pathways (4). One convenient subclassification depends upon the ability of the normal kidney to release large quantities of cAMP following a PTH challenge (12,13). Thus, PTH resistance may be due to a defective cAMP response which is usually referred to as the syndrome of pseudohypoparathyroidism (PHP) type I (12). Alternatively the defect can occur at sites distal to cAMP, as in pseudohypoparathyroidism type II (14).

PTH type I, which is inherited in various Mendelian patterns, is not a single nosological entity. One subgroup comprises patients who have a typical phenotypic appearance, which includes short metacarpals and metatarsals and is known as Albright's Hereditary Osteodystrophy (15). Many patients in this subgroup are said to have abnormal G subunit activity (16). Since other hormone receptors also interact with the same G subunits, these patients are also variably resistant to the action of these hormones (16). Anti-PTH receptor antibodies have been found by 2 groups (17,18). Other receptor abnormalities will presumably be described in patients whose resistance is limited to PTH.

Post cAMP resistant states (called PHP type II) are also thought to be of several types. A single patient has been described in whom PTH was unable to activate vitamin D 1-hydroxylase (19). Antibodies presumably to the renal tubular phosphate transporter have been described in a patient with PHP II (20). However the majority of hypoparathyroid patients with this rare syndrome have been diagnosed by the failure of PTH injections to augment urinary phosphate excretion despite an adequate cAMP response (4,14). Post-cyclase PTH resistance occurs in hypocalcaemic states (21) and some case reports purporting to show a return of PTH responsiveness in PHP type II following therapy may have been describing vitamin D deficient subjects (22).

Breslau et al. (23) studied PHP subjects who attained normocalcaemia spontaneously in spite of markedly impaired cAMP responses to PTH. This can be thought of as similar to the variability of hormone resistance between hormones, which is seen in G subunit deficient pseudohypoparathyroid patients. It may simply be that PTH acts via second messengers other than cAMP and that these vary from cell to cell and from pseudohypoparathyroid patient to pseudohypoparathyroid patient.

Hypoparathyroidism (iii) Due to Combined PTH Deficiency and Resistance

PTH deficiency and resistance may coexist. For example hypomagnesaemia which may inhibit PTH release from the parathyroid gland has also been associated with PTH resistance (10). However, it is our current view that in many cases hypomagnesaemia is the result and not the cause of hypoparathyroidism.

Hypoparathyroidism (iv) Due to Abnormal PTH

We have recently studied a family with clinical and biochemical hypoparathyroidism who had circulating immunoreactive PTH but whose PTH sensitivity was normal to both long (p.4) and short hPTH infusions. In this family much circumstantial evidence

including immunologic and HPLC examinations of the immunoreactive
circulating PTH suggests that it is abnormal and that it lacks
biological activity. A second family with this syndrome is
currently under investigation. Nusynowicz and Klein (24)
presented a single patient who may have had abnormal PTH.

Diagnosis

A diagnosis of hypoparathyroidism should be considered in all
hypocalcaemic patients especially in the presence of
hyperphosphataemia. While the serum inorganic phosphate may be
normal in hypoparathyroidism the values are rarely low except in
association with vitamin D deficiency. Some conditions such as
CRF, vitamin D deficiency, hypomagnesaemia and malabsorption must
be excluded. Although these conditions may cause the
"hypoparathyroidism", as defined, they are generally regarded as
separate entities.

Serum PTH estimation divides the patients into those with PTH
deficiency who have no circulating hormone and those with
presumptive PTH resistance in whom circulating PTH is detected.

This simplistic classification is liable to result in
misdiagnosis. A review of 30 patients with surgical hypoparathyroidism studied over a number of years with many PTH
measurements showed that 5 of these patients had detectable PTH on
at least one occasion and that in 3 others the values were higher
than normal on at least one occasion. Dynamic tests are therefore
required for a definitive diagnosis of PTH resistance and for an
understanding of the mechanism underlying the resistance.

The classic diagnostic test for PTH resistance involves a
PTH injection over a short period of time with measurements of
changes in urinary cAMP and phosphate (12,13). Flat cAMP
responses confirm the diagnosis of PHP type I. The phosphaturic
response whether expressed as mmol phosphate/mmol creatinine (13)
or as $TmPO_4$/GFR (unpublished) does not separate patients with
pseudohypoparathyroidism from those with idiopathic hypoparathyroidism. The overlap makes the phosphaturic response to PTH an
unsatisfactory criterion for the diagnosis of PHP type II.

There have been several reports describing "normal"
hypercalcaemic responses to PTH injections in patients with
defective cyclase responses (25) and at least one such patient was
untreated at the time of the test (26). This phenomenon is
compatible with partial PTH resistance with the observed
hypercalcaemia actually representing a diminished response either
in terms of absolute increments or with a dose response curve
which is shifted to the right. Since on ethical grounds repeated
PTH injections are not given to normal subjects, no comparisons
are possible. The increasing availability of hPTH 1-34 may make
the assessment of serum calcium responses to PTH one of the
investigations required for the study of PTH resistance.

We have recently described a 6 hour hPTH infusion protocol
(27) in which the changes in serum calcium and $1,25(OH)_2D$ and the
urinary changes in calcium, phosphate and cAMP are monitored. The
increases in $1,25(OH)_2D$ during this test clearly separate
previously defined (short PTH infusion) pseudohypoparathyroid

patients from both normal subjects and idiopathic hypoparathyroid patients. Serum calcium changes also separate the two hypoparathyroid groups. The other parameters obtained during the 6 hour test are less reliable on an individual patient basis in separating the groups. We hope that this test may eventually be useful for assessing post cAMP PTH resistant states.

In summary, the diagnosis of hypoparathyroidism requires two steps. The confirmation of hypocalcaemia due to hypoparathyroidism, followed by attempts to define the underlying aetiology.

Clinical Features

In our series patients with surgical hypoparathyroidism (28-31) the prevalence of various clinical features was as follows: tetany 88%; cataracts 50%; abnormal EEG 49%; vocal cord paralysis 41%; epileptiform seizures 34%; hypothyroidism 30%; and basal ganglia calcification 6%. This 6% prevalence of basal ganglia calcification was based on plain X-ray appearances and is likely to be a significant underestimate. Computerised tomographic (CT) scans suggest that the prevalence of cerebral calcification approximates that of cataracts (about 50%) (31). We believe that cerebral calcification increases with increasing duration of hypocalcaemia but we have no controlled study to validate this impression. The reason why a hypocalcaemic condition should be associated with ectopic calcification is unknown. Similarily, the reason why the basal ganglia is a site of predilection for calcification in hypoparathyroidism and other unrelated diseases is not known.

Electroencephalographic (EEG) findings in hypoparathyroid patients (Table 1) suggest that patients with EEG abnormalities are significantly more likely to experience fits and conversely, that fits are less likely to occur in patients with normal EEG's (30). It is not our experience that EEG returns to normal with normalisation of serum calcium.

Table 1
Epilepsy/EEG and Surgical Hypoparathyroidism

EEG at Time of Normocalcaemia	No.	History of Seizure at Time of Hypocalcaemia
Normal	21	3
Abnormal	20	11

$$(p < 0.001, X^2)$$

The claim is often made that surgical hypoparathyroidism is associated with psychiatric disease. We have compared a group of patients with surgical hypoparathyroidism to an appropriate control group composed of age and sex matched individuals who had undergone thyroidectomy at the same time as the affected group but who were normocalcaemic. The results of the Minnesota Multiple Personality Inventory suggest that hypochondriasis, depression and hysteria are no more common in hypocalcaemic patients than in normocalcaemic patients (Table 2) even when hypocalcaemia is prolonged. All three groups of patients had a greater prevalence of psychiatric symptoms than a normal population and we believe these symptoms may have been responsible for the initial thyroidectomy.

Table 2
Psychiatric Disturbances in Chronic Surgical Hypoparathyroidism
Mean Raw Scores Minnesota Multiple Personality Inventory

| | Patients | | Controls |
	N=28	N=12*	N=15
Hypochondriasis	18 ± 7	19 ± 6	19 ± 7
Depression	28 ± 9	27 ± 5	26 ± 6
Hysteria	25 ± 5	26 ± 5	25 ± 6

* A subgroup with presumed hypocalcaemia of greater than 11 years' duration

Patients with untreated surgical hypoparathyroidism had a significantly increased incidence of macroscopic cataracts as compared to the control group (Table 3). However, scattered lenticular opacities were seen by slit lamp examination with equal frequency in controls and hypoparathyroid patients (29). These lenticular opacities are common in the general population and the concept (based on the presence of such opacities) that patients with spasmophilia have latent or subclinical hypoparathyroidism should be viewed sceptically.

Table 3
Lens Opacities in Hypoparathyroidism

	Patients	Controls
Macroscopic*	16	2
Microscopic	13	16
None	3	7

* Presence of macroscopic cataracts vs the absence of macroscopic cataracts (microscopic + none) ($p < 0.0001$, X^2)

Dupruytren's contractures were present in 6/33 female hypoparathyroid patients compared with 1/29 controls ($p = 0.02$, X^2).

Patients with idiopathic hypoparathyroidism, which is less common that surgical hypoparathyroidism, are generally younger at the time of presentation (6) and some of them are mentally retarded. The calcium related problems are often overshadowed by the associated endocrine or non-endocrine problems.

Patients with pseudohypoparathyroidism may be indistinguishable from idiopathic hypoparathyroidism on clinical grounds. PHP may be associated with the typical skeletal phenotype (Albright's hereditary osteodystrophy). We have only seen one patient with PHP (defined by a flat cAMP response to PTH) who had the classical syndrome of Albright's hereditary osteodystrophy. This patient was the only one of five individuals with short metacarpals whom we studied who had any demonstrable abnormalities of calcium metabolism.

We have not encountered any patients with PHP type II. We have seen two patients in whom this diagnosis might have been entertained but both had very mild renal osteodystrophy impairment and both were vitamin D deficient.

The prognosis of treated hypoparathyroidism (of all varieties) is good and many of our patients have lived into their 70's and 80's.

Treatment

Treatment of all forms of hypoparathyroidism consists of vitamin D or one of its metabolites in pharmacological doses with or without calcium supplementation. This is likely to remain the case even with the increasing availability of hPTH which at present needs to be given by injection. In some patients the calcaemic response varies from time to time, in spite of the fact that the prescribed dose of vitamin D has remained unaltered. This phenomenon has been observed with vitamin D_2 as well as with the newer vitamin D metabolites.

The availability of potent compounds such as $1,25(OH)_2D_3$ or 1-alpha-OHD_3 with their relatively short biological half lives (32) has led to the belief that these substances are better than ergocalciferol (vitamin D_2). For example, $1,25(OH)_2D_3$, a "naturally" occurring metabolite with rapid onset of action, can be advantageous in acute situations. However, the newer compounds are more expensive, they require more frequent administration and compliance cannot be easily monitored (33). We see no advantage in changing over from vitamin D_2 to the newer analogues in patients who are well controlled on the older preparation. We do not use combinations of long acting and short-acting vitamin D metabolites.

It is customary to prescribe calcium supplementation for patients on pharmacological doses of vitamin D, so that fluctuations in dietary calcium have less effect on calcium absorption and hence serum calcium. It is our impression that calcium supplementation helps to reduce the vitamin D dose required to maintain normocalcaemia. However to our knowledge there are no controlled studies on this point.

Summary

Hypoparathyroidism comprises a fascinating group of syndromes, many of them incompletely understood. However the tools are now becoming available which will allow us to examine these disorders in considerable detail. Since the treatment of hypoparathyroidism is not entirely satisfactory at present an improved understanding of the pathophysiology may help to develop strategies for the improved care of these patients.

References

1. Parfitt, A.M. (1976) Metabolism 25, 909.
2. Hino, M. (1986) Calcif. Tissue Int. 38, 193.
3. Puschett, J.B. (1982) Min. Electro. Metab. 7, 281.
4. Aurbach, G.D. et al. (1985) In Williams Textbook of Endocrinology (W.B. Saunders), p.1137-1217.

5. Blizzard, R.M. et al. (1966) Clin. Exp. Immunol. 1, 119.
6. Kleerekoper, M. et al. (1974) Arch. Intern. Med. 134, 944.
7. McMahon, M.J. et al. (1978) Br. J. Surg. 65, 216.
8. Albright, F. et al. (1942) Endocrinol. 30, 922.
9. Kruse, K. et al. (1987) Acta Paed. Scand. 76, 115.
10. Estep, H. et al. (1969) J. Clin. Endocr. 29, 842.
11. Kidd, G.S. (1980) Am. J. Med. 68, 772.
12. Chase, L.R. et al. (1969) J. Clin. Invest. 48, 1832.
13. Furlong et al. (1986) Aust. N.Z.J. Med. 16, 794.
14. Drezner, M. et al. (1973) N. Engl. J. Med. 289, 1056
15. Mann, J.B. et al. (1962) Annal Int. Med. 56, 315.
16. Spiegel et al. (1982) N.E.J.M. 307, 679.
17. Juppner, H. et al. (1978) Lancet 2, 1222.
18. Audran, M. et al. (1987) J. Clin. Endocrinol. Metab. 64, 937.
19. Metz, S.A. et al. (1977) N.E.J.M. 297, 1084.
20. Yamada, K. et al. (1984) J. Clin. Endocrinol. Metab. 58, 339.
21. Rao, D.S. et al. (1985) J. Clin. Endocrinol. Metab. 61, 285.
22. Rodriguez, H.J. et al. (1974) J. Clin. Endocrinol. Metab. 39, 693.
23. Breslau, N.A. et al. (1980) Am. J. Med. 68, 856.
24. Nusynowitz, M.L. et al. (1973) Am. J. Med. 55, 677.
25. Stogmann, W. et al. (1975) Am. J. Med. 59, 140.
26. Lawoyin, S. et al. (1979) J. Clin. Endocrinol. Metab. 49, 783.
27. McElduff et al. (1987) Calcif. Tissue Int. (in press).
28. Shearman, B.T. et al. (1965) B.M.J. 2, 619.
29. Ireland, A.W. et al. (1968) Arch. Intern. Med. 122, 408.
30. Basser, L.S. et al. (1969) Annal Intern. Med. 71, 507.
31. Posen, S. et al. (1979) Annal Intern. Med. 91: 415.
32. Kanis, J.A. et al. (1977) B.M.J. 1, 78.
33. Mason, R.S. et al. (1979) Clin. Endocrinol. 10, 265.

INHIBITION OF PARATHYROID HORMONE BIOACTIVITY IN PSEUDOHYPOPARATHYROIDISM TYPE I AND BY HUMAN PTH(3-84) PRODUCED IN E.COLI

Walter Born, Nigel Loveridge, Charles Nagant de Deuxchaisnes, and Jan A. Fischer

University of Zurich, CH-8008 Zurich (Switzerland) (W.B., J.A.F.); Rowett Research Institute, Aberdeen, AB2 9SB (Scotland) (N.L.); University of Louvain, 1200 Brussels (Belgium) (C.N.D.)

Parathyroid hormone(1-84) (PTH(1-84)), synthesized in the parathyroid gland as a larger mol wt precursor protein, prepropPTH (1), functions as an important regulator of calcium and phosphate homeostasis through interaction with receptors in the kidney and in bone (2).

Upon completion of the amino acid sequence analysis of bovine PTH(1-84) (3), in vivo and in vitro studies with synthetic fragments and analogues of the hormone demonstrated that the amino-terminal PTH(1-34) fragment exhibits full biological activity (4). PTH bioactivity was reduced in vitro and in vivo by the deletion of the amino-terminal alanine of bovine PTH(1-34) and abolished in vitro when the valine in the second position was removed (5).

These observations directed the design of PTH antagonists (6, 7). PTH(3-34) still bound, although weakly, to PTH receptors (8, 9). Receptor binding and stability of this PTH(3-34) fragment was improved with methionines in positions 8 and 18 substituted by norleucines, and the carboxyl-terminal phenylalanine by a tyrosineamide. [Nle^{8,18}, Tyr^{34}]PTH(3-34)amide inhibited receptor binding of [^{125}I]PTH(1-84) to renal membranes at a one to one molar ratio (7). This analogue has so far been recognized as the most potent antagonist of the PTH responses in kidney, bone and skin derived tissues in vitro (10-14). However, it failed, in a 10- to 200-fold molar excess, to inhibit the effects of PTH(1-34) and -(1-84) on renal phosphate transport in dogs and chickens, and on the rise of plasma calcium in chickens (15, 16). It even had weak agonist properties (17-19). Residual agonist activity was eliminated by additional deletions at the amino-terminus. [Tyr^{34}]PTH(7-34)amide was devoid of any agonist activity, but still bound to PTH receptors. This analogue, at a molar ratio of 100 to 1000 with respect to PTH(1-34), antagonized the urinary cAMP and phosphate, and the hypercalcemic responses to PTH in the rat in vivo (20, 21).

Endogenous PTH inhibitor activity in Pseudohypoparathyroidism Type I

Pseudohypoparathyroidism type I (PSPI) is a form of clinical hypoparathyroidism with reduced biological activity of exogenously administered parathyroid hormone at its target organs (22-24). The patients exhibit a form of secondary hyperparathyroidism with high levels of endogenous bioactive and immunoreactive PTH (25). The nature of the deficient response to PTH has been controversial. In most patients with the clinical signs of Albright's osteodystrophy the defect has been attributed to the reduced activity of a guanine nucleotide regulatory protein (N- or G-protein) (26, 27). However, N-protein activity is equally reduced in siblings of PSPI patients with absent overt clinical hypoparathyroidism (28, 29). Moreover, in some patients the decreased or absent phosphaturic and hypercalcemic responses to PTH can be restored after treatment with vitamin D and normalisation of circulating endogenous PTH levels (30, 31). N-protein deficiency is therefore not necessarily related to the impaired PTH responses of target organs seen in PSPI patients with overt clinical hypoparathyroidism.

In view of these inconsistent observations we have proposed an alternative pathogenic mechanism and have documented the presence of a PTH-inhibitory activity in the plasma of PSPI patients (25, 32). When PSPI plasma was analyzed by gel permeation chromatography, two PTH inhibitory components were separated from intact endogenous PTH(1-84). The latter had the biological activity of synthetic human PTH(1-84), when assayed in a renal cytochemical bioassay which is based on the stimulation of glucose-6-phosphate dehydrogenase activity in distal convoluted tubules (33). The PTH inhibitory components were slightly larger than intact PTH(1-84) and of the apparent size of PTH(1-34). Immunoreactive PTH, when measured with an anti-amino-terminal and an anti-midregion PTH(1-84) radioimmunoassay, was undetectable in these samples. When the two components were individually rechromatographed on reversed phase high performance liquid chromatography (HPLC), the elution profiles were heterogenous. A minor fraction coeluted with human PTH(3-84) synthesized in E.coli (34).

In unextracted plasma of PSPI patients PTH inhibitory activity was transiently reduced in response to intravenous calcium infusions which also suppressed PTH secretion, but restored circulating bioactive PTH activity (35). In a PSPI patient who had undergone total parathyroidectomy, PTH inhibitory activity was absent (36). These findings together with the observed postoperative normalisation of some of the responses to PTH in the same patient, indicated that the PTH inhibitory activity may originate from the parathyroid glands.

PTH inhibitory properties of human PTH(3-84) synthesized in E.coli

Complementary DNA endocing human preproPTH directs the synthesis of the authentic hormone precursor, and of human PTH(3-84) and -(8-84) in E.coli when fused to the E.coli lac promoter on a multicopy plasmid (37). Human preproPTH was localized at the surface of the cytoplasmic membrane but was not processed to mature PTH(1-84). Human PTH(3-84) and -(8-84) were found in the cytoplasm and appeared as independent translation products derived from the fusion gene in pulse-chase experiments (37).

PTH bioactivity and PTH inhibitory activity of PTH-like proteins produced in E.coli were also assessed in the renal cytochemical bioassay (submitted for publication). When cell extracts of transformed E.coli cells were subjected to reversed phase HPLC, PTH inhibitory activity was detected in effluent fractions containing human PTH(3-84). Cell extracts from PTH negative control cells were devoid of PTH inhibitory activity. PTH(3-84) was 100-times more active as PTH inhibitor than the synthetic [$Nle^{8,18}$,Tyr^{34}]PTH(3-34)amide, and at a 5-fold molar excess over PTH(1-84) completely blocked the biological action of intact PTH(1-84). PTH(8-84) had only 1% of the PTH inhibitory activity of synthetic [$Nle^{8,18}$,Tyr^{34}]PTH(3-34)amide. PTH(3-84) and -(8-84) had less than 0.1% of the biological activity of synthetic human PTH(1-84) which retained its bioactivity when chromatographed on the same reversed phase HPLC system. The results suggest that the carboxyl-terminal portion of the intact human PTH(1-84) molecule contributes importantly to the inhibitory potency of amino-terminally truncated PTH fragments.

Summary and Conclusions

The hypercalcemic and phosphaturic activities of PTH(1-84) reside within the (1-34) portion of the molecule. Sequential deletion of the first and second amino acid residues of bovine PTH(1-84) result in a progressive loss of PTH bioactivity in vivo and in vitro. However, human PTH (3-84), which was identified in cell extracts of E.coli carrying a fusion gene between the E.coli lac promoter and complementary DNA encoding human preproPTH on a multicopy plasmid, was a potent PTH antagonist in the cytochemical bioassay. On a molar basis, it had 100 times higher PTH inhibitory activity than the synthetic [Nle^{8,18},Tyr^{34}]PTH(3-34)amide. PTH inhibitory activity was also detected in the renal cytochemical bioassay in unextracted plasma samples of PSPI patients. Endogenous intact PTH(1-84) in PSPI plasma was found to have the biologic activity of synthetic human PTH(1-84) when separated, on gel permeation chromatography, from two distinct PTH inhibitory components which eluted slightly ahead of intact PTH (1-84) and with synthetic human PTH(1-34, respectively. The two PTH inhibitory components, which were not detected by two independent anti-PTH radioimmunoassay systems, were heterogenous when individually rechromatographed on reversed phase HPLC. A minor component eluted from the column with the retention time observed for human PTH(3-84) synthesized in E.coli. These observations in combination with the fact that immunologically undetectable amounts of human PTH(3-84) efficiently inhibited PTH bioactivity in the renal cytochemical bioassay, suggest that low amounts of circulating PTH-like proteins may antagonize endogenous, biologically active PTH(1-84) in PSPI patients.

References

1. J. F. Habener, M. Rosenblatt, B. Kemper, H. M. Kronenberg, A. Rich, and J. T. Potts, Jr., Pre-proparathyroid hormone: Amino acid sequence, chemical synthesis and some biological studies of the precursor region, Proc. Natl. Acad. Sci. (USA) 75:2616 (1978).
2. M. Rosenblatt, Parathyroid hormone: intracellular transport, secretion and receptor interaction, in: "Peptide and Protein Reviews", M. T. W. Hearn, ed., Dekker, New York (1984).
3. H. D. Niall, H. T. Keutmann, R. T. Sauer, M. L. Hogan, B. F. Dawson, G. D. Aurbach and J. T. Potts, Jr., The amino sequence of bovine parathyroid hormone, Hoppe Seyler's Z.Physiol. Chem. 351:1586 (1970).
4. J. T. Potts, Jr., G. W. Tregear, H. T. Keutmann, H. D. Niall, R. Sauer, L. J. Deftos, B. F. Dawson, M. L. Hogan and G. D. Aurbach, Synthesis of a biologically active N-terminal tetratriacontapeptide of parathyroid hormone, Proc. Natl. Acad. Sci. (USA) 68:63 (1971).
5. G. W. Tregear, J. Van Reitschoten, E. Greene, H. T. Keutmann, H. D. Niall, B. Reit, J. A. Parsons and J. T. Potts, Jr., Bovine parathyroid hormone: Minimum chain length of synthetic peptide required for biological activity, Endocrinology 93:1349 (1973).
6. M. Rosenblatt, G. V. Segre, G. A. Tyler, G. L. Shepard, S. R. Nussbaum and J. T. Potts, Jr., Identification of a receptor binding region in parathyroid hormone, Endocrinology 107:545 (1980).
7. M. Rosenblatt, E. N. Callahan, J. E. Mahaffey, A. Pont and J. T. Potts, Jr., Parathyroid hormone inhibitors: design, synthesis, and biologic evaluation of hormone analogues, J. Biol. Chem. 252:5847 (1977).
8. D. Goltzman, A. Peytremann, E. Callahan, G. W. Tregear and J. T. Potts, Jr., Analysis of the requirements for parathyroid hormone action in renal membranes with the use of binding analogues, J. Biol. Chem. 250:3199 (1975).
9. G. V. Segre, M. Rosenblatt, B. L. Reiner, J. E. Mahaffey and J. T.

Potts, Jr., Characterization of parathyroid hormone receptors in canine renal cortical plasma membranes using radioiodinated sulfur-free hormone analogue: correlation of binding with adenylate cyclase activity, J. Biol. Chem. 254:6980 (1979).

10. T. C. Chen, M. Rosenblatt and J. B. Puschett, Effects of calcium on a parathyroid hormone-sensitive adenylate cyclase inhibitor, Biochem. Biophys. Res. Commun. 94:1227 (1980).

11. S. R. Goldring, J.E. Mahaffey, M. Rosenblatt, J.-M. Dayer, J. T. Potts, Jr. and S. M. Krane, Parathyroid hormone inhibitors: comparison of biological activity in bone- and skin-derived tissue, J. Clin. Endocrinol. Metab. 48:655 (1979).

12. S. R. Goldring, J.-M. Dayer and M. Rosenblatt, Factors regulating the response of cells cultured from human giant cell tumors of bone to parathyroid hormone, J. Clin. Endocrinol. Metab. 53:295 (1981).

13. T. Takano, M. Takigawa, E. Shirai, F. Suzuki and M. Rosenblatt, Effects of synthetic analogues and fragments of bovine parathyroid hormone on adenosine 3',5'-monophosphate level, ornithine decarboxylase activity, and glycosaminoglycan synthesis in rabbit costal chondrocytes in culture: structure-activity relations, Endocrinology 116:2536 (1985).

14. M. P. M. Hermann-Erlee, J. N. M. Heersche, J. W. Hekkelman, P. J. Gaillard, G. W. Tregear, J. A. Parsons and J. T. Potts, Jr., Effects on bone in vitro of bovine parathyroid hormone and synthetic fragments representing residues 1-34, 2-34, 3-34, Endocr. Res. Commun. 3:21 (1976).

15. D. A. Gray, J. A. Parsons, J. T. Potts, Jr., M. Rosenblatt and R. W. Stevenson, In vivo studies on an antagonist of parathyroid hormone [Nle^{8,18},Tyr^{34}]bPTH-(3-34)amide, Br. J. Pharmacol. 76:259 (1982).

16. J. A. McGowan, T. C. Chen, J. Fragola, J. B. Puschett and M. Rosenblatt, Parathyroid hormone: effects of the 3-34 fragment in vivo and in vitro, Science 219:67 (1983).

17. G. V. Segre, M. Rosenblatt, G. L. Tully III, J. Laugharn, B. Reit and J. T. Potts, Jr., Evaluation of an in vitro parathyroid hormone antagonist in vivo in dogs, Endocrinology 116:1024 (1985).

18. N. Horiuchi, M. Rosenblatt, H. T. Keutmann, J. T. Potts, Jr. and M. F. Holick, A multiresponse parathyroid hormone assay: an inhibitor has agonist properties in vivo, Am. J. Physiol. 244:E589 (1983).

19. K. J. Martin, E. Bellorin-Font, J. Freitag, M. Rosenblatt and E. Slatopolski, The arterio-venous difference for immunoreactive parathyroid hormone and the production of adenosine 3',5'-monophosphate by isolated perifused bone: studies with analogues of parathyroid hormone, Endocrinology 109:956 (1981).

20. N. Horiuchi, M. F. Holick, J. T. Potts, Jr. and M. Rosenblatt, A parathyroid hormone inhibitor in vivo: design and biological evaluation of a hormone analogue, Science 220:1053 (1983).

21. S. H. Doppelt, R. M. Neer, S. R. Nussbaum, P. Federico, J. T. Potts, Jr. and M. Rosenblatt, Inhibition of the in vivo parathyroid hormone-mediated calcemic response in rats by a synthetic hormone antagonist, Proc. Natl. Acad. Sci. (USA) 83:7557 (1986).

22. F. Albright, C. H. Burnett, P. M. Smith and W. Parson, Pseudo-Hypoparathyroidism, an example of "Sebright-Bantam-Syndrome". Report of three cases, Endocrinology (Baltimore) 30:922 (1942).

23. L. R. Chase, G. L. Melson and G. D. Aurbach, Pseudohypoparathyroidism: Defective excretion of 3',5'-AMP in response to parathyroid hormone, J. Clin. Invest. 48:1832 (1969).

24. E. A. Werder, J. A. Fischer, R. Illig, S. Bernasconi, A. Fanconi and A. Prader, Pseudohypoparathyroidism and idiopathic hypoparathyroidism: Realtionships between serum calcium and parathyroid hormone levels and the urinary cyclic andenosine3',5'-monophospate response to parathyroid extract, J. Clin. Endocrinol. Metab. 46:872 (1978).

25. N. Loveridge, F. Tschopp, W. Born, J.-P. Devogelaer, C. Nagant de Deuxchaisnes and J. A. Fischer, Separation of inhibitory activity from biologically active parathyroid hormone in patients with pseudohypoparathyroidism type I, Biochim. Biophys. Acta 889:117 (1986).

26. A. M. Spiegel, M. A. Levine, S. J. Marx and G. D. Aurbach, Pseudo-hypoparathyroidism: the molecular basis for hormone resistance - a retrospective, New Engl. J. Med. 307:679 (1982).

27. C. Van Dop and H. R. Bourne, Pseudohypoparathyroidism. Ann. Rev. Med. 34:259 (1983).

28. J. A. Fischer, H. R. Bourne, M. A. Dambacher, F. Tschopp, R. De Meyer, J.-P. Devogelaer, E. A. Werder and C. Nagant de Deuxchaisnes, Pseudohypoparathyroidism: Inheritance and expression of deficient receptor-cyclase coupling protein activity, Clin. Endocrinol. (Oxford) 19:747 (1983).

29. M. A. Levine, T.-S. Jap, R. S. Mauseth, R. W. Downs and A. M. Spiegel, Activity of the stimulatory guanine nucleotide-binding protein is reduced in erythrocytes from patients with pseudohypoparathyroidism and pseudopseudohypoparathyroidism: Biochemical, endocrine, and genetic analysis of Albright's hereditary osteodystrophy in six kindreds, J. Clin. Endocrinol. Metab. 62:497 (1986).

30. S. M. Suh, D. Fraser and S. W. Koor, Pseudohypoparathyroidism: Responsiveness to parathyroid extract induced by vitamin D_3 therapy, J. Clin. Endocrinol. Metab. 30:609 (1970).

31. W. Stögmann and J. A. Fischer, Pseudohypoparathyroididsm: Disappearance of the resistance to exogenous parathyroid extract during treatment with vitamin D, Am. J. Med. 58:140 (1975).

32. N. Loveridge, J. A. Fischer, C. Nagant de Deuxchaisnes, M. A. Dambacher, F. Tschopp, E. Werder, J.-P. Devogelaer, R. De Meyer, L. Bitensky and J. Chayen, Inhibition of cytochemical bioactivity of parathyroid hormone by plasma in pseudohypoparathyroidism type I, J. Clin. Endocrinol. Metab. 54:1274 (1982).

33. G. N. Kent, N. Loveridge, J. Reeve and J. M. Zanelli, Pharmacokinetics of synthetic human parathyroid hormone 1-34 in man measured by cytochemical bioassay and radioimmunoassay, Clin. Sci. 68:171 (1985).

34. W. Born, N. Loveridge, C. Nagant de Deuxchaisnes, J.B. Petermann and J. A. Fischer, Comparison of biological and biochemical properties of a PTH-inhibitor in pseudohypoparathyroidism type I and of human PTH(3-84) synthesized in E.coli, in: Calcium regulation and bone metabolism: Basic and clinical aspects, D. V. Cohn, F. J. Martin, P. J. Meunier, eds., Excerpta Medica, Amsterdam (1987)

35. N. Loveridge, J. A. Fischer, J.-P. Devogelaer and C. Nagant de Deuxchaisnes, Suppression of parathyroid hormone inhibitory activity of plasma in pseudohypoparathyroidism type I by iv calcium, Clin. Endocrinol. (Oxford) 24:549 (1986).

36. C. Nagant de Deuxchaisnes and S. M. Krane, Hypoparathyroidism, in: "Metabolic Bone Disease", L. V. Avioli, S. M. Krane, eds., Academic Press, New York, (1978).

37. W. Born, M. Freeman, G. N. Hendy, A. Rapoport, A. Rich. J. T. Potts, Jr. and H. M. Kronenberg, Human preproparathyroid hormone synthesized in E.coli is transported to the surface of the bacterial inner membrane but not processed to the mature hormone, Mol. Endocrinol. 1:5 (1987).

MISCELLANEOUS

POLYMORPHONUCLEAR LEUCOCYTES ARE A TARGET FOR PARATHYROID HORMONE: AN EFFECT ON THEIR RANDOM MIGRATION

Ciaran C. Doherty, Patrice LaBelle, John F. Collins, Nachman Brautbar, Dean Moyer and Shaul G. Massry

Division of Nephrology and the Department of Medicine
University of Southern California, School of Medicine
Los Angeles, California 90033

Defective leukocyte function manifested by impaired migration (1,2) and reduced phagocytic (3-5) and bactericidal activity (6) has been observed in patients with uraemia. Also, sera from dialysis patients contain a heat stable factor that inhibited granulocyte chemotaxis (7). The mechanisms and/or the potential uraemic factors underlying these defects in leukocyte functions are not known.

Patients with renal failure have secondary hyperparathyroidism (8-10) and markedly elevated blood levels of parathyroid hormone (PTH) (11-13). Certain data suggest that PTH may affect leukocyte function. Khan et al (14) reported that patients with primary hyperparathyroidism and normal renal function displayed an impairment in random migration and chemotaxis of leukocytes and these abnormalities disappeared after the removal of the parathyroid adenoma. Also, Tuma et al (15) found that sera from uraemic patients with high blood levels of PTH stimulated chemiluminesence of polymorphonuclear leukocytes and this effect was reduced or reversed after the decrease in the blood levels of PTH produced by parathyroidectomy.

It is theoretically possible that the state of secondary hyperpara-thyroidism of uraemia contributes at least partially to the defects in leukocyte functions. The present study was undertaken to examine the effects of PTH on random migration of polymorphonuclear leukocyte (PMNL) and investigate the pathways through which PTH may interact with PMNL.

METHODS

Venous blood was withdrawn from healthy subjects in heparinized test tubes containing 10 U of heparin for each one milliliter of blood. The blood samples were layered onto an equal volume of Ficoll/Hypaque (Pharmacia Fine Chemicals Inc., Piscataway, N.J.) and allowed to separate into clearly defined layers, a process which required 45-60 minutes. The top layer containing granulocytes and monocytes was aspirated, washed three times in Hank's balanced salt solution (HBSS) consisting of KCL 5.4mM (40 mg/100ml), KH_2PO4 4.4 mM (60mg/100ml), NaCl 137 mM (800 mg/100ml), Na_2HPO4. $7H_2O$ 3.6 mM (90mg/100 ml), glucose 0.56 mM (100 mg/100ml) Grand Island Biological Co., Grand Island, N.Y.) and calcium and magnesium were added as $CaCl_2$ and $Mg Cl_2$ to provide for calcium and magnesium concentrations of 2.5 and 2.2 mM respectively.

New Actions of Parathyroid Hormone
Edited by S. G. Massry and T. Fujita
Plenum Press, New York

The cells were then suspended in HBSS fortified with 2% bovine serum albumin which contains sodium azide (HBSS/BSA) (Sigma Chemical Co. St. Louis, MO) to provide a concentration of 2.5×10^6 cells/ml. This gave a mixed leukocyte suspension made of 65-70% PMNL, with the rest being mononuclear cells. Since PMNL are the only blood cells which migrate into micropore filters of 3 u pore size, and since micropore filters of this size were used in the study, no further separation of PMNL from other blood cells was required for the purpose of measuring PMNL motility.

Random motility of PMNL was investigated utilizing the Boyden technique (16). The cell suspension was placed in the upper compartment of a modified Boyden Chamber (Bellco Glass Co., Vineland, N.J.) and HBSS without bovine serum albumin in the lower compartment. PMNL random motility was assessed using the leading front method of Zigmond and Hirsch (17) and PMNL random migration (u per 60 minutes at 37°c) was measured as the distance travelled by the leading front of cells that migrated into cellulose ester micropore filters (Millipore Corp., Bedfore, Mass.) with pores of 3.0 u diameter. The measurement of the migration was made as follows: filters were stained with hematoxylin, mounted on microscope slides, coded and read blind by one observer. Five high power fields were randomly chosen from each filter and the distance between the cells located at the top of the filter and the leading front of the cells was determined with the microtome fine adjustment of the microscope. Measurements were made in duplicates (two filters) for each study.

The effect of 1-84 PTH on cAMP and GMP production by PMNL was examined. For these studies 98% pure PMNL preparation was used. This was obtained by a two step separation procedure involving Ficoll/Hypaque centrifugation followed by dextran sedimentation and hypotonic lysis of erythrocytes (18). 99% of the cells were viable as determined by the Trypan blue dye test.

Random migration of PMNL obtained from uraemic patients were also examined and the results were correlated with the serum levels of PTH. Also the effects of 50 U/ml of 1-84 PTH on random migration of PMNL from uraemic patients were evaluated.

The concentration of PTH in serum was measured by radioimmunoassay using sheep antiserum 478 (kindly supplied by Dr. Claude Arnaud), ^{125}I-labelled bovine PTH, and pooled sera from patients with renal failure as standard. This antibody reacts predominantly with an immunologic deter-minant in the carboxyl region of PTH and will detect both the intact hormone and its carboxy-terminal fragment. The values for this in 63 blood samples from normal subjects ranged from undetectable to 15 uleq/ml (mean $\pm$SE 7.5 $\pm$0.7), and PTH was detectable in 33 of 63 (52%) normal subjects. Elevated blood levels of PTH were found in 60 patients with chronic renal failure. The lower limit of detectability was 1 uleq/ml.

RESULTS

The effects of various concentrations of 1-84 PTH and 1-34 PTH on random migration of human PMNL are shown in figure 1 and those of 53-84 PTH are given in Table I. The intact 1-84 PTH stimulated random migration of PMNL. This stimulatory effect became significant at 20 U/ml of the hormone when random migration increased from 22.9 $\pm$ 1.6 to 31.2 $\pm$ 1.5 u/60 min (p<0.01). The maximum effect was achieved at a concentration of 50 U/ml of the hormone with the random migration being 41.1 $\pm$ 2.5 u/60 min. There was no further increment in random migration with higher doses of the hormone. Thus, there was a dose response relationship between random migration of PMNL and 1-84 PTH for the concentration range of 10-50 U/ml. In contrast both 1-34 PTH and 53-84 PTH did not affect random migration of PMNL. The same batch of 1-34 PTH exerted biological activity in another system as evidenced by stimulating the beating of the isolated heart cells of rat (20). Inactivation of 1-84 PTH abolished its stimulatory effect on random migration (23 $\pm$ 1.5 vs control of 24 $\pm$ 1.3 u/60 min).

The effects of prolonged exposure of PMNL to 1-84 PTH on their random migration are depicted in Figure 2. The hormone produced the stimulation of random migration described above but the effect declined with prolonged prior incubation of the cells with the hormone. Random migration decreased from 48.9 $\pm$ 2.9 to 34.7 $\pm$ 3.1 u/60 min after 2 hours of preincubation; however, random migration was still significantly higher than control (34.7 $\pm$ 3.1 vs. 25.7 $\pm$ 0.5 u/60 min, p<0.01). Random migration was not different from control after preincubation of the cells with 1-84 PTH from 4-6 hours. Finally, random migration was impaired after preincubation with the hormone for 8-20 hours with the values being significantly (p<0.05 - 0.025) lower than control.

Figure 3 provides the data on the effect of various peptide hormones on random migration of PMNL. None of the peptide hormones studied (calcitonin, vasopressin, glucagon and insulin) produced a significant stimulation of random migration. In addition, calcitonin did not abolish the stimulatory effect of 1-84 PTH on random migration (table II).

The effects of various concentrations of calcium on random migration of PMNL in the absence of PTH are shown in figure 4. It is evident that the presence of calcium in the media is not required for random migration and increasing calcium concentrations of up to 2.5 mM do not stimulate random migration.

The interaction between 1-84 PTH and the various calcium concentrations in media on random migration of PMNL are given in table III. The hormone produced significant stimulation of random migration from 24.7 $\pm$ 1.0 to 36.8 $\pm$ 2.0 u/60 min (p<0.01) in the absence of calcium in the media. Random migration after exposure of the cells to the hormone in the presence of 0.5 to 1.5 mM calcium was not different from that observed in the absence of calcium. However, random migration after addition of 1-84 PTH was modestly but significantly (p<0.025) higher in media containing 2.5 mM calcium (43.1 $\pm$ 2.5 u/60 min) than in the absence of calcium (36.8 $\pm$ 2.9 u/60 min).

The effects of calcium ionophore in the presence of 2.5 mM calcium on random migration of PMNL are given in table IV and the interactions between calcium ionophore and 1-84 PTH in the absence of calcium and in the presence of 2.5 mM calcium on random migration are depicted in figure 5. Calcium ionophore (10^{-4} mM) in the presence of 2.5 mM calcium did not stimulate random migration (table IV). In the absence of calcium in the media, there was no significant difference between random migration of PMNL induced by 1-84 PTH whether the cells were preincubated with calcium ionophore or not. However, in the presence of 2.5 mM calcium and 1-84 PTH, the preincubation of the cells with calcium ionophore resulted in slightly but significantly greater random migration. The latter was 37.5 $\pm$ 1.5 u/60 min without preincubation with ionophore and 42.3 $\pm$ 1.1 u/60 min (p < 0.02) by cells preincubated with the ionophore.

TABLE 1   EFFECT OF 50 U/ml OF THE CARBOXYTERMINAL FRAGMENT OF
PARATHYROID HORMONE (53-84 PTH) ON RANDOM MIGRATION
OF HUMAN POLYMORPHONUCLEAR LEUKOCYTES.

Random Migration (u/60 min.)	
Control	53-84 PTH
26.4	24.7
32.0	31.5
32.5	34.4
25.0	25.6
23.6	22.5
Mean $\pm$ SE 27.9 $\pm$ 1.8	27.7 $\pm$ 2.2

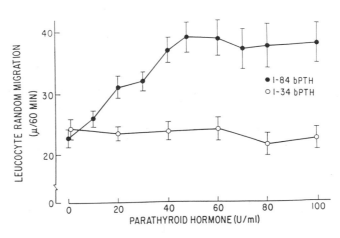

Figure 1.

The effects of 1-84 PTH and 1-34 PTH on random migration of
polymorphonuclear leukocyte. Each data point represents the
mean value of six studies and the brackets 1 SE

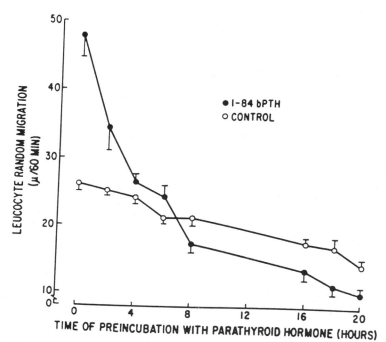

Figure 2. The effects of prolonged exposure of polymorphonuclear leukocytes to 1-84 PTH as compared to control. The data at "O" time
were obtained after incubation of the cells for one hour with
1-84 PTH or with vehicle only. Each data point represents the
mean value of five studies and the brackets 1 SE.

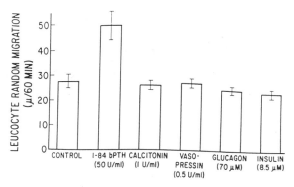

Figure 3. The effects of various peptide hormones on random migration of
polymorphonuclear leukocytes. Each column represents the mean
value of four studies and the brackets 1 SE.

TABLE II   THE EFFECT OF CALCITONIN ALONE, 1-84 PTH ALONE OR
           TOGETHER WITH CALCTONIN ON RANDOM MIGRATION OF
           HUMAN POLYMORPHONUCLEAR LEUKOCYTES

		Random Migration (u/60 minutes)		
	Control	Calcitonin 1 U/ml	1-84 PTH 50 U/ml	Calcitonin + PTH
	24.5	23.1	30.8	30.9
	32.0	28.6	48.3	49.0
	25.0	29.7	43.1	43.4
	34.6	26.3	44.4	50.0
	31.4	37.3	44.3	40.9
Mean $\pm$ SE	29.5$\pm$2.0	29.0$\pm$2.4	42.2$\pm$3.0	42.8$\pm$3.4
P vs Control		NS	$<$0.01	$<$0.01

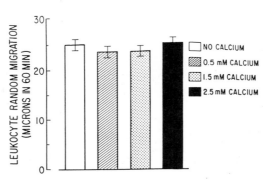

Figure 4.   Effects of various concentrations of calcium on random migra-
            tion of polymorphonuclear leukocytes. Each column represents
            mean value and the brackets denote 1 SE.

TABLE III   INTERACTION BETWEEN 1-84 PTH AND CALCIUM ON RANDOM MIGRATION OF POLYMORPHONUCLEAR LEUKOCYTES

	Random Migration (u/60 min)			
Calcium mM	0	0.5	1.5	2.5
-PTH	24.7 ± 1.0	23.9 ± 1.0	23.5 ± 1.2	24.8 ± 1.2
+PTH	36.8 ± 2.0	39.4 ± 2.5	38.0 ± 2.0	43.1 ± 2.5
P	< 0.01	< 0.01	< 0.01	< 0.01

Results are presented as mean $\pm$ SE of 6-8 experiments.

TABLE IV   EFFECT OF CALCIUM IONOPHORE A23187 ON RANDOM MIGRATION OF HUMAN POLYMORPHONUCLEAR LEUKOCYTES IN THE PRESENCE OF 2.5 mM CALCIUM

	Random Migration (u/60 min.)
Control	Calcium Ionophore
24.7	26.2
22.7	21.4
21.7	22.4
27.6	29.0
22.8	24.4
Mean $\pm$ SE 23.9 ± 1.0	24.7 ± 1.0

TABLE V   EFFECT OF PARATHYROID HORMONE AND NOREPINEPHRINE ON CYCLIC AMP AND CYCLIC GMP OF HUMAN POLYMORPHONUCLEAR LEUKOCYTES

	Control	5 Seconds	30 Seconds
CYCLIC AMP (fmole/10^6 cells)			
Vehicle	756 ± 218		826 ± 196
1-84 PTH (50 U/ml)		782 ± 84	867 ± 127
Norepinephrine (1×10^{-3} M)		1514 ± 192*	2700 ± 408*
CYCLIC GMP (fmole/10^6 cells)			
Vehicle	25 ± 3.6		24 ± 3.5
1-84 PTH (50 U/ml)		28 ± 3.3	24 ± 3.9
Norepinephrine (1×10^{-3} M)		29 ± 1.5	31 ± 3.2

Data are Mean $\pm$ SE of 6 studies.

*P<0.01 from control and PTH

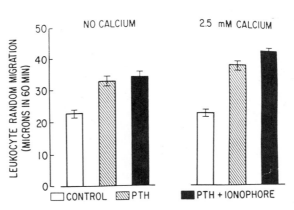

Figure 5.   The interaction between PTH and calcium ionophore in the presence and absence of calcium. Each column represents the mean value and the brackets denote 1 SE.

The effects of verapamil and its interaction with 1-84 PTH on random migration of PMNL are given in figure 6. Verapamil in a concentration of 5×10^{-2} mM did not affect random migration and did not abolish the stimulatory effect of 1-84 PTH on random migration.

Quinidine (10^{-4} M) produced a modest but significant (p<0.02) stimulation of random migration of PMNL, from 24.1 $\pm$ 0.8 to 29.0 $\pm$ 7 per u/60 min. The migration after quinidine and 1-84 PTH (38.5 $\pm$ 1.8 u/60 min) was significantly higher than quinidine alone (p<0.02) but not different from that observed after 1-84 PTH alone (39.4 $\pm$ 1.7 u/60 min), figure 7.

Stimulation of PMNL random motility by an agonist may be due to chemotactic activity of the agent. Therefore, potential chemotactic property of 1-84 PTH was sought by placing the hormone in the lower compartment of the Boyden Chamber. Under these circumstances, the random migration of PMNL was 25.1 $\pm$ 1.8 u/60 min without PTH and 25.0 $\pm$ 1.7 u/60 min with PTH. However, the BSA used in our study contained sodium azide and this compound may interfere with chemotaxis; this was confirmed in our hands with 10% zymosan activated serum as a chemotactic agent; the increase in random motility was 17.4 $\pm$ u/60 min in the presence of azide and 58.5 $\pm$ u/60 min in the absence of azide, p<0.01. To rule out the possibility that the failure to demonstrate chemotactic activity for PTH was due to the presence of azide, the chemotactic property of PTH was examined utilizing azide-free BSA. In this system, PMNL random migration was 63 $\pm$ 2.8 u/60 min without PTH and 61 $\pm$ 2.8 u/60 min with PTH. The increment in random migration produced by zymosan activated serum was 65 $\pm$ 3.5 u/60 min in the presence of PTH and 69 $\pm$ 3.3 u/60 without PTH. It appears that 1-84 PTH has no chemotactic activity.

The effects of 50 U/ml of 1-84 PTH and 1×10^{-3} M norepinephrine on cAMP and cGMP are shown in Table V. 1-84 PTH produced no significant change in the 5 second and the 30 minute levels of cAMP and cGMP of the PMNL. Norepinephrine on the other hand produced a significant rise in the levels of cAMP (from 756 $\pm$ 218 to 1514 $\pm$ 192 (5 seconds) to 2700 $\pm$ 408 (30 minutes) f mol/10^6 cells, p<0.01) but not in that of cGMP.

The values of random migration of PMNL obtained from uraemic patients and the effects of 50 U/ml of 1-84 PTH on the random migration of these cells are shown in table VI. The random migration of PMNL from uraemic patients are significantly lower than those from normal subjects (16.9 $\pm$ 1.0 vs 26.4 $\pm$ 0.99 u/60 min, p<0.001). Furthermore, 50 U/ml of 1-84 PTH produced only modest but significant (p<0.02) increment in random motility of PMNL from uraemic patients (from 16.9 $\pm$ 1.0 to 20.2 $\pm$ 0.7 u/60 min). However, this change of 3.3 $\pm$ 0.64 u/60 min was markedly and significantly (p<0.001) less than that observed in the PMNL of the normal subjects (16.1 $\pm$ 1.3 u/60 min). There was a significant and inverse relationship between the values of random migration and the serum levels of PTH in the uraemic patients (r=-0.87, p<0.01), figure 8.

DISCUSSION

The results of the present study demonstrate that human PMNL are target cells for the intact PTH molecule (1-84 PTH) and not for its amino-terminal (1-34 PTH) or its carboxy-terminal (53-84 PTH) fragments. The acute exposure of PMNL to 1-84 PTH produced significant stimulation of their random migration in a dose dependent fashion. This action of the hormone appears to be a direct one on random migration and not mediated via a chemotactic effect of PTH since the hormone did not stimulate chemotaxis.

The demonstration that the inactivation of the hormone abolished its effect on PMNL motility is consistent with the notion that this action is related to the biologic activity of the hormone and not due to a contaminant of the hormone preparation. Furthermore, it appears that this action is specific to PTH since other peptide hormones failed to exert a similar effect.

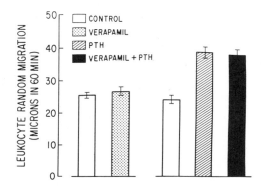

Figure 6. Effects of verapamil, PTH, and verapamil and PTH on random migration of polymorphonuclear leukocytes. Each column represents mean value and brackets denote 1 SE.

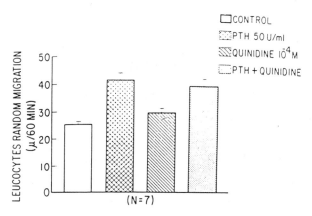

Figure 7. The effects of quinidine, 1-84 PTH and 1-84 PTH plus quindine on random migration of polymorphonuclear leukocytes. Each column represents the mean value of seven studies and brackets 1 SE.

TABLE VI   RANDOM MIGRATION OF HUMAN POLYMORPHONUCLEAR LEUKOCYTE OBTAINED
FROM PATIENTS WITH ADVANCED RENAL FAILURE

| | Random Migration (u/60 min.) | | |
	Base Line	PTH (50 U/ml)	$\triangle$
Normal n = 28	26.4$\pm$0.99	42.5$\pm$2.06*	16.1$\pm$1.34
Uraemic n = 10	16.9$\pm$1.00	20.2$\pm$0.70**	3.3$\pm$0.64
P	<0.001	<0.001	<0.001

*   P<0.001 from baseline

**   P<0.02   from baseline

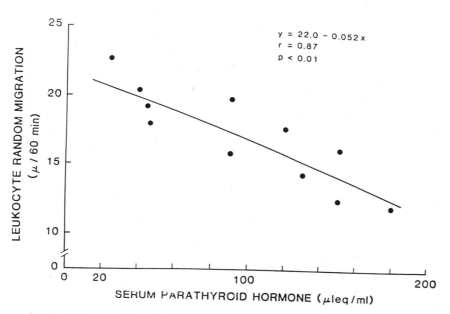

Figure 8.   The relationship between random migration of polymorphonuclear
leukocytes and serum levels of PTH in patients with advanced
uremia.   Each point represents one patient.

It is generally accepted that the amino-terminal fragment of PTH is the biologically active moiety of the hormone (21). This notion is based on the ability of this fragment to increase cAMP production by the kidney (22) and mobilize calcium from bone (23). However, these observations do not necessarily mean that the 1-34 fragment has all the biologic effects of the hormone. Our data show that 1-34 PTH does not exert the effect that 1-84 PTH does on PMNL. A corollary of our observations are the findings that 1-34 PTH does not enhance glucose release by the liver (24), does not inhibit erythropoiesis (25), and does not impair platelet aggregation (26) as 1-84 PTH does. Our finding that 53-84 PTH did not affect the motility of PMNL would suggest that either the intact hormone or a bigger or other carboxy-terminal fragment is needed for the action on random migration of PMNL. However, if the carboxy-terminal fragment(s) is the moiety that affects PMNL motility, its accumulation in large quantities in the blood of uraemic patients (27) may play an important role in the pathogenesis of PMNL dysfunction in uraemia.

Our studies also demonstrate that prolonged exposure to 1-84 PTH inhibits random migration of the PMNL. This finding of a difference between an acute and a chronic effect of PTH on PMNL function is not surprising. Similar observations have been noted in other systems. For example, PTH acutely stimulates the chronotropic (20) and inotropic (28) properties of the myocardium but chronic exposure to the hormone impairs both myocardial metabolism and function (29). The demonstration that chronic exposure to PTH inhibits random migration of PMNL has important clinical implications in uraemia. Uraemic patients have a chronic state of secondary hyperparathyroidism (8-13) and have impaired PMNL random migration (1,2). Our data confirm that patients with advanced uraemia have impaired random migration of PMNL and the severity of the defect is directly related to the blood levels of PTH. Our observations, therefore, are consistent with a cause and effect between secondary hyperparathyroidism in uraemia and the impairment in leukocyte motility.

The mechanism through which PTH acts on the PMNL is not fully elucidated. PTH increases entry of calcium into many mammalian cells (30-35) and is considered a potent ionophore. It also enhances production of cAMP via the stimulation of an adenylate cyclase system (22). Both of these actions mediate its effect on many organs. However, our studies showed that PTH exerts its effect in the absence of calcium in the media, and only at a calcium concentration of 2.5 mM was a slightly greater effect of PTH noted. Further, the calcium ionophore A23187 does not have a similar effect on PMNL and verapamil, a calcium channel blocker, does not affect random migration nor abolish the effect of PTH. In addition, the hormone does not stimulate the production of cAMP or cGMP by PMNL. Thus, it appears that the action of PTH on PMNL motility is not related to the ionophoric effect of the hormone nor is it due to stimulation of an adenylate cyclase system.

PTH also affects phospholipid turnover of mammalian cells (36-39) and may inhibit mitochondrial oxygen consumption (29,40) and oxidative phosphorylation (41). Although such actions of the hormone on PMNL have not been evaluated in our studies, it is theoretically possible that they may mediate the observed influence of the hormone on random migration. Some of these actions of the hormone may cause redistribtuion of calcium between various cell compartments. Indeed, the effect of quinidine, an agent that causes a rise in cytosolic calcium by redistribution of this ion among cell organelles (42,43), on the random migration of PMNL is consistent with such a hypothesis. Also chronic exposure to PTH inhibits energy production by the mitochondria of the myocardium (29) and the skeletal muscle (40), and a similar effect on the mitochondrial of PMNL may account for their impaired function after chronic exposure to PTH.

REFERENCES

1. Baum, J., V. Rafael, M. Cestero and R.B. Freeman. 1975. Chemotaxis of the polymorphonuclear leukocyte and delayed hypersensitivity in uraemia. Kidney Int:6:S147-S153

2. Greene, W.H., R. Cassan, S.M. Marver, and P.G. Quie. 1976. The effect of haemodialysis on neutrophil chemotactic responsiveness. J.Lab. Clin.Med:88:971-983

3. Brogan, T.D. 1967. Phagocytosis of polymorphonuclear leukocytes from patients with renal failure. Br.Med J:3:596-599

4. Burlesson, R.L. 1974. Reversible inhibition of phagocytosis in anephric uraemic patients. Surg. Forum:15:75-77

5. Montgomerie, J.Z., G.M. Kalmanson and L.B. Guze. 1972. Leukocyte phagocytosis and serum bactericidal activity in chronic renal failure. Amer.J.Med.Sci:264:385-393

6. Salant, D.J., A.M. Glover, R. Anderson, A.M. Meyers, R. Rabbin, J.A. Myburgh and A.R. Rabson. 1975. Polymorphonuclear leukocyte function in chronic renal failure and after renal transplantation. Proc.Europ.Dial.Transpl.Assoc:12:370-379

7. Goldblum, S.E., D.E. Van Epps, and W.P. Reed. 1979. Serum inhibitor of C_5 fragment-mediated polymorphonuclear leukocyte chemotaxis associated with chronic haemodialysis. J.Clin.Invest:64:255-274

8. Pappenheimer, A.M., and S.L. Wilens. 1935. Enlargement of the parathyroid glands in renal disease. Amer.J.Pathol:11:37-91

9. Roth, S.I., and R.B. Marshall. 1969. Pathology and ultrastructure of the human parathyroid glands in chronic renal failure. Arch. Intern.Med:124:397-407

10. Katz, A.I., C.L. Hampers, and J.P. Merrill. 1979. Secondary hyperparathyroidism and renal oesteodystrophy in chronic renal failure. Medicine (Baltimore):48:333-374

11. Berson, S.A., and R.S. Yalow. 1966. Parathyroid hormone in plasma in adenomatous hyperparathyroidism, uraemia, and bronchogenic carcinoma. Science:154:907-909

12. Massry, S.G., J.W. Coburn, M. Peacock, and C.R. Kleeman. 1972. Turnover of endogenous parathyroid hormone in uraemic patients and those undergoing haemodialysis. Trans.Am.Soc.Artif.Intern.Organs: 18:416-422

13. Arnaud, C.D. 1973. Hyperparathyroidism and renal failure. Kidney Int: 4:89-95

14. Khan, F., A.J. Khan, C. Papagaroufalls, J. Warman, P. Khan, H.E. Evans. 1979. Reversible defect of neutrophil chemotaxis and random migration in primary hyperparathyroidism. J.Clin.Endocrinol.Metab: 48:582-584

15. Tuma, S.N., R.R. Martin, L.E. Mallette, and G. Eknoyan. 1981. Augmented polymorphonuclear leukocyte chemiluminescence in uraemic patients with secondary hyperparathyroidism. J.Lab.Clin.Med:97: 291-298

16. Boyden, S.V. 1962. The chemotactic effect of mixtures of antibody and antigen on polymorphonuclear leucocytes. J.Exp.Med:155:453-466

17. Zigmond, S.H., and J.G. Hirsch. 1973. Leucocyte locomotion and chemotaxis. New methods for evaluation and demonstration of a cell-derived chemotactic factor. J.Exp.Med:137:387-410

18. Boyum, A. 1968. Isolation of Mononuclear cells and granulocytes from human blood. Scand.J.Clin.Lab.Invest:21(suppl):77-89

19. Steiner, A.L., A.S. Pagliara, L.R. Chase, and D.M. Kipnis. 1972. Radioimmunoassay for cyclic nucleotides. II Adenosine, 3'5'-monophosphate in mammalian tissue and body fluids. J.Biol.Chem:247: 1114-1120

20. Bogin, E., S.G. Massry, and I. Harary. 1981. Effect of parathyroid hormone on rat heart cells. J.Clin.Invest:67:1215-1227

21. Aurbach, G.D., H.T. Keutmann, H.D. Naill, G.W. Tregear, J.L.H. O'Riorda R. Marcus, S.J. Marx, and J.T. Potts, JR. 1972. Structure, synthesis and mechanism of action of parathyroid hormone. Recent Prog.Horm. Res:28:353-398

22. Canterbury, J.M., G.S. Levey, and E. Reiss. 1973. Activation of renal cortical adenylate cyclase by circulating immunoreactive parathyroi hormone fragments. J.Clin.Invest:52:524-527

23. Kleeman, C.R., S.G. Massry, and J. Coburn. 1971. The clinical physiology of calcium homeostasis, parathyroid hormone and calcitonin. Calif.Med:114:16-43

24. Hruska, K.A., J. Blondin, R. Bass, J. Santiago, T. Lorraine, P. Altsheler, K. Martin, and S. Klahr. 1979. Effect of intact parathyroid on the hepatic glucose release in the dog. J.Clin.Invest: 64:1016-1023

25. Meytes, D., E. Bogin, A. Ma, P.P. Dukes, and S.G. Massry. 1981. Effec of parathyroid hormone on erythropoiesis. J.Clin.Invest:69:1017-1025

26. Remuzzi, G., P. Dodesini, M. Livio, G. Mecca, A. Benigni, A. Scheepati, E. Poletti, and G. DeGaetano. 1982. Parathyroid hormone inhibits human platelet function. Lancet:2:1321-1324

27. Freitag, J., K.J. Martin, K.A. Hruska, C. Anderson, M. Conrads, J. Land erson, S. Klahr, and E. Slatopolsky. 1978. Impaired parathyroid hormone metabolism in patients with chronic renal failure. N.Engl J.Med:298:29-32

28. Kohot, Y., K.L. Klein, R.A. Kaplan, W.G. Sanborn, and K. Kurokawa. 198 Parathyroid hormone has a positive inotropic action on the heart. Endocrinology:109:2252-2254

29. Baczynski, R., S.G. Massry, R. Kohan, Y. Saglikes, and N. Brautbar. 1985. Effect of parathyroid hormone on myocardial energy metabolism in the rat. Kid.Int:27:718-725

30. Wallach, S., J.V. Bellovia, J. Schorr, and J. Schaffers. 1966. Tissue distribution of electrolytes, Ca^{47} and Mg^{28} in experimental hyper and hypoparathyroidism. Endocrinology:78:16-28

31. Borle, A.B. 1968. Calcium metabolism in Hela cells and the effect of parathyroid hormone. J.Cell.Biol:36:567-582

32. Borle, A.B. 1968. Effects of purified parathyroid hormone on the calcium metabolism of monkey kidney cells. Endocrinology:83: 1316-1322

33. Chausmer, A.B., B.S. Sherman, and S. Wallach. 1972. The effect of parathyroid hormone on hepatic cell transport of calcium. Endocrinology:90:663-672

34. Borle, A.B. 1973. Calcium metabolism at the cellular level. Fed.Proc 30:1944-1950

35. Bogin, E., S.G. Massry, J. Levi, M. Djaldeti, G. Bristol, and J. Smith. 1982. Effect of parathyroid hormone on osmotic fragility of human erythrocytes. J.Clin.Invest:69:1017-1025

36. Lo, H., D.C. Lehotay, D. Katz, G.S. Levey. 1976. Parathyroid hormone-mediated incorporation of ^{35}P orthophosphate into phosphatidic aci and phosphotidylinositol in renal cortical slices. Endocrinol. Res.Comm:3:377-385

37. Molitoris, B.A., K.A. Hruska, N. Fishman, and W.H. Daughaday. 1979. Effects of glucose and parathyroid hormone on renal handling of myoinositol by isolated perfused dog kidney. J.Clin.Invest:63: 1110-1118

38. Farese, R.B., P. Bidot-Lopez, A. Sabir, J.S. Smith, B. Schinbreckler, R. Larson. 1980. Parathyroid hormone acutely increases polyphosphoinositides of the rabbit kidney cortex by a cycloheximide-sensitive process. J.Clin.Invest:65:1523-1530

39. Brautbar, N., J. Chakraborty, J. Coates, and S.G. Massry. 1985. Calcium, parathyroid hormone and phospholipid turnover of human red blood cells. Miner.Elect.Metab:11:111-116

40. Baczynski, R., S.G. Massry, M. Magott, S. El-Belbessi, R. Kohan, and N. Brautbar. 1985. Kidney Int:28:722-727

41. Bogin, E., J. Levi, I. Harary, and S.G. Massry. 1982. Effects of parathyroid hormone on oxidative phosphorylation of heart mitochondria. Miner.Elect.Metab:7:151-156

42. Batra, S. 1976. Mitochondrial calcium release as a mechanism for quinidine contracture in skeletal muscle. Biochem.Pharmacol: 25:2631-2633

43. Harrow, J.A.C., and N.S. Dhalla. 1976. Effects of quinidine on calcium transport activities of the rabbit heart mitochondria and sarcotubular vesicles. Biochem.Pharmacol:25:897-902.

PATHOGENESIS OF SECONDARY HYPERPARATHYROIDISM IN RENAL FAILURE

Eduardo Slatopolsky. Silvia Lopez-Hilker, Adriana Dusso, Alex Brown, and Kevin Martin

Renal Division, Department of Medicine
Washington University School of Medicine
St. Louis, Missouri 63110

In the last five years, investigators have made substantial progress in the understanding of the factors involved in the regulation of parathyroid hormone secretion in renal insufficiency. Chief cell hyperplasia of the parathyroid glands and high levels of immunoreactive parathyroid hormone (iPTH) are among the earliest alterations of mineral metabolism observed in patients with chronic renal failure. Although many factors are responsible for the regulation of the secretion of PTH, it appears that in patients with renal insufficiency, the most important factor for the development of secondary hyperparathyroidism is a reduction in the serum-ionized calcium. However, recent experimental work in dogs (1) indicates that hypocalcemia may not be essential for the development of secondary hyperparathyroidism in chronic renal failure.

Altered secretion of parathyroid hormone in renal failure

An alteration in the suppression of parathyroid hormone by calcium has been shown in glands obtained from patients with chronic renal failure (2,3). This observation suggests that the mechanism for increased parathyroid hormone levels in chronic renal failure may be a shift in the set point for calcium-regulated PTH secretion as well as an increase in the parathyroid tissue mass. The set point for calcium in normal parathyroid cells is approximately 1.0 mM calcium ion whereas in patients with secondary hyperplasia, the set point was found to be increased to 1.26 mM calcium ion (2,3). The shift in the set point for calcium-regulated parathyroid hormone secretion is also manifested as an increase in the calcium concentration required for the inhibition of the adenylase cyclase activity in membranes prepared from hyperplastic parathyroid glands obtained from patients with chronic renal insufficiency (4). Thus, normal concentration of serum calcium may not be sufficient to suppress hyperplastic parathyroid glands and serum calcium may have to be increased to the upper limits of normal in order to control the release of PTH in patients with secondary hyperparathyroidism.

Regulation of PTH by vitamin D metabolites: alterations in uremia

Investigators (5-7) have provided evidence that vitamin D metabolites directly affect regulation of PTH secretion. Oldham et al (8) isolated a calcium-binding protein from porcine parathyroid glands with properties similar to those of the calcium-binding protein found in mammalian intestine mucosa. Subsequently, Brumbaugh et al (9) demonstrated specific binding of $1,25(OH)_2D_3$ to cytosolic and nuclear receptors of the chief parathyroid glands *in vitro*. In studies by Oldham et al (10) in vitamin D-deficient dogs, indicated that higher concentrations of calcium were necessary to suppress the release of parathyroid hormone in these animals. When similar studies were performed in the same animals after $1,25(OH)_2D_3$ administration, the parathyroid glands appeared to be more sensitive to mild increments in serum calcium.

The low levels of $1,25(OH)_2D_3$ observed in patients with advanced renal insufficiency (11) may potentially play a role in the abnormal behavior of the parathyroid glands. To further clarify the role of $1,25(OH)_2D_3$ in the development of secondary hyperparathyroidism, we performed studies in 20 patients on maintenance hemodialysis with the use of an intravenous form of $1,25(OH)_2D_3$ (12). In the control part of the studies, blood was obtained before dialysis three times a week for a period of three weeks. In the treatment period, $1,25(OH)_2D_3$ was given intravenously at the end of each dialysis for a period of eight weeks. The starting dose was 0.5 μg and gradually was increased to a maximum of 4.0 μg/treatment. Finally, a second post-treatment control period was continued for an additional three weeks. Blood samples were obtained for total and ionized calcium, magnesium and phosphorus. PTH was measured with our chicken antibody CH9. This antibody recognizes the C-terminal, mid-region and intact PTH molecule. The mean serum calcium increased from 8.5 mg/dl to 9.4 mg/dl with a peak response of 10.9 mg/dl during $1,25(OH)_2D_3$

administration. In the post-treatment period, serum calcium decreased to a mean of 9.0 mg/dl. In general, there was a tendency for serum phosphorus to increase during $1,25(OH)_2D_3$ administration. Every single patient had a substantial decrease in the levels of PTH during $1,25(OH)_2D_3$ administration. A mean decrement in serum PTH levels was 70.1%. After three weeks of treatment, there was a gradual rise in the levels of ionized calcium. Concomitantly, there was a significant decrease in the levels of iPTH. After $1,25(OH)_2D_3$ was discontinued, PTH increased in every single patient. Thus, the present studies demonstrated that $1,25(OH)_2D_3$ has a remarkable suppressive effect on the release of PTH. Likely, the effects are mainly due to elevation in serum calcium to the upper limits of normal. However, it will seem that in addition to the calcemic effect, $1,25(OH)_2D_3$ per se modify the secretion of PTH. Early, during the administration of $1,25(OH)_2D_3$, before there was a significant increase in ionized calcium, already there was a decrease in the levels of iPTH. Temporal studies show a $20.1 \pm 5.2\%$ decrease in PTH without significant change in serum calcium with intravenous $1,25(OH)_2D_3$ (Figure 1).

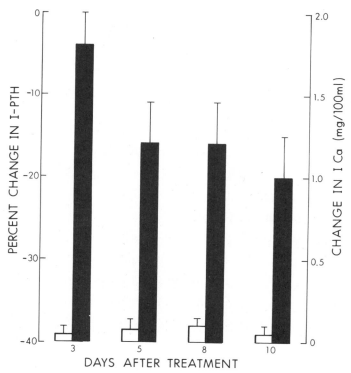

Fig. 1   Temporal relationship between iPTH and ionized Ca during calcitriol treatment (Adapted from Ref. 12).

In five patients, the serum calcium was increased by the oral administration of calcium carbonate. The decrement in serum iPTH was only $25 \pm 6.6\%$ when compared with 73.5% obtained by the administration of $1,25(OH)_2D_3$. Thus, a similar serum calcium achieved administration of $1,25(OH)_2D_3$, rather than calcium carbonate has a greater suppressive effect on the release of PTH.

These studies indicate that $1,25(OH)_2D_3$ administered intravenously rather than orally may result in a greater delivery of vitamin D metabolite to peripheral target tissues other than the intestine and allow a greater expression of biological effect of $1,25(OH)_2D_3$ in peripheral tissues, i.e. parathyroid glands. The use of intravenous $1,25(OH)_2D_3$ provides a simple and extremely effective way to suppress secondary hyperparathyroidism in dialysis patients.

Potential role of vitamin D on the abnormal set point for calcium in renal failure

Since studies with parathyroid cells obtained from uremic patients indicate that there is a shift in the set point for calcium-regulated parathyroid hormone secretion and $1,25(OH)_2D_3$ has a direct suppressive effect on PTH release, we (1) perform further studies to determine if *in vivo* changes in vitamin D metabolism may affect the set point for calcium. Studies were performed before and after the induction of renal failure in dogs. Hypocalcemia was prevented by the administration of a high calcium diet. Initially, ionized calcium was 4.79 ± 0.09 mg/dl and gradually increased to 5.3 ± 0.5 mg/dl after the development of renal insufficiency. Despite a moderate increase in ionized calcium produced by a high calcium diet, amino terminal PTH increased from 65 to 118 pg/ml. Serum $1,25(OH)_2D_3$ decreased from 25 to 12 pg/ml. Further studies were performed in a group of dogs receiving 75 to 100 ng of $1,25(OH)_2D_3$ twice daily. In this group of dogs the levels of serum $1,25(OH)_2D_3$, and amino-terminal iPTH, did not increase after nephrectomy, (Figure 2).

Thus, the low levels of $1,25(OH)_2D_3$, independent of changes in ionized calcium may have a direct effect on the abnormal secretion of parathyroid hormone.

In chronic renal failure, the parathyroid glands are hyperplastic. In addition, a shift in the set point for calcium and an altered adenylate cyclase activity have been demonstrated. Both mechanisms may be related to a decrease in the serum levels of $1,25(OH)_2D_3$. Since in our uremic dogs we avoided the fall in serum concentration of $1,25(OH)_2D_3$ by its exogenous administration, it is possible that with the administration of this hormone we prevented the altered synthesis and secretion of PTH associated with low levels of $1,25(OH)_2D_3$.

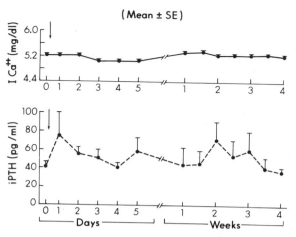

Fig. 2   Serum ionized calcium and amino-terminal PTH before and after the induction of renal fialure. (Arrow denotes nephrectomy. Adapted from Ref. 1)

Recent evidence for direct action of 1,25(OH)$_2$D$_3$ on PTH synthesis and secretion

Recent studies in our laboratory (13) with primary monolayer cultures of bovine parathyroid cells demonstrated a direct suppressive effect on PTH release during addition of 1,25(OH)$_2$D$_3$ into the medium. Furthermore, Cantley et al (14) showed that the reduction of pre-pro PTH messenger RNA levels correlated with a similar reduction in PTH secretion. Recently, Silver et al (15) demonstrated that 1,25(OH)$_2$D$_3$ plays an important role in the regulation of parathyroid hormone gene transcription *in vivo* in the rat. Rats were administered 100 pMOL of 1,25(OH)$_2$D$_3$ metabolite intraperitoneally and the levels of pre-pro PTH messenger RNA were determined. Pre-pro PTH mRNA levels were < 4% of basal at 48 hours at which time there were no increases in serum calcium. *In vitro* nuclear transcriptions show that in 1,25(OH)$_2$D$_3$-treated rats, PTH transcription was 10% of control. Similar results were obtained by Russell and collaborators (16). Thus, it will seem from the above mentioned studies, that 1,25(OH)$_2$D$_3$ has a direct effect on the regulation and secretion of PTH. The main action may be related to inhibition of synthesis of pre-pro PTH mRNA. Moreover, Korkor (17) found that the number of receptors for 1,25(OH)$_2$D$_3$ in parathyroid glands, was reduced in patients with chronic renal failure as compared to patients with transplanted kidneys or primary hyperparathyroidism. Korkor suggested that $1,25(OH)_2D_3$ binding by parathyroid tissue is decreased in chronic renal failure and may contribute to the pathogenesis of secondary hyperparathyroidism by reducing the inhibition by $1,25(OH)_2D_3$ on PTH secretion. Further studies are necessary to fully characterize the role of parathyroid receptor of $1,25(OH)_2D_3$ on the pathogenesis of secondary hyperparathyroidism in chronic renal failure.

Additional evidence for a role of phosphate retention in the genesis of secondary hyperparathyroidism

Since phosphate regulates the conversion of $25(OH)D_2$ to $1,25(OH)_2D_3$, it has been postulated that the low phosphate diet in chronic renal failure suppresses PTH release by increasing the production of $1,25(OH)_2D_3$ (18,19). To gain further information into the mechanism by which low phosphate diets prevent secondary hyperparathyroidism, we performed studies in seven normal dogs before and after the induction of uremia (20). The dogs were fed a low phosphorus diet for one month. In the first month of a low phosphorus diet, ionized calcium did not change significantly. In spite of renal insufficiency, amino terminal iPTH became undetectable in 94% of 148 samples. Of interest, serum levels of $1,25(OH)_2D_3$ decreased from a mean of 21.1 ± 1.8 pg/ml (normal GFR) to 8.8 ± 0.9 pg/ml (one month of renal failure). The suppression of PTH was not due to an increase in the levels of $1,25(OH)_2D_3$. Thus, a low phosphate diet prevented the development of secondary hyperparathyroidism in dogs with renal insufficiency. In addition to the well known effect of phosphate in the regulation of $1,25(OH)_2D_3$, a low phosphate diet may have an effect on the secretion of parathyroid hormone on a long term basis. Potentially, phosphorus may affect phospholipid composition of parathyroid cell membrane, cytosolic calcium and calcium fluxes in the parathyroid cells and/or regulation of $1,25(OH)_2D_3$ receptors in the parathyroid glands, thus, indirectly phosphorus may regulate the secretion of PTH. Further studies are necessary to precisely characterize the mechanism by which phosphate contributes to the regulation of PTH secretion in chronic renal failure.

References

1. Lopez-Hilker, S., Galceran, T., Chan, Y., Rapp, N, Martin, K.J. and Slatopolsky, E., 1986, Hypocalcemia may not be essential for the development of secondary hyperparathyroidism in chronic renal failure. J. Clin. Invest. 78:1097.

2. Brown, E.M., Brennan, M.F., Hurwitz, S., Windeck, R., Marx, S.J., Spiegel, A.M., Koehler, J.O.., Gardner, D.G., and Aurbach, G.D., 1978, Dispersed cell prepared from human parathyroid glands: distinct calcium sensitivity of adenomas vs primary hyperplasia. J. Clin. Endocrinol. Metab. 46:267.

3. Brown, E.M., Wilkson, R.E., Eastman, R.C., Pallota, J. and Marynick, S.P., 1982, Abnormal regulation of parathyroid hormone release by calcium in secondary hyperparathyroidism due to chronic renal failure. Clin. Endocrinol. Metab. 54:172.

4. Bellorin-Font, E., Martin, K.J., Feitag, J.J., Anderson, C., Sicard, G., Slatopolsky, E. and Klahr, S., 1981, Altered adenylate cyclase kinetics in hyperfunctioning human parathyroid glands. J. Clin. Endocrinol. Metab. 52:499.

5. Chertow, B.S., Baylink, D.J., Wergedal, J.E., Su, M.H.H. and Norman, A.W., 1975, Decrease in serum immunoreactive parathyroid hormone in rats and in parathyroid hormone secretion *in vivo* by 1,25-dihydroxycholecalciferol. J. Clin. Invest. 56:668.

6. Au, W.Y.W. and Bukowsky, A., 1976, Inhibition of PTH secretion by vitamin D metabolites in organ cultures of rat parathyroids. Fed. Proc. 35:530.

7. Dietel, M., Dorn, G., Montz, R., Altenahr, E., 1979, Influence of vitamin D_3, 1,25-dihydroxyvitamin D_3 and 24,25-dihydroxyvitamin D_3 on parathyroid hormone secretion, adenosine 3', 5'-monophosphate release, and ultrastructure of parathyroid glands in organ culture. Endocrinol. 105:237.

8. Oldham, S.B., Fischer, J.A., Shen, L.H., Arnaud, C.D., 1974, Isolation and properties of a calcium-binding protein from porcine parathyroid glands. Biochem. 13:4790.

9. Brumbaugh, P.F., Hughes, M.R. and Haussler, M.R., 1975, Cytoplasmic and nuclear binding components for $1\alpha,25$-dihydroxyvitamin D_3 in chick parathyroid glands. Proc. Natl. Acad. Sci. USA 72:4871.

10. Oldham, S.B., Smith, R., Hartenbower, D.L., Henry, H.L., Norman, A.W. and Coburn. J.W., 1979, The acute effects of 1,25-dihydroxycholelcalciferol on serum immunoreactive parathyroid hormone in the dog. Endocrinol. 104:248.

11. Slatopolsky, E., Gray, R., Adams, N.D., Lewis, J., Hruska, K., Martin K.J., Klahr, S., DeLuca, H. and Lemann, J., 1979, The pathogenesis of secondary hyperparathyroidism in early renal failure. Walter deGruyter, Publishers, Berlin-New York.

12. Slatopolsky, E., Weerts, C., Thielan, J., Horst, R., Harter, H. and Martin, K.J., 1984, Marked suppression of secondary hyperparathyroidism by intravenous administration of 1,25-dihydroxycholecalciferol in uremic patients. J. Clin. Invest. 74:2136.

13. Chan, Y.L., McKay, C., Dye, E., and Slatopolsky, E., 1986, The effect of 1,25-dihydroxycholecalciferol on parathyroid hormone secretion by monolayer cultures of bovine parathyroid cells. Calcif. Tissue Int. 38:27.

14. Cantley, L.K., Russell, J., Lettieri, D., and Sherwood, L.M., 1985, 1,25-dihydroxyvitamin D_3 suppresses parathyroid hormone secretion from parathyroid cells in tissue culture. Endocrinol. 117:2114.

15. Silver, J., Naveh-Many, T., Mayer, H., Schmeizer, H.J. and Popovtzer, M.M., 1986, Regulation by vitamin D metabolites of parathyroid hormone gene transcription *in vivo* in the rat. J. Clin. Invest. 78:1296.

16. Russell, J., Lettieri, D. and Sherwood, L.M., 1986, Suppression by $1,25(OH)_2D_3$ of transcription of the pre-pro parathyroid hormone gene. Endocrinol. 119:2864.

17. Korkor, A.B., 1987, Reduced binding [^{3}H] 1,25-dihydroxyvitamin D_3 in the parathyroid glands of patients with renal failure. New Eng. J. Med. 316:1573.

18. Portale, A.A., Booth, B.S., Halloran, B.P., and Morris Jr., R.C., 1984, Effect of dietary phosphorus on circulating concentrations of 1,25-dihydroxyvitamin D and immunoreactive parathyroid hormone in children with moderate renal insufficiency. J. Clin. Invest. 73:1580.

19. Llach, F. and Massry, S.G., 1985, On the mechanism of secondary hyper-parathyroidism in moderate renal insufficiency. J. Clin. Metab. 61:601.

20. Lopez-Hilker, S., Rapp, N., Martin, K. and Slatopolsky, E., 1986, On the mechanism of the prevention of secondary hyperparathyroidism by phosphate restrictions. Kidney Internat. 29:164 (Abstract).

SIGNAL PATHWAYS FOR PTH DEGRADATION IN THE CLONAL
OSTEOGENIC UMR106 CELL

Toru Yamaguchi, Masaaki Fukase and Takuo Fujita

Third Division, Department of Medicine, Kobe
University School of Medicine
7-5-1 Kusunoki-cho, Chuo-ku, Kobe 650, Japan

Introduction

A clonal osteogenic UMR106 cell line, derived from rat osteosarcoma, is known to have morphological and biochemical characteristics of mature osteoblasts in its response to PTH. In this cell, PTH was shown to stimulate cAMP production as a second messenger (1) and also stimulate the breakdown of phospholipids in the cell membrane (2,3). One product, diacylglycerol, activates protein kinase C and the other product, inositol 1,4,5-triphosphate induces Ca^{2+} mobilization from an intracellular stored pool to the cytoplasm, activating Ca^{2+}-receptive proteins (4). Taken together, these observations suggest that the possible mechanism of signal pathway activation by PTH in this cell might be mediated through protein kinase A, protein kinase C and Ca^{2+}-receptive proteins.

In previous work, we reported the existence of a limited PTH-hydrolyzing activity in UMR106 cells (5). In the present study, using this cell line, the effects of activators and inhibitors of signal pathways on the PTH-degrading activity were examined to clarify the roles of these signal transduction systems for PTH degradation.

Methods

PTH fragments and cAMP were measured as described elsewhere (5). In brief, the monolayer of the cells (approximately 4×10^6 cells/9.6 cmm^2 dish) were preincubated in the 1.5 ml of serum free DMEM with various agents for 60 min, then 75 ng hPTH-(1-84) was added to the medium. PTH fragments in the medium produced by degradation of hPTH-(1-84) during the subsequent 60 min incubation were separated from intact PTH by adding trichloroacetic acid (TCA) and bovine serum albumin to yield final concentrations of 5 % and 0.25 %, respectively. PTH fragments in TCA non precipitate were measured by Yamasa PTH-RIA kits. Cyclic AMP in the medium was also measured by RIA.

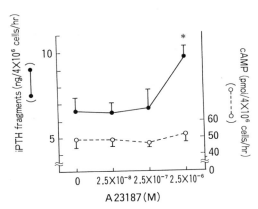

Fig 1.   Dose-dependent effect of A23187 on PTH degradation and PTH-stimulated cAMP production.

Results and Discussion

The effect of a protein kinase C activator, phorbol 12-myristate 13-acetate (PMA) on PTH degradation and PTH-stimulated cAMP production was investigated. Dose-dependent increase of PTH fragments and cAMP production in the medium occured in response to PMA. 1-oleoyl-2-acetyl-glycerol (OAG), another protein kinase C activator, also stimulated PTH degradation and PTH-stimulated cAMP production in a dose-dependent manner (data not shown).

The dose-dependent effect of the calcium ionophore A23187 was examined as shown in Fig 1. An increase of PTH fragments was evident at the concentration of 2.5 μM, but the PTH-stimulated cAMP production was not affected by A23187 at or below this concentration in UMR106 cells.

These data indicate that selective activation of either of two pathways in the calcium messenger system by protein kinase C activators or by the calcium ionophore enhances PTH-degrading activity. In addition, activation of the protein kinase C-mediated pathway by PMA or OAG enhances PTH-stimulated cAMP production. However, Ca^{2+}-receptive proteins-mediated pathway by itself appears to have no ability to control PTH-stimulated cAMP production since the calcium ionophore exerted no effect on it.

Table 1 shows the combined effect of PMA and A23187 on PTH degradation and PTH-stimulated cAMP production. When 2.5 μM A23187 was used in combination with 20, 50 and 100 ng/ml PMA, respectively, PTH degradation and cAMP production were synergistically increased.

In order to investigate the effect of protein kinase C inhibitors on PTH degradation, we used H-7, a potent inhibitor of protein kinase C and HA1004, its weak inhibitor. H-7 suppressed PTH degradation in a dose-dependent manner and caused a marked inhibition by 75 % when the concentration was 200 μM. On the other hand, no inhibition by HA1004 was observed at concentrations of 20 and 50 μM, respectively, and even at 200 μM, the inhibition was only 29 %. This data further indicates the involvement of protein kinase C in PTH degradation by UMR106 cells.

Table 1. Combined effects of PMA and A23187 on PTH degradation and PTH-stimulated cAMP production.

Production of iPTH fragments (% of control)

PMA (ng/ml)	0	20	50	100
-A23187	100.0±2.9	95.6±3.0	116.4±1.9	128.3±4.3
+A23187 (2.5µM)	140.7±2.6	164.4±3.1	173.5±7.6	185.6±18.0

PTH-stimulated cAMP production (% of control)

PMA (ng/ml)	0	20	50	100
-A23187	100.0±17.1	190.6±7.6	193.3±9.0	175.3±10.2
+A23187 (2.5µM)	156.9±25.6	314.7±33.3	314.8±22.1	336.4±79.8

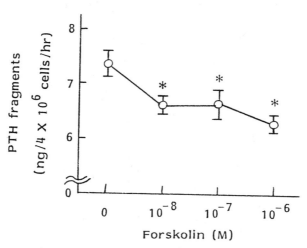

* P<0.01 significantly different from the control

Fig 2. Dose-dependent effect of forskolin on PTH degradation.

We examined the role of cAMP-mediated pathway using forskolin and (Bu)2cAMP. Although both forskolin and (Bu)2cAMP failed to influence PTH degradation in the absence of isobutyl-methyl-xanthine (IBMX), , in the presence of 1 mM IBMX, forskolin suppressed PTH degradation (Fig 2) and (Bu)2cAMP also inhibited it (data not shown). These data might suggest an inhibitory effect of cAMP-mediated pathway on PTH degradation.

The present results indicate that the PTH-degrading process in UMR106 cells appears to be controlled by a bidirectional mode: Two pathways in the calcium messenger system, protein kinase C-mediated pathway and Ca^{2+}-signaling pathway, enhances PTH-degrading activity but the cAMP-mediated pathway suppresses it. Protein kinase C-mediated pathway, nevertheless, potentiates a PTH-stimulated cAMP production, which in turn, activates the cAMP-mediated pathway in a monodirectional fashion. Taken together, the UMR106 cell might have a feedback mechanism to control the PTH-degrading process. At present, it is not clear whether or not this control system plays any role in modulating physiological responses in UMR106 cells. Further studies are required to elucidate this point.

References

1. Martin TJ, Ingleton PM, Underwood JCE, Michellangelli VP and Hunt NH (1976) Nature 260:436-438.
2. Lerner UH, Sahlberg K and Frdholm BB (1986) IXth International Conference on Calcium Regulating Hormones and Bone Metabolism, Nice, France. Abstract No 28.
3. Civitelli R, Reid I, Dobre V, Shen V, Halstead L, Avioli K and Hruska K (1987) Ninth Annual Scientific Meeting American Society for Bone and Mineral Research, Indianapolis, Indiana. Abstract No 233.
4. Nishizuka Y (1986) Science 233:305-312.
5. Yamaguchi T, Baba H, Fukase M, Kinoshita Y, Fujimi T and Fujita T (1986) Biochem.Biophys.Res.Commun. 141:762-768.

PARATHYROID HORMONE-RESPONSIVE CLONAL CELL LINES

FROM MOUSE GROWTH CARTILAGE

Masaharu Takigawa, Eiji Shirai, Motomi Enomoto, Akihiro
Kinoshita and Fujio Suzuki

Department of Biochemistry and Calcified-Tissue Metabolism
Faculty of Dentistry, Osaka University, Suita, Osaka, Japan

INTRODUCTION

The major target organs for parathyroid hormone (PTH) are the bone and kidney. PTH regulates or influences metabolism of calcium and phosphate in these tissues and its action is presumably mediated by 3',5'-cyclic AMP (cAMP) (Rosenblatt, 1982). For investigation of the role of cAMP in mediating the action of PTH, several PTH-responsive clonal cell lines have been established from bone (Aubin et al., 1982; Nakatani et al., 1984) and osteosarcoma (Majeska et al., 1980; Partridge et al., 1983). However, no PTH-responsive cell line has yet been established from cartilage, which is another target organ for PTH (Takigawa et al., 1979; 1980; Kawashima et al., 1980). We have shown that PTH increases the intracellular cAMP level in rabbit costal chondrocytes grown in primary culture (Takigawa et al., 1981) but that the cells lose the abilities to proliferate and to respond to PTH during successive passages (Takigawa et al., 1987). This paper reports the establishment from mouse growth cartilage (GC) of a cell line, and derivative clonal lines that respond to PTH.

MATERIALS AND METHODS

Cell Culture

Mouse chondrocytes were isolated from GC of the ribs of young C57BL/6N mice weighing about 15 g by treatment with EDTA, trypsin and collagenase as described (Takigawa et al., 1980; 1981). Inocula of 1 x 10^5 cells were introduced into 35 mm dishes and cultured in 2 ml of Eagle's minimum essential medium (MEM) containing 10 % fetal bovine serum (FBS). The cultures were kept at 37°C in a humidified atmosphere of 5% CO_2 in air. On day 17, inocula of 5 x 10^5 cells were transferred to four 60 mm dishes and fed twice a week with the same medium without further subcultivation. After 2 months, six colonies composed of rapidly proliferating, morphologically fibroblast-like cells (about 20 cells per colony) appeared on sheets of polygonal, but degenerating cells. When the number of cells per colony became >1000, the colonies were transferred to 35 mm culture dishes and grown in MEM containing 20 % FBS. The cells in three of the six colonies transferred proliferated well. When the cells reached confluence, they were subcultured at a ratio of 1:3-5 in medium containing 20 % FBS. Of these cell lines, only one, named MGC/T1, grew during many

New Actions of Parathyroid Hormone
Edited by S. G. Massry and T. Fujita
Plenum Press, New York

serial passages. Clones were isolated by distributing trypsin-treated MGC/T1 cells (at passage 27) into 96-well microwell plates at an average dilution of one cell/well. Wells containing only one cell were maintained until a monolayer was formed, and then the cells were transferred to 35 mm culture dishes and grown in the same medium. Mouse skin fibroblasts were obtained from new born ICR/Crj mice by treatment with EDTA and trypsin by a reported procedure (Pfefferkorn and Hunter, 1963) and rabbit costal GC cells were isolated as described previously (Takigawa et al., 1980). These cells were cultured in MEM containing 10 % FBS. Normal rat kidney (NRK) cells and Swiss 3T3 fibroblasts were also cultured in MEM containing 10 % FBS.

Assays

The bovine PTH-active fragment (synthetic 1-34, 6,000 IU/mg; Peninsula Laboratories, Belmont, California) was dissolved in 20 µl of phosphate-buffered saline (PBS) and added to the cultures. After an appropriate time, the intracellular cAMP level was determined with a Yamasa cAMP assay kit as described previously (Takigawa et al., 1981).

Glycosaminoglycan (GAG) synthesis was monitored by determining the incorporation of [^{35}S]sulfate into cetylpyridinium chloride-precipitable materials after treatment with Pronase E, as described previously (Takigawa et al., 1980).

Alkaline phosphatase (ALP) activity was assayed by the method of Bessey et al. (1946). Briefly, cells in 35 mm dishes were washed 3 times with saline, scraped into 1 ml of 0.02 % Nonidet P-40, and sonicated at 20 KHz for 60 sec at 0°C. The sonicates were centrifuged for 10 min at 1,600 x g at 4°C and ALP activity in the supernatant was assayed with p-nitrophenylphosphate as substrate.

Protein was determined by the method of Lowry et al. (1951) with bovine serum albumin as a standard.

Calcium deposits were stained with alizarin red S by the method of Dahl (1952).

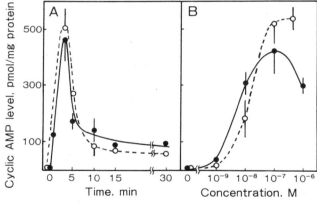

Fig. 1. Stimulation by PTH of the intracellular cAMP level in MGC/T1 cells (●) and rabbit GC cells (O). A. PTH was added at a concentration of 10^{-7} M to confluent cultures of MGC/T1 cells (passage 25) or primary cultures of rabbit GC cells, and the cultures were harvested at the times shown. B. PTH was added to confluent cultures of these cells at the concentrations indicated and the cultures were harvested 2 min later. Points and bars are means ± S.D. for 4 dishes.

424

Table 1. Effect of PTH on the cAMP level in cell lines from mouse costal growth cartilage

Cell line	Passage No.	Cyclic AMP level (pmol/mg protein)		Extent of stimulation (+PTH/−PTH)
		−PTH	+PTH	
Primary culture		$9.4 \pm 2.3^{*}$	773 ± 197	82
Uncloned line				
MGC/T1	25	3.7 ± 0.3	461 ± 63	125
Cloned lines				
MGC/T1.4	70	4.6 ± 0.6	670 ± 29	146
MGC/T1.17	40	10.9 ± 1.9	153 ± 43	14
MGC/T1.18	40	8.1 ± 1.8	1403 ± 145	173

The cells were plated at a density of 2×10^5 cells/35 mm dish. When they became confluent, PTH (10^{-7} M) or PBS was added to the cultures, and the cells were harvested 2 min later. *Values are means $\pm$ S.D. for 4 dishes.

RESULTS

When 10^{-7} M PTH was added to cultures of the uncloned line, MGC/T1 cells, at passage 25, the intracellular cAMP level increased very rapidly to a maximum after 2 min, and then decreased abruptly. PTH had a detectable effect at a concentration of 10^{-9} M and a maximum effect at 10^{-7} M, inducing about 125-fold the control level. The change in the level of cAMP after addition of PTH to MGC/T1 cells was similar to that in primary cultures of rabbit costal GC cells (Fig. 1). The dose-response curve of change in the cAMP level in response to PTH was also similar to that in primary cultures of rabbit GC cells (Fig. 1). The stimulated level in MGC/T1 cells was lower than that in primary cultures of mouse GC cells, but the extent of stimulation was greater than that of the latter cells (Table 1). This stimulation has been observed until at least passage 80. PTH increased the cAMP level in all 16 clonal lines derived from MGC/T1 cells. The basal and stimulated levels of cAMP in some of these lines are shown in Table 1. As with MGC/T1 cells, the maximal stimulation was observed 2 min after addition of 10^{-7} M PTH in all the clonal lines listed in Table 1 (data not shown). However, the responses of the clones to PTH differed. The PTH-stimulated cAMP level and the extent of stimulation ("foldness") in MGC/T1.18 were higher than those in MGC/T1 cells and primary cultures of GC cells. The PTH-stimulated cAMP level in MGC/T1.4 was almost the same as that in primary cultures of mouse GC cells and higher than that in MGC/T1 cells. The extent of stimulation in MGC/T1.4 cells was greater than that in MGC/T1 and primary cultures of GC cells. On the other hand, the PTH-stimulated cAMP level and the extent of stimulation in MGC/T1.17 cells were lower than those in MGC/T1 and primary cultures of GC cells.

GAG synthesis is a marker of the cartilage phenotype. However, the incorporations of [^{35}S]sulfate into GAG in MGC/T1 cells and all the clonal lines were less than that into primary cultures of mouse GC cells (Table 2). The GAG syntheses in MGC/T1 and MGC/T1.18 cells were higher than those in cells derived from other tissues, but the GAG syntheses in MGC/T1.4 and MGC/T1.17 cells were almost the same as those in cells derived from other tissues.

Since primary cultures of rabbit costal GC cells have about 10 times higher ALP activity than that of rabbit costal resting cartilage cells (unpublished) and primary cultures of mouse GC cells also have high ALP activity (Table 2), we also determined the ALP activities of the MGC/T1 line and its clonal lines. As shown in Table 2, the ALP activity of

Table 2. GAG synthesis and ALP activity of MGC/T1 cells and their clonal
cell lines, and cells derived from other tissues.

Type of cells		Days after inoculation	GAG synthesis (dpm/µg protein)	ALP activity (nmol/mg prot./30 min)
MGC/T1	(passage 25)	8	12.3 + 1.1	625 + 59
		15	13.5 + 0.9	1821 + 81
		28	10.5 + 1.4	4741 + 43
MGC/T1.4	(passage 70)	8	3.9 + 0.4	1182 + 582
MGC/T1.17	(passage 40)	8	4.8 + 0.1	3504 + 321
MGC/T1.18	(passage 40)	8	9.8 + 1.9	198 + 12
Mouse GC	(primary)	15	28.9 + 6.6	2000 + 70
Mouse skin	(primary)	8	4.3 + 0.7	75 + 2
NRK		8	2.7 + 1.1	19 + 5
Swiss 3T3		8	5.4 + 1.9	53 + 6

MGC/T1 and its clonal lines were inoculated at a density of 2×10^5 cells
/35 mm dish at the indicated passages. Mouse GC cells, mouse skin fibroblasts, NRK cells and Swiss 3T3 fibroblasts were inoculated at a density
of 1×10^5 cells/ 35 mm dish. On the indicated days, these cells were
labeled with 1 µCi/ml of [^{35}S]sulfate for 2 h or harvested for determination of ALP activity. Values are means + S.D. for 4 dishes.

MGC/T1 cells increased time-dependently, being comparable with that of
primary cultures of mouse costal GC cells on day 15, increasing during
culture to about 7 times the activity on day 8. The ALP activity in
MGC/T1 cells was much higher than those of cells derived from other tissues on day 8. The enzyme activity was heat labile and was inhibited by
L-homoarginine but not by L-phenylalanine, suggesting that the ALP was of
the liver-bone-kidney type. On day 8, the ALP activities of clonal lines
MGC/T1.4 and MGC/T1.17 were higher than that of clone MGC/T1, while that
of clonal line MGC/T1.18 was much lower, but significantly higher than
those of cells derived from other tissues.
    The morphology of MGC/T1 cells in the logarithmic growth phase was
fibroblast-like but they became polygonal as they became confluent. When
the cells were fed with growth medium for 8 weeks without subcultivation,
they formed refractile nodules. The morphologies of sparse cultures of
the clonal lines were also fibroblast-like but their morphologies in
confluent cultures differed. MGC/T1.4 cells became polygonal as they
became confluent and then became multilayered. MGC/T1.18 became polygonal
as they became confluent and showed contact inhibition. MGC/T1.17 cells
were still fibroblastic in confluent cultures and formed nodules like
mountain ranges when cultured for more than 2 weeks without subcultivation. Interestingly, when MGC/T1.17 cells were cultured for 2 months in
the presence of 50 µg/ml of vitamin C and 5 mM β-glycerophosphate, these
nodules stained markedly with alizarin red, indicating calcification.

DISCUSSION

    We reported previously that PTH increases the intracellular cAMP
level in rabbit costal chondrocytes grown in primary culture, but that the
cells lose the ability to respond to PTH during succesive passages (Takigawa et al., 1987). In contrast, the PTH-responsiveness of MGC/T1 and all
the clonal lines listed in Table 1 has been maintained during more than 40
passages. Since PTH increased the cAMP level very much in GC cells, but
little in resting cartilage cells from the nasal septum (Takano et al.,
1987), which does not calcify throughout life, this stimulation is a
marker of GC cells. But, responsiveness to PTH is also a marker of

osteoblastic cells (Luben et al., 1976; Aubin et al., 1982; Majeska et al., 1980). ALP activity is also high in GC cells and low in resting cartilage cells, so this enzyme activity is a marker of both GC cells and osteoblastic cells. Therefore, the MGC/T1 line and clonal lines, MGC/T1.4, T1,17 and T1.18 have typical phenotypes of GC cells, which are in some measure common to those of osteoblastic cells.

The GAG synthesis in MGC/T1.4 and MGC/T1.17 cells were almost the same as those in cells derived from other tissues, although the MGC/T1 and MGC/T1.18 lines had higher activity for GAG synthesis than cells derived from other tissues. However, the ratio of α_1 and α_2 chains of [^{3}H]proline labeled collagen synthesized by MGC/T1.4 and MGC/T1.17 cells were much higher than 2:1, suggesting that these lines produce type II collagen which is also a marker of the cartilage phenotype (unpublished). Therefore, these clonal lines were of cartilage cell origin, but they may have lost these phenotypes during serial passage or may have originated from cartilage cells that did not express these phenotypes, such as hypertrophic chondrocytes.

To obtain the MGC/T1 cells, we exposed secondary cultures of mouse GC cells to a temperature sensitive mutant of Rous sarcoma virus (Schmidt-Ruppin strain) using polyethyleneglycol. However, MGC/T1 cells did not show temperature-dependent changes in responsiveness to PTH, they did not produce a virus inducing transformation of chick embryo fibroblasts when fused with chick embryo fibroblasts infected with Rous sarcoma associated virus, and when a cell extract was treated with anti-pp60^{v-src} the precipitate did not contain tyrosine kinase activity. These findings show that this cell line was not established because of the v-src gene.

We have subcultured these cell lines at an average ratio of 1:4 and lines MGC/T1 are now in passage 85. Therefore, MGC/T1 have now been cultured for at least 170 cell generations from the start of culture, indicating that the line is a so called "established cell line". Lines MGC/T1.4, MGC/T1.17 and MGC/T1.18 are now in passages 78, 50 and 50, respectively, from the start of culture (51, 23 and 23 passages, respectively, after cloning), and are also thought to be immortalized. Since these cell lines have high ALP activity and show high responsiveness to PTH, they undoubtedly originated from skeletal cells. However, further investigations are necessary on their differentiated properties to determine their exact origin. Scince MGC/T1.4 and MGC/T1.18 are highly responsive to PTH, they should be useful in studies on PTH receptors of skeletal cells and/or the role of cAMP in mediation of the action of PTH on cells. MGC/T1.17 may also be useful in studies on endochondral ossification, because it has high ALP activity and ability to calcify.

ACKNOWLEDGEMENTS

We thank Dr. Akira Hakura for his providing Rous sarcoma viruses and for helpful discussion and Dr. Hirokazu Inoue for tyrosine kinase assay. We also thank Mrs. Elizabeth Ichihara for assistance in the preparation of this manuscript, Miss Yoshie Endo and Mrs. Midori Adachi for technical assistance and Miss Hiroko Chuganji for secretarial assistance. This work was supported in part by Grants-in-Aid for Scientific Research from the Ministry of Education, Science and Culture of Japan (to M.T. and F.S.), the Research Foundation for Cancer and Cardiovascular Diseases (to M.T.) and the Osaka Anti-Cancer Society (to M.T.), and Kudo Scientific Research Foundation (to M.T.)

REFERENCES

Aubin, J. E., Heersche, J. N. M., Merrilees, M. J., and Sodek, J., 1982, Isolation of bone cell clones with differences in growth, hormone

responses, and extracellular matrix production, J. Cell Biol.,
92:452.

Bessey, O. A., Lowry, O. H., and Brock, M. J., 1946, A method for the rapid
determination of alkaline phosphatase with five cubic millimeters of
serum, J. Biol. Chem., 164:321.

Dahl, L. K., 1952, A simple and sensitive histochemical method for calcium,
Proc. Soc. Exp. Biol. Med., 80:474.

Kawashima, K., Iwata, S., and Endo, H., 1980, Selective activation of
diaphyseal chondrocytes by parathyroid hormone, calcitonin and
N^6,O^2-dibutyryl adenosine 3',5'-cyclic monophosphoric acid in
proteoglycan synthesis of chick embryonic femur cultivated in vitro,
Endocrinol. Jpn., 27:357.

Lowry, O. H., Rosebrough, N. J., Farr, A. L., and Randall, R. J., 1951,
Protein measurement with the Folin phenol reagent, J. Biol. Chem.,
193:265.

Luben, R. A., Wong, G. L., and Cohn, D. V., 1976, Biochemical characterization with parathormone and calcitonin of isolated bone cells:
Provisional identification of osteoclasts and osteoblasts. Endocrinology, 99:526.

Majeska, R. J., Rodan, S. B., and Rodan, G. A., 1980, Parathyroid hormone-
responsive clonal cell lines from rat osteosarcoma, Endocrinology,
107:1494.

Nakatani, Y., Tsunoi, M., Hakeda, Y., Kurihara, N., Fujita, K, and
Kumegawa, M., 1984, Effects of parathyroid hormone on cAMP production
and alkaline phosphatase activity in osteoblastic clone
MC3T3-E1 cells, Biochem. Biophys. Res. Commun., 123:894.

Partridge, N. C., Alcorn, D., Michelangeli, V. P., Ryan, G., and Martin,
T. J., 1983, Morphological and biochemical characterization of four
clonal osteogenic sarcoma cell lines of rat origin, Cancer Res.,
43:4308.

Pfefferkorn, E. R., and Hunter, H. S., 1963, Purification and partial
chemical analysis of Sindbis virus, Virology, 20:433.

Rosenblatt, M., 1982, Pre-proparathyroid hormone, proparathyroid hormone,
and parathyroid hormone. The biological role of hormone structure,
Clin. Orthop. Relat. Res., 170:260.

Takano, T., Takigawa, M., Shirai, E., Nakagawa, K., Sakuda, M., and Suzuki,
F., 1987, The effect of parathyroid hormone (1-34) on cyclic AMP
level, ornithine decarboxylase activity, and glycosaminoglycan
synthesis of chondrocytes from mandibular condylar cartilage, nasal
septal cartilage, and spheno-occipital synchondrosis in culture,
J. Dent. Res., 66:84.

Takigawa, M., Watanabe, R., Ishida, H., Asada, A., and Suzuki, F., 1979,
Induction by parathyroid hormone of ornithine decarboxylase in rabbit
costal chondrocytes in culture, J. Biochem., 85:311.

Takigawa, M., Ishida, H., Takano, T., and Suzuki F., 1980, Polyamine and
differentiation: Induction of ornithine decarboxylase by parathyroid hormone is a good marker of differentiated chondrocytes,
Proc. Natl. Acad. Sci. USA, 77:1481.

Takigawa, M., Takano, T., and Suzuki, F., 1981, Effects of parathyroid
hormone and cyclic AMP analogues on the activity of ornithine
decarboxylase and expression of the differentiated phenotype of
chondrocytes in culture, J. Cell. Physiol., 106:259.

Takigawa, M., Shirai, E., Fukuo, K., Tajima, K., Mori, Y., and Suzuki, F.,
1987, Chondrocytes dedifferentiated by serial monolayer culture
form cartilage nodules in nude mice, Bone and Mineral, 2:449.

PARATHYROID HORMONE STIMULATES COLONY FORMATION

OF CHICK EMBRYO CHONDROCYTES IN SOFT AGAR

Tatsuya Koike, Yukio Kato, Masahiro Iwamoto, and Fujio Suzuki

Osaka University, Faculty of Dentistry, Department of
Biochemistry. Suita Yamadaoka 1-8, Osaka, 565, Japan

SUMMARY

Chondrocytes isolated from 16- to 19-day-old chick embryos were seeded and maintained for 3 weeks in soft agar. No colony formation was observed without added hormones or growth factors even in the presence of 10 % serum. PTH induced colony formation by the cells. This effect was detected at PTH concentrations as low as 10^{-10} M. The maximal stimulation of colony formation was observed at 10^{-8} M. The colony-forming efficiency of PTH-maintained cultures was 6-9 %. Dibutyryl cyclic-AMP (0.1 mM) also stimulated soft agar growth of chick embryo chondrocytes. However, Prostaglandin I_2 (30 μM) did not stimulate colony formation, although it increased cyclic-AMP levels in chondrocytes. Thus, the growth-promoting effect of PTH is not mediated by cyclic-AMP. PTH had lesser effect on soft agar growth of chondrocytes that were isolated from sternal cartilages of postnatal 14-day-old chickens and rib cartilages of 28-day-old rabbits.

INTRODUCTION

Previous studies have shown that PTH increases cyclic-AMP levels, ornithine decarboxylase activity, and proteoglycan synthesis in monolayer cultures of rabbit growth-cartilage cells (Takigawa et al., 1980, 1981). Further, PTH stimulates the growth of chick embryo cartilage (Kawashima et al., 1980; Burch and Lebovitz, 1983) and chondroprogenitor cells of new born mouse mandibular chondyle in organ culture (Lewinson and Silbermann, 1986). However, there have been no studies demonstrating the mitogenic effect of PTH in a chondrocyte culture system. No stimulation of thymidine uptake nor cell division by PTH was observed in rabbit chondrocyte cultures on plastic culture dishes. Although chondrocytes are ordinarily maintained on plastic dishes, these cells readily lose their phenotypic characteristics after proliferating for several generations. In contrast, chondrocytes in suspension culture maintain their phenotypic expression for a long culture period (Benya and Shaffer, 1982; Kato et al., 1987). We have therefore tested the effect of PTH on chondrocyte growth in soft agar.

MATERIALS AND METHODS

Chondrocytes were isolated from sternal cartilages of chick embryos and chickens and from rib cartilages of 4-week-old rabbits by trypsin and collagenase digestion (Kato et al., 1987; Suzuki et al., 1976). Isolated cells

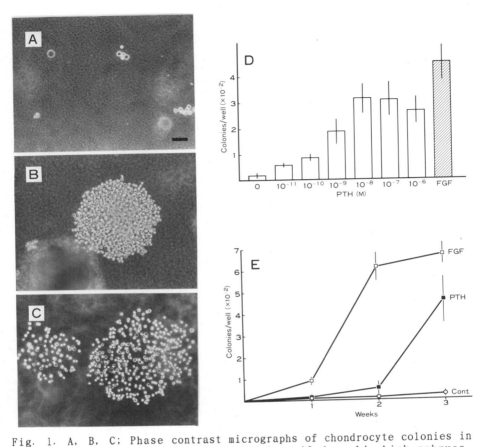

Fig. 1. A, B, C; Phase contrast micrographs of chondrocyte colonies in soft agar. Chondrocytes were isolated from 16-day-old chick embryos. Chick embryo chondrocytes (5000 cells/ 0.5ml/13 mm well) were seeded and maintained without (A), with FGF (0.16ng/ml) (B) or with PTH (10^{-8} M) (C) in soft agar. After 3 weeks in culture, pictures were taken with a Olympus phase contrast photomicroscope. Bar, 100μm.

D; Effect of increasing concentrations of PTH on soft agar colony formation by chick embryo chondrocytes. Cells were seeded and maintained for 3 weeks in soft agar with various concentrations of PTH. PTH and FGF (0.16 ng/ml) were added every fourth day. Values are averages ± S.D. for two to four cultures in two independent experiments.

E; Time course for the PTH- and FGF-induction of colony formation by chick embryo chondrocytes in soft agar. Cells were seeded and maintained in soft agar with PTH (10^{-8} M) or FGF (0.16 ng/ml), as described above. Values are averages ± S.D. for two to four cultures in two independent experiments.

were suspended in Ham's F-12 medium supplemented with 0.41 % Bacto agar and 10 % fetal bovine serum. The suspension (5000 cells in 0.5 ml) was overlaid onto 13-mm wells which were precoated with 0.5 ml of semiliquid Ham's F-12 medium supplemented with 0.72 % Bacto agar and 10 % fetal bovine serum. Mitogenic and metabolic agents were added 3 days after cell seeding. PTH, fibroblast growth factor (FGF), and prostaglandin I$_2$ were added every fourth day. Dibutyryl cyclic-AMP was added once 3 days after cell seeding.

RESULTS

Chick embryo chondrocytes proliferated poorly in soft agar without added hormones or growth factors even in the presence of 10 % fetal bovine serum (Fig. 1A). However, FGF induced remarkable colony formation. Colonies formed in FGF-maintained cultures were large and compact (Fig. 1B). PTH also induced colony formation. Colonies in PTH-maintained cultures were loose clusters of cells (Fig. 1C). In the present study, a cell colony was defined as either a compact cluster of cells with a diameter of more than 0.1 mm or a loose cluster of more than 40 cells. Fig. 1D shows the effect of increasing concentrations of PTH on colony formation by chick embryo chondrocytes. Colonies could be seen at PTH concentrations as low as 10^{-10} M. The maximal stimulation of colony formation was observed at 10^{-8} M. Fig. 1E shows the time course for the PTH- and FGF-induction of colony formation in soft agar. In FGF-maintained cultures, colonies were easily identified 5-7 days after cell seeding. The colonies rapidly grew up to large colonies. The number of colonies reached a maximum 2 weeks after cell seeding. The size of colonies continued to increase for more than 4 weeks. In contrast, PTH induced colony formation more slowly. Only after 2 weeks in culture, colony formation was observed. The number of colonies in PTH-maintained cultures reached a maximum 3 weeks after cell seeding. The colony-forming efficiency (3 weeks) of FGF- and PTH-maintained cultures was 13 and 9 %, respectively (Fig. 1E).

Table 1 shows the effect of PTH (10^{-8} M), FGF (0.16 ng/ml), dibutyryl cyclic-AMP (0.1 mM), and prostaglandin I_2 (30 μM) on soft agar growth of chick embryo chondrocytes and rabbit costal chondrocytes. Dibutyryl cyclic-AMP, as well as PTH and FGF, stimulated colony formation of chick embryo chondrocytes. However, PTH and dibutyryl cyclic-AMP did not induce colony formation by rabbit chondrocytes. FGF was strongly mitogenic for both chick embryo and rabbit chondrocytes. Prostaglandin I_2 did not stimulate soft agar growth of chick embryo and rabbit chondrocytes, although it markedly increased intracellular cyclic-AMP levels in chondrocytes.

Table 1. Effects of mitogens and hormones on soft agar colony formation by chick embryo chondrocytes and rabbit chondrocytes

Agents	Colonies per well	
	Chick embryo chondrocytes	Young rabbit chondrocytes
Control	31± 4	0
FGF	479±30	128±23
Dibutyryl cyclic-AMP	187±15	0
PTH	329±13	0
Prostaglandin I_2	28± 4	0

Chondrocytes were isolated from sternal cartilages of chick embryos and rib cartilages of 4-week-old rabbits by trypsin and collagenase digestion. Cells were seeded in soft agar at a density of 5,000 cells per well. All agents were added 3 days after cell seeding. FGF (0.16 ng/ml), PTH (10^{-8} M), and prostaglandin I_2 (30 μM) were added every fourth day. Dibutyryl cyclic-AMP (0.1 mM) was added once 3 days after cell seeding. Colonies were counted 3 weeks after cell seeding. Values are averages ± S.D. for four to six cultures in three independent experiments.

DISCUSSION

PTH and dibutyryl cyclic-AMP induced soft agar colony formation by chick embryo chondrocytes. Because PTH increases cyclic-AMP levels in chondrocytes (Suzuki et al., 1976; Takigawa et al., 1980, 1981; Takano et al., 1985), the growth-promoting effect of PTH might be mediated by cyclic-AMP. However, prostaglandin I_2 did not stimulate soft agar growth of chondrocytes, although the agent, as well as PTH, increased cyclic-AMP levels in chondrocytes (Kato et al., unpublished). Furthermore, PTH did stimulate colony formation at very low concentrations (10^{-10} to 10^{-9} M), which did not have any effect on cyclic-AMP levels in rabbit chondrocytes (Takano et al., 1985) and chick limb bud mesenchymal cells (Zull et al., 1981). Therefore, it is unlikely that cyclic-AMP plays a second messenger role in the PTH stimulation of chondrocyte growth.

The present study also shows that PTH does not stimulate soft agar growth of chondrocytes isolated from rib cartilages of 4-week-old rabbits. Our preliminary experiments have also shown that PTH induces only a low level of colony formation by chondrocytes from sternal cartilages of postnatal 2-week-old chickens. These observations, taken together with those in previous studies, suggest that PTH has a significant effect on chondrocyte growth during the development of embryos, whereas it had lesser effect on chondrocyte growth in the postnatal life. It is interesting to note that PTH is capable of stimulating proteoglycan synthesis by chick embryo (Kawashima et al., 1980) and adult rat cartilages (Guri and Bernstein, 1964), and 4-week-old rabbit chondrocytes (Takigawa et al., 1980, 1981) in vitro. Further studies are needed to understand the age-dependent response of chondrocytes to the mitogenic stimulus provided by PTH. Chondrocyte cultures in agarose gels will be useful in studying the mechanism by which PTH stimulates cartilage growth.

REFERENCES

Benya, P. D. and Shaffer, J. D., 1982, Dedifferentiated chondrocytes re-express the differentiated collagen phenotype when cultured in agarose gels, Cell, 30:215.

Burch, W. M. and Lebovitz, H. E., 1983, Parathyroid hormone stimulates growth of embryonic chick pelvic cartilage in vitro, Calcif. Tissue Int., 35:526.

Guri, C. D. and Bernstein, D. S., 1964, Effect of parathyroid hormone on mucopolysaccharide synthesis in rachitic rat cartilage in vitro, Proc. Soc. Exp. Biol. Med., 116:702.

Kato, Y., Iwamoto, M., and Koike, T., 1987, Fibroblast growth factor stimulates colony formation of differentiated chondrocytes in soft agar, J. Cell. Physiol., (in press)

Kawashima, K., Iwata, S., and Endo, H., 1980, Growth stimulative effect of parathyroid hormone, calcitonin and $N^6,O^{2'}$-dibutyryl adenosine $3';5'$-cyclic monophosphoric acid on chick embryonic cartilage cultivated in a chemically defined medium, Endocrinol. Japon., 27:349.

Lewinson, D. and Silbermann, M., 1986, Parathyroid hormone stimulates proliferation of chondroprogenitor cells in vitro, Calcif. Tissue Int., 38:155.

Suzuki, F., Yoneda, T., and Shimomura, Y., 1976, Calcitonin and parathyroid-hormone stimulation of acid mucopolysaccharide synthesis in cultured chondrocytes isolated from growth cartilage, FEBS Lett., 70:155.

Takano, T., Takigawa, M., Shirai, E., Suzuki, F., and Rosenblatt, M., 1985, Effects of synthetic analogs and fragments of bovine parathyroid hormone on adenosine $3',5'$-monophosphate level, ornithine decarboxylase activity, and glycosaminoglycan synthesis in rabbit costal chondrocytes in culture: Structure-activity relations, Endocrinology, 116:2536.

Takigawa, M., Isida, H., Takano, T., and Suzuki, F., 1980, Polyamine and differentiation: Induction of ornithine decarboxylase by parathyroid hormone is good marker of differentiated chondrocytes, Proc. Natl. Sci. U.S.A., 77:1481.

Takigawa, M., Takano, T., and Suzuki, F., 1981, Effects of parathyroid hormone and cyclic AMP analogues on the activity of ornithine decarboxylase and expression of the differentiated phenotype of chondrocytes in culture, J. Cell. Physiol., 106:259.

Zull, J. E., Youngman, K., and Caplan, A. I., 1981, The development of hormonal responses of cultured embryonic chick limb mesenchymal cells, Develop. Biol., 86:61.

EFFECT OF PARATHYROID HORMONE ON ORNITHINE DECARBOXYLASE ACTIVITY

IN HUMAN OSTEOGENIC SARCOMA CELLS

Hitoshi Goto, Shuzo Otani, Isao Matsui-Yuasa, Seiji
Morisawa, Kazuhiko Yukioka,* Yoshiki Nishizawa,* and
Hirotoshi Morii*

Osaka City Medical School, Department of Biochemistry
*2nd Department of Internal Medicine, Osaka, Japan

INTRODUCTION

Ornithine decarboxylase (ODC; EC 4.1.1.17) is a rate-limiting enzyme of the biosynthesis of polyamines (putrescine, spermidine, and spermine), which are related to the growth and differentiation of eukaryotic cells (1). Takigawa et al. have shown that PTH induces ODC activity, that polyamines are involved in glycosaminoglycan biosynthesis in rabbit chondrocytes, and that cAMP is involved in PTH-induced biochemical events (2). In concerning osteoblasts, PTH affects the alkaline phosphatase activity (3), collagen synthesis (4), and cell proliferation (5,6). PTH also affects ODC activity in bone cells isolated from mice (7) and chicken (8). These results and others have suggested that PTH action is mainly mediated by cAMP. However, PTH also elevates the intracellular ionized calcium level (9) and induces phosphatidyl inositol turnover (10). Thus, these events also are candidates for the signal transduction of PTH. We are interested in whether PTH affects ODC activity and DNA synthesis and whether cAMP is the second messenger of PTH action in the human osteoblast-like osteosarcoma cell line SaOS2.

MATERIALS AND METHODS

Materials

Synthetic human 1-34 parathyroid hormone (1-34hPTH) was kindly supplied by the Toyo Jozo Co. (Tokyo).

Methods

Cell culture. The SaOS2 cell line (ATCC HTB-85) was established from an osteosarcoma of an 11-year-old Caucasian girl by Fogh in 1975. The cells were plated at 5 x 10^5/5 ml in Falcon 3002 tissue culture plates in McCoy 5A medium containing 10% heat inactivated fetal calf serum and maintained at 37°C in a humified 95% air, 5% CO_2 environment for 7-9 days. When cells had grown to confluence, the medium was changed and 1-34hPTH or other agents were added. After culture for 15 min - 72 h, depending on the experiment, the cells were harvested.

New Actions of Parathyroid Hormone
Edited by S. G. Massry and T. Fujita
Plenum Press, New York

Assay of ODC activity. ODC activity was measured by estimation of the $^{14}CO_2$ released from $[1-^{14}C]$ornithine (Amersham, UK) by the method of Siimes and Jänne (11) with some modifications.

Assay of cAMP content. The cAMP content was measured by radioimmuno-assay with a cAMP assay system (Amersham).

Assay of polyamine level. The intracellular polyamine level was estimated by HPLC with a cation exchange column. Polyamines separated by the column were reacted with o-phthalaldehyde and measured with a fluorescence detector.

Assay of DNA synthesis. DNA synthesis was measured by estimation of $[^3H]$thymidine incorporation into the acid-insoluble fraction after labelling of the cells with 1 μCi of $[6-^3H]$thymidine (Amersham) for the last 6 h.

Assay of protein content. The protein content was measured with the Bio-Rad protein assay system (Richmond, CA).

RESULTS

1. Effect of change of medium on ODC activity

ODC activity in SaOS2 cells at confluent culture was not detected. The ODC activity was increased by fresh medium, but not by conditioned medium; it peaked at 6 h after the change of medium, and then decreased rapidly. The levels of putrescine, spermidine, and spermine also increased parallel to the ODC activity, peaked at 6 - 9 h after the change of medium and decreased slowly.

2. Effect of PTH on ODC activity

Cells were incubated with various concentrations of PTH and fresh medium for 6 h, and then the ODC activity of the cells was assayed. ODC activity was augumented by addition of PTH in a dose-dependent manner at 10^{-9} to 10^{-8} M; the effect was maximum at 10^{-8} and 10^{-7} M. Concentrations of PTH of 10^{-10} M or less had no effect on ODC activity (Fig. 1). Augmentation of ODC activity by PTH did not occur in conditioned medium.

3. Effect of dibutyryl cAMP, cholera toxin, and 3-isobutyl-1-methyl-xanthine in ODC activity

Incubation of cells in conditioned medium with or without PTH or dibutyryl cAMP (dbcAMP) did not increase the ODC activity. In contrast, fresh medium caused an increase in the ODC activity, and the addition of dbcAMP augmented the increase in a dose-dependent manner. The effect of 2.0 mM dbcAMP was equal to that of 10^{-8} M PTH (Fig. 2). Cholera toxin (0.25 μg/ml) and 0.2 mM 3-isobutyl-1-metyl-xanthine (IBMX) as well as PTH (10^{-8} M) also caused augmentation of the increase in ODC activity caused by fresh medium.

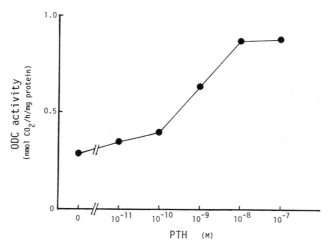

Fig. 1. Effect of PTH on ODC activity in SaOS2 cells. Cells were incubated with fresh medium in the presence of various concentrations of PTH for 6 h. Then the ODC activity of the cells were measured.

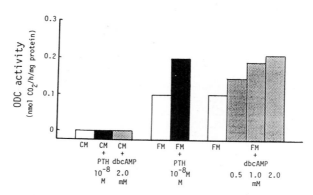

Fig. 2. Effect of PTH and dbcAMP on ODC activity in SaOS2 cells. Cells were incubated in conditioned medium (CM) or in fresh medium (FM) in the presence or absence of PTH or dbcAMP for 6 h. Then the ODC activity of the cells were measured.

4. Effect of PTH on cAMP level

Fresh medium alone did not increase the cAMP level. However, fresh medium with PTH caused a marked increase in the cAMP level after 15 - 30 min of incubation. When cells were incubated with conditioned medium in the presence of PTH, the cAMP level was increased (Fig. 3). PTH at the concentration of 10^{-10} M caused no effect on the cAMP level, but at the concentration of 10^{-8} M, it increased the cAMP level (Fig. 4).

5. Effect of PTH on DNA synthesis

PTH at the concentration of 10^{-8} M inhibited [^{3}H]thymidine incorporation into DNA at 48 h and 72 h after the change of medium. Such inhibition was not caused by the addition of 10^{-10} M PTH.

DISCUSSION

Fresh medium increased ODC activity in confluent SaOS2 cells, but conditioned medium did not. Fresh medium did not elevate the intracellular cAMP level. Therefore, some growth factors in fresh medium, probably in the fetal calf serum, caused an increase in ODC activity via a cAMP-independent pathway.

PTH did not affect the ODC activity of cells incubated with conditioned medium, but augmented the increase in ODC activity caused by fresh medium in a dose-dependent manner. The PTH concentrations that augmented ODC activity coincided with those that elevated the intracellular cAMP level. dbcAMP, cholera toxin, and IBMX, which all increase the intracellular cAMP level, augmented the increase in ODC activity caused by fresh medium; and the extent of augmentation was similar to that of PTH. These results suggest that the action of PTH are mediated by cAMP. Thus, PTH activates adenylate cyclase and elevates the intracellular cAMP level, and in turn augments the increase in ODC activity caused by fresh medium (Fig. 5).

ODC activity increases in many growing cells in parallel to the growth rate (1). However, in this study, we showed that PTH inhibited [^{3}H]thymidine incorporation into DNA in SaOS2 cells. In rabbit chondrocytes, PTH inhibits DNA synthesis via the cAMP-dependent pathway (2). The mechanism of inhibition of DNA synthesis by PTH in SaOS2 cells is not known, but cAMP may be involved in the inhibition of DNA synthesis.

In conclusion, this study showed that the increase in ODC activity caused by fresh medium is not mediated by cAMP, and that PTH augmented the increase in ODC activity by raising the intracellular cAMP level. The biochemical significance of this augmentation of ODC activity by PTH is not clear now; further study is necessary to answer this question.

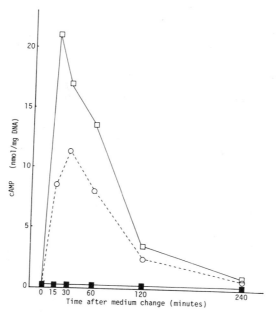

Fig. 3. Effect of PTH on the cAMP level in SaOS2 cells. ○--·-○, conditioned medium + PTH (10^{-8} M): □——□, fresh medium + PTH (10^{-8} M): ■——■, fresh medium alone.

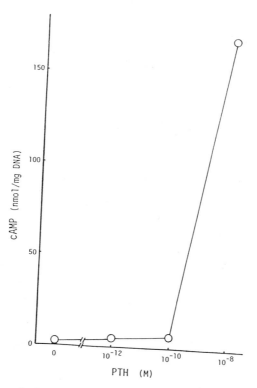

Fig. 4.   Effect of PTH concentration on cAMP level in SaOS2 cells. Cells were incubated with fresh medium and various concentrations of PTH for 30 min.   The intracellular cAMP level was measured.

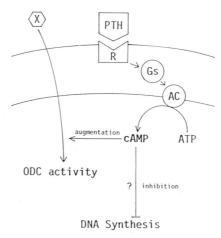

Fig. 5. Scheme of augmentation mechanism of ODC activity by PTH. R, receptor: Gs, G-protein: AC, adenylate cyclase.

REFERENCES

1. Heby, O. (1981) Differentiation 19, 1
2. Takigawa M., Ishida H., Takano T. and Suzuki F. (1980) Proc. Natl. Acad. Sci. USA 77, 1481
3. Luben R. A., Wong G. L. and Chon D. V. (1976) Endocrinology 99 : 526
4. Kream B. E., Rowe D., Smith M. D., Maher V. and Majeska R. (1986) Endocrinology 119 : 1922
5. Partridge N. C., Opie A. L., Opie R. T. and Martin T. J. (1985) Calcif. Tissue Int. 37 : 519
6. MacDonald B. R., Gallagher J. A. and Russel R. G. G. (1986) Endoclinology 118 : 2445
7. Löwik C. W. G. M., van Zeeland J. K. and Herrmann-Eelee M. P. M. (1983) Calcif. Tissue Int. 35 : 5151
8. Boonekamp P. M. (1985) Bone 6 : 37
9. Löwik C. W. G. M., van Leeuwen J. P. T. M., van der Meer J. M., van Zeeland J. K., Scheven B. A. A. and Herrmann-Erlee M. P. M. (1985) Cell Calcium 6 : 311
10. Rappaport M. S. and Stem P. H. (1986) J. Bone Min. Res. 1 : 173
11. Siimes M. and Jänne J. (1967) Acta Chem. Scand. 21 : 815

ENHANCED MINERALIZATION WAS OBSERVED BY

MICROCARRIERS IN CLONAL OSTEOBLASTIC CELL LINE

Masaaki Shima, Kanji Yamaoka and Yoshiki Seino

Department of Pediatrics, Osaka University Hospital
Osaka University School of Medicine
Fukushima-ku, Osaka 553, Japan

SUMMARY

MC3T3-E1 cells showed mineral deposits after about one week of
culture when incubated in the presence of microcarrier beads. These
deposits appeared as white spots on the dish surface, and under light
microscopy the cells showed multiple cell layers and mineralization
around the microcarriers. The deposits stained positively with calcium-
specific Von Kossa's method. Using conventional assay, alkaline phosphatase activity (ALP) and parathyroid hormone-stimulated intracellular
c-AMP production were lower in the microcarrier cultures than in the
control, but using cytochemical methods high alkaline phosphatase
activity was found around the microcarriers. These results indicate
that microcarriers facilitated the formation of multiple cell layers
and provided a culture environment for mineralization.

INTRODUCTION

Recently Kodama et al. established a clonal osteoblastic cell line,
MC3T3-E1, derived from newborn c57BL/6 mouse calvaria (1,2). This cell
line retains alkaline phosphatase activity (ALP), the ability to produce
collagen fibers, and to produce and mineralize ground substance in vitro.
The cells also respond to parathyroid hormone (PTH), prostaglandin E_2 and
1,25-dihydroxyvitamin D_3 by increasing ALP activity. Thus, they retain
many osteoblastic functions and are a useful model for the investigation
of osteoblastic cells.

van Wezel (3) introduced a method for culturing in suspension
anchorage-dependent animal cells on small spheres (microcarriers).
Since its introduction, microcarrier technique has been applied to a
wide variety of different cells enabling the attainment of high yields
of cells, viruses and cell products (4).

Applying microcarrier culture technique to MC3T3-E1 cells, mineralization was observed as early as one week of culture, when the cells
were incubated and plated with the microcarriers. This interesting
finding was the basis for the following experiments designed to study
the mechanism of mineralization induced by the microcarriers.

New Actions of Parathyroid Hormone
Edited by S. G. Massry and T. Fujita
Plenum Press, New York

MATERIALS AND METHODS

Cell Culture

The cells were cultivated in alpha MEM supplemented with 10% fetal calf serum (FCS) at 37.0°C in a humidified atomosphere of 95% air and 5% CO_2 and subcultured every 3 days at a dilution of 1:3 using 0.003% pronase. In experiments, 5×10^4 cells and 4 mg of microcarriers were mixed and plated in 35-mm Corning plastic dishes in 2 ml of medium supplemented with 10% serum, and cultured for 5, 7, 10 and 14 days. In the control, 5×10^4 cells were cultured without the microcarriers in the same manner. Culture medium was exchanged every 3 days. In these experiments, the microcarriers used were Cytodex 3 (Pharmacia Fine Chemicals). Cytodex 3 microcarriers consist of a surface layer of denatured collagen bound to a matrix of cross-linked dextran, and have surface area of 4.6 cm^2/mg dry weight. The denatured collagen of Cytodex 3 microcarriers is derived from pig skin type 1 collagen.

Light Microscopy

MC3T3-El cells were stained with a Ca-specific Von Kossa's method which improved the sensitivity and specificity for demonstrating calcium by initial treatment with oxalic acid (5). ALP activity was localized by incubating with AS-BI phosphate as a substrate and fast blue RR salt as a coupler at room temperature for 15 minutes (6).

Determination of Intracellular c-AMP

On the day before the experiments, the FCS-containing culture medium was replaced with alpha MEM containing 0.3% bovine serum albumin. For measurement of intracellular c-AMP level, cells were preincubated in 2.0 ml of the same medium containing 1.0 mM isobutyl methylxanthine (IBMX) for 15 minutes at 37.0°C, and then incubated with or without 5×10^{-8} M 1-34 hPTH dissolved in alpha MEM containing 0.3% BSA and 1.0 mM IBMX at 37°C for 5 minutes. After incubation, the medium was aspirated and 1.0 ml of ice-cold 5% trichloroacetic acid was added. The cells were disrupted by sonication and centrifuged at 4000 rpm for 10 minutes. The supernatant was washed three times with water-saturated ethyl ether and then used for the c-AMP assay. After acetylation c-AMP was determined using a radioimmunoassay kit (New England Nuclear). The trichloroacetic acid precipitate was used for the determination of protein content.

Assay of ALP Activity, Protein and DNA Content

After the desired period of cultivation, cells were washed three times with Ca-, Mg-free phosphate-buffered saline, collected into 2.0 ml of 0.2% Nonidet P-40 (Sigma) containing 1 mM $MgCl_2$, and sonicated in an ice bath for 5 minutes. After centrifugation at 3000 rpm for 10 minutes, the supernatant was used for enzyme assay. ALP activity was assayed by the method of Lowry et al., using p-nitrophenolphosphate as the substrate (7). DNA content was measured by the method of Labarca et al. (8), and protein content was estimated by the method of Bradford (9).

RESULTS

The control MC3T3-El cells formed a confluent monolayer by 4 days of culture. Although it took 5-6 days for cells incubated with microcarriers to reach confluency, the cells produced mineral deposits by the 7th day of culture (Fig. 1). These deposits appeared as white spots on the dish surface and stained positively using the Ca-selective Von Kossa

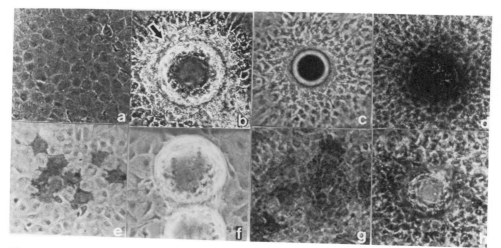

Fig. 1. Phase-contrast microscopic appearance of MC3T3-El cells in day 7 cultures. ×82 control (a) and incubated with microcarriers (b). Staining pattern of Ca using von Kossa method in 7 (c) and 10 (d) days of culture. Mineralization (arrow) was found around microcarriers and was stained with von Kossa method. Cytochemistry of ALP activity. (e) and (f), 4 days of cultivation and (g) and (h) 7 days of cultivation. ×82 (e) and (g), control culture and (f) and (h), microcarrier culture.

method. Light microscopy of cultures with microcarriers showed multi-layers of cells with many inclusion bodies around the microcarriers. The mineralization areas progressively increased with time, and by 14 days of culture covered the microcarriers. Cells not associated with the microcarriers had no mineral deposits. In the control, the cell margins became obscure because the cells piled up and produced ground substance, but no mineral deposits were evident on the 7th day of culture. The control cells continued to pile up and produce ground substance, and mineralization was found on the dish surface by the 14th day of culture.

In the presence of microcarriers cellular protein content increased more rapidly and was significantly higher than the controls on days 7, 10, and 14 of culture (Fig. 2). In the control cultures, protein content increased progressively with time, whereas in the microcarrier cultures,

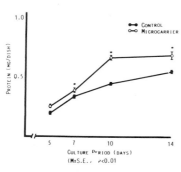

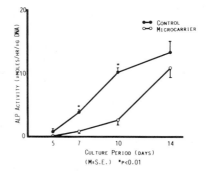

Fig. 2. Time course of protein content in MC3T3-El cells in control (●) and incubated with microcarriers (○). Each point shows the mean±S.E. of 7 cultures.

Fig. 3. Time course of ALP activity in MC3T3-El cells in control (●) and incubated with microcarriers (○). Each point shows the mean±S.E. of 3 cultures.

Table 1. Basal and PTH Stimulated Intracellular c-AMP Levels

Culture Period (Days)	Basal c-AMP level (pmol/mg pr.)		PTH stimulated intracellular c-AMP (pmol/mg pr.)	
	Control	Microcarrier	Control	Microcarrier
5	17.5 ± 0.6	13.42 ± 2.1	885.2 ± 75.3	308.0 ± 33.1*
7	15.2 ± 0.9	11.51 ± 1.0	1680.7 ± 164.8	1101.72 ± 109.7*
10	19.1 ± 5.7	12.93 ± 2.0	2694.9 ± 174.6	1547.85 ± 208.6*
14	20.5 ± 0.4	11.27 ± 0.5	4058.7 ± 113.5	2514.14 ± 231.5*
		(N = 3)		(N = 4)

Values are presented M ± S.E.
* p<0.05, significantly lower than control

protein content increased rapidly for the first 10 days of culture and
then plateaued.

ALP activity was low during the logarithmic phase of cell growth,
but began to increase after the cells formed confluent monolayers.
Values reached 13.3±3.9 µmol/hr/µg DNA by the 14th day in the control
culture (Fig. 3). In microcarrier culture, ALP activity increased more
slowly but was detectable by day 7 of culture. ALP increased at a lower
rate than in the control until day 10, but then increased more rapidly
reaching 10.9±1.6 µmol/hr/µg DNA at the day 14.

Basal c-AMP levels were relatively constant for all culture periods,
the control levels being somewhat higher than cultures incubated with
microcarriers (Table 1). PTH-stimulated intracellular c-AMP production
was increased progressively with time between the 5th and 14th days of
the control and microcarrier cultures. In the control, c-AMP levels
correlated closely with ALP activity (Fig. 4). Cells grown with microcarriers have decreased the intracellular c-AMP production as shown in
Table 1.

In cytochemical studies, ALP activity was detectable in only a
limited number of the control cells after 4 days of culture (Fig. 1e).
The stained cells formed clusters, and with increased length of culture
more cells stained positively (Fig. 1g). In microcarrier cultures, ALP

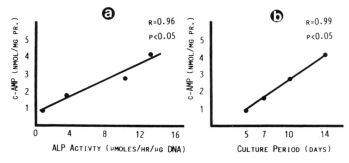

Fig. 4. Relationship between PTH stimulated intracellular c-AMP and
ALP activity (a) and culture period (b) in the control cells.
Correlation coefficient (r) and significance value (p) are
presented in the graph.

activity was not detected after 4 days of cultivation (Fig. 1f), but intense ALP activity was found mainly around the microcarriers after the 7th day of culture (Fig. 1h). ALP activity determined by the Lowry method correlated well with the intense of ALP staining in both control and microcarrier culture.

DISCUSSION

ALP activity has been reported to be a good marker for the differentiation of osteoblastic cells, i.e. the activity increases after the cells form confluent monolayers and correlates with collagen production (12). In our results, ALP activity seemed to correlate with differentiation; activity was not detected before confluency, but was detected after formation of confluent monolayers in both control and microcarrier cultures. In the control, ALP activity increased linearly after confluency. In contrast with the microcarriers, the rate of increase of ALP activity was lower for first 10 days of culture. On the other hand, the rate of increase in protein content was higher in the microcarriers than controls during the period. This may be because the cells continued to proliferate three-dimensionally around the microcarriers after they attained a confluent monolayer. Because the cells remained at the stage of exponential growth during this period, ALP activity would be suppressed. However, ALP activity increased remarkably in the microcarrier cultures when protein content reached a plateau (Fig. 2). Recently, Hakeda et al. (11) showed that forskolin, PTH and prostaglandin E_2 elevated intracellular c-AMP level and that the c-AMP seemed to act as a stimulator of osteoblastic cell maturation in vitro. The present study demonstrates that although the basal levels of intracellular c-AMP remained relatively constant thought the culture period, PTH-stimulated c-AMP production increased progressively with culture period and correlated closely with ALP activity. Therefore, the intracellular c-AMP production may be also a reflection of differentiation in these cells. The same finding was reported by Kumegawa et al. (12), showing that PGE_2 increased c-AMP and ALP activity in a dose-dependent fashion in MC3T3-E1 cells. In addition, Majeska and Rodan (13) documented the same observation by two c-AMP-stimulatory hormones, PTH and isoproterenol, in ROS 17/2 cell line.

The cells cultured with microcarrier beads showed mineral deposits as early as day 7 of culture, but ALP activity and PTH-stimulated c-AMP production were lower than in the control. Because microcarriers increased the effective culture surface by three-fold more than that of in the control, it took another 1-2 days longer to form confluent monolayers, and the cells continued to proliferate much longer than in the control after confluency (Fig. 2). This may explain why differentiation was delayed as a whole. Although total ALP activity was lower than in the control, higher ALP activity was found locally around the microcarriers (Fig. 1). As reported by Ecarot-Charrier et al. (14), mineralization of osteoblastic cells in culture occurred only in multilayer areas. MC3T3-E1 cells have been shown to differentiate at the monolayer stage when collagen production is prevented using ascorbic acid-deficient conditions (2). Cell interaction and compaction may be important in inducing mineralization. ALP activity also began to increase after formation of the confluent monolayer, that is, compaction. The control MC3T3-E1 cells grow to form multiple cell layers at a slow pace after the formation of a confluent monolayer (Fig. 2). In contrast, the cells incubated with microcarriers easily formed multiple layers and readily differentiated around the microcarriers as early as one week of culture. At least in part, this may explain why the cultures show mineralization at 7 days of culture.

In conclusion, MC3T3-E1 cells produced mineral deposits when incubated with microcarriers as early as one week. This may be related to the fact that microcarriers facilitated the formation of multiple layers and differentiation of the cells around the microcarriers.

REFERENCES

1. H. Kodama, Y. Amagai, H. Sudo, S. Kasai and S. Yamamoto, Establishment of a clonal osteogenic cell line from newborn mouse calvaria, Jpn J Oral Biol 23:899 (1981).
2. H. Sudo, H. Kodama, Y. Amagai, S. Yamamoto and S. Kasai, In vitro differentiation·and calcification in a new clonal osteogenic cell line derived from newborn mouse calvaria, J Cell Biol 98:191 (1983).
3. A. L. van Wezel, Growth of cell stains and primary cells on microcarriers in homogenous culture, Nature 216:64 (1967).
4. P. van Hemert, D. G. Kilburn and A. L. van Wezel, Homogenous cultivation of animal cells for production of virus and virus products, Biotechnol Bioeng 11:875 (1969).
5. F. Gallyas and J. R. Wolff, Oxalate pretreatment and use of a physical developer render the Kossa method selective and sensitive for calcium, Histochemistry 83:423 (1985).
6. M. S. Burstone, Histochemical observation on enzymatic processes in bone and teeth, Ann N Y Acad Sci 85:431 (1960).
7. O. H. Lowry, N. R. Roberts, M. L. Wu, W. S. Hixon and E. J. Crawford, The quantitative histochemistry of brain, J Biol Chem 207:19 (1954).
8. C. Labarca and K. Paigen, A simple, rapid and sensitive DNA assay procedure, Anal Biochem 102:344 (1980).
9. M. M. Bradford, A rapid and sensitive method for the quantitation of microgram quantities of utilizing the principle of protein-dye binding, Anal Biochem 72:248 (1976).
10. M. Kumegawa, M. Hiramatsu, K. Hatakeyama, T. Yajima, H. Kodama, T. Osaki and K. Kurisu, Effects of epidermal growth factor on osteoblastic cells in vitro, Calcif Tissue Int 35:542 (1983).
11. Y. Hakeda, E. Ikeda, Y. Nakatani, N. Maeda and M. Kumegawa, Induction of osteoblastic cell differentiation for forskolin. Stimulation of cyclic AMP and alkaline phosphatase activity, Biochim Biophys Acta 838:49 (1985).
12. M. Kumegawa, E, Ikeda, S. Tanaka, T. Haneji, T. Yora, Y. Sakagishi, N. Minami and M. Hiramatsu, The effects of prostaglandin E$_2$, parathyroid hormone, 1.25 dihydroxycholecalciferol, and cyclic nucleotide analog on alkaline phosphatase activity in osteogenic cells, Calcif Tissue Int 36:72 (1984).
13. R. J. Majeska and G. A. Rodan, Alkaline phosphatase inhibition by parathyroid hormone and isoproterenol in a clonal rat osteosarcoma cell line. possible mediation by cyclic AMP, Calcif Tissue Int 34:59 (1982).
14. B. Ecarot-Charrier, F. H. Glorieux, M. Rest and G. Pereira, Osteoblasts isolated from mouse calvaria initiate matrix mineralization in culture, J Cell Biol 96:639 (1983).

PTH CONTROL OF OSTEOBLASTIC FUNCTION

R. Civitelli, I.R. Reid, K.A. Hruska, and L.V. Avioli

Division of Bone and Mineral Diseases, Washington Univ.
School of Medicine at the Jewish Hospital of St. Louis
St. Louis, Mo. USA

INTRODUCTION

The aging of human bone has been characterized by a variety of acquired hormonal and cellular aberrations not the least of which are hypotheses which detail an "imbalance" between osteoblastic and osteoclastic function due to either osteoblastic senescence and/or alterations in the "coupling" between osteoclasts and osteoblasts. Age-related decrements in osteoblastic activation when coupled with age-related increments in osteoclastic activity could readily account for a steady and progressive loss of bone with age. Intracellular calcium ($Ca^{2+}i$) has been established as "the" pivotal factor in controlling the behavior of eukaryotic cells, and senescent cells from extraskeletal tissues have been characterized by acquired alterations in calcium content and/or homeostasis (1).

The most recent models describing the cellular mechanisms of bone remodeling assign to the osteoblast the role of mediator in the transduction of bone resorption signaling from local and general factors to the osteoclasts (2). This view is supported by the experience of Chambers and co-workers who discovered that bone resorption signaling can be transferred to osteoclasts through the medium conditioned by osteoblasts incubated with general and local bone resorbing factors, such as parathyroid hormone (PTH) (3), and in interleukin-1 (4); and by a previous observation that the osteoclasts do not respond directly to PTH (5). On this basis, we have designed studies with the purpose to define the regulation of osteoblast function by PTH, using animal and human cells expressing an osteoblast phenotype.

RESULTS AND DISCUSSION

Recent studies in renal cells (6) demonstrated that PTH can elicit a transient increase of $Ca^{2+}i$, associated to inositol 1,4,5-tris-phosphate [IP_3] and diacylglycerol (DAG) production. These products derive from phosphatidylinositol 4,5-bisphosphate [$PIns\ (4,5)-P_2$] hydrolysis by phospholipase C, and constitute messages which in turn activate protein kinase C (DAG) and mobilize calcium from intracellular stores (IP_3). We extended these studies to osteoblastic cells. First, using the fluorescent Ca^{2+}-sensitive probes Indo-1 and Fura-2, we examined the effect of PTH on $Ca^{2+}i$ in normal and transformed osteoblasts. In suspensions of osteogenic sarcoma cells (UMR 106) loaded with Indo-1, PTH triggered a transient increase of $Ca^{2+}i$, with a return to baseline within one minute (7). To date, at least two other groups reported this finding in transformed osteoblastic cell lines (8,9). The dose response curve of PTH-induced $Ca^{2+}i$ transients and cAMP production were quite similar; with ED_{50} being approximately $5/10^{-8}M$ PTH for both. The PTH effect on $Ca^{2+}i$, was reproduced in cell monolayers of normal human osteoblasts obtained by collagenase digestion of rib fragments and loaded with Fura-2, confirming that the mobilization of $Ca^{2+}i$ is an event following PTH interaction with its receptor in cells expressing an osteoblast phenotype.

The PTH-induced transient rise in $Ca^{2+}i$ could be almost entirely blocked by pretreatment with inhibitors of sarcoplasmic reticulum Ca^{2+} release such as dantrolene and TMB-8. In addition, chelation of extracellular Ca^{2+} by EGTA did not prevent the $Ca^{2+}i$ increase produced by PTH exposure in UMR 106-01 cells. These experiments suggested that an intracellular source of the Ca^{2+} contributed to the $Ca^{2+}i$ transients.

This latter hypothesis was confirmed in further experiments which revealed that PTH can elicit a rapid increase of inositol trisphosphate and tetrakiaphosphate (IP_4) in UMR 106 cells, with a peak at 30 seconds, and a return to baseline within 1 minute. Using an HPLC procedure, we could demonstrate that the IP_3 generated after PTH exposure was almost entirely represented by inositol 1,4,5 trisphosphate, and only in part by the isomer inositol 1,3,4 trisphosphate, which derives from dephosphorylation of IP_4 (10). Thus, it seems that the $Ca^{2+}i$ transients induced by PTH are, in most part, derived from IP_3-stimulated release of $Ca^{2+}i$ from an IP_3-sensitive endoplasmic reticulum $Ca^{2+}i$ pool.

We subsequently found that in UMR 106 cells, PTH produced an increase of DAG which was detectable at 5 min after hormonal stimulation. This finding confirms the hypothesis that the PTH-receptor is associated with an activation of phospholipase C, the latter hydrolyzing PIns (4,5)-P2 with consequent release of IP_3 and DAG. In this regard, we subsequently identified a phospholipase C enzyme in the plasma membrane of osteoblasts with a pH optimum of 7.0 and an apparent Km for PIP_2, PIP, and PI of 28 µM, 34 µM, and 120 µM, respectively. The accumulated data suggest the existence of an intracellular second message system(s) alternative to cAMP production, which are activated by PTH in target cells. Subsequently, other experiments were designed in the attempt to understand the role of the cAMP, $Ca^{2+}i$, and DAG message systems in osteoblast function.

PTH-induced changes in $Ca^{2+}i$ were associated with a slight hyperpolarization in single cell recordings of membrane potential using the voltage-sensitive fluorescent probe di-BA-C4. However, no effect was detected in bulk cell suspensions (Civitelli, R., Avioli, L.V., and Hruska, K.A., unpublished observation). A difference in sensitivity may explain this discrepancy. In any case, the importance of membrane potential changes in PTH control of osteoblasts is still to be elucidated.

Activation of protein kinase C by DAG leads to cytosolic alkalinization through activation of the Na^+/H^+ exchanger which is thought to be permissive to cell replication. Thus, we investigated the hormonal control of intracellular pH (pHi) in osteoblast-like cells using the fluorescent pH-indicator BCECF. Contrarily to what would be expected from the previous assumption, PTH inhibited the amiloride-sensitive Na^+/H^+ exchange, producing cell acidification (11). This result correlated with the observed inhibition of [^3H]-thymidine incorporation in the same cell line (11). In both cases the effects of PTH were mimicked by forskolin and cAMP analogues. Addition of ionomycin in doses that reproduced the PTH-induced $Ca^{2+}i$ increments potentiated the cAMP dependent effects on pHi and mitogenesis. The antimitogenic effect of PTH may suggest that activation of the Ca^{2+}-message system by PTH is primarily utilized for control of stimulus-response coupling (12). Since the primary action of PTH in bone is to stimulate resorption, studies were designed to evaluate the potential role of these intracellular message systems on bone resorption. Both cAMP analogues and ionomycin (to a lesser extent) were able to stimulate ^{45}Ca release from rat fetal limb bones prelabeled with ^{45}Ca, whereas phorbol esters were not. As observed for pHi and mitogenesis, the effects of ionomycin and cAMP analogues were additive, and fully mimicked the effect of PTH, suggesting that the Ca message system is additive to cAMP in inducing bone resorption (12).

CONCLUSION

In conclusion, the hormonal control of osteoblastic function by PTH appears to be mediated by receptor coupling to both adenylate cyclase and phospholipase C. A complex pattern of interactions among the various intracellular biochemical pathways results in a variety of cellular activities, including ionic changes, DNA synthesis and secretion product synthesis, which characterizes the cellular response to the hormonal stimulus. All of these factors must be anticipated and reconciled in studies designed to evaluate age-related changes in osteoblastic function per se and/or alterations in the coupling between osteoblasts and osteoclasts.

REFERENCES

1. Avioli, LV. Am. J. Nephrol. 1986; 6 Suppl 1:151-154.
2. Rodan GA, Martin TJ. Calcif. Tiss. Int. 1981; 33:349-351.
3. McSheehy PMJ, Chambers TJ. Endocrinology 1986; 118:824-828.
4. Thomson BM, Saklatvala J, Chambers TJ. Exp. Med. 1986; 164:104-112.
5. Braidman IP, Anderson DC, Jones CJP, Weiss JB. J. Endocrinol. 1983; 99:387-399.
6. Hruska KA, Moskowitz D, Esbrit P, Civitelli R, Westbrook S, Huskey M. J. Clin. Invest. 1987; 79:230-239.
7. Reid Ir, Civitelli R, Halstead LR, Avioli LV, Hruska KA. Am. J. Physiol. 1987; 252:E45-E51.
8. Lowick CWGM, van Leeuwen JPTM, van der Meer JM, van Zeeland JK, Scheven BAA, Herrmann-Eriee MPM. Cell Calcium 1985; 6:311-326.
9. Yamaguchi DT, Hahn TJ, Iida-Klein A, Kleeman CR, Mualeem S. J. Biol. Chem. 1987; 262:7711-7718.
10. Batty IR, Nahorski SR, Irvine RF. Biochem. J. 1985; 232:211-215.
11. Reid IR, Civitelli R, Avioli LV, Hruska KA. J. Bone. Min. Res. 1987; 2(S1):127A.
12. Civitelli R, Reid IR, Dobre V, Shen V, Halstead LR, Avioli LV, Hruska KA. J. Bone. Min. Res 1987; 2(S1):233A.

DEVELOPMENT OF SIMPLE AND SENSITIVE SYSTEM FOR DETECTION OF

BONE SEEKING SUBSTANCES EMPLOYING CHICK EMBRYO TIBIAE

Masaei Kurokawa, Akitoshi Kawakubo, Masahiro Yoneda, Kensuke Takatsuki
and Akio Tomita*

1st. Dept. of Internal Medicine, Nagoya University School of Medicine
*Central Laboratory for Clinical Investigation, Aichi Medical University
65 Tsuruma-cho, Showa-ku, Nagoya, 466 Japan

INTRODUCTION

Hypercalcemia is one of the most common complications of malignant diseases. Besides metastatic bone lesions, systemic bone resorption mediated by humoral factors which are produced by tumors causes hypercalcemia. Among many factors attributed to the "humoral hypercalcemia of malignancy", the adenylate cyclase stimulating factor (ACSF), first described by Stewert et al. (1) in 1980, has been most extensively studied. Recently an ACSF isolated from a lung carcinoma was purified by Martin et al. (2). It is a polypeptide of 18,000 daltons having a remarkable homology with human parathyroid hormone (hPTH). However, ACSFs with different molecular weight have been reported by other investigators, suggesting that there may be multiple ACSF species.

To study ACSFs in tumor extracts, cultures of renal cortical cells or osteoblastic cells are commonly used. The cultures however, are time- and cost-consuming and require sterile procedures. To solve these problems, we have developed a simple, rapid and sensitive bioassay system for ACSFs employing fragments of embryonic chick tibiae, which does not require sterile procedures.

METHOD

Tibiae from 18 day old chick embryo were finely minced with scissors. The bone fragments were filtered through 800 μm stainless steel mesh and preincubated for 60 min at 37°C in Earle's medium under 5% CO_2. The fragments were then rinsed twice and stirred in Earle's medium containing 20mM HEPES, 2mM isobutyl methylxanthine and 2% bovine serum albumine. Four hundred μl aliquots of the suspension were transfered to 24 well culture dish, to which 100 μl of medium containing test materials was added. After 120 min incubation at 37°C, cAMP in the medium was determined by RIA.

RESULT

The effects of hPTH1-34, Prostaglandin E_1 and E_2 on cAMP production in the system are compared on the molar basis (Fig. 1) When hPTH1-34 was added to the bone fragments, significant increase of cAMP production was observed at concentrations higher than 10^{-9}M. Prostaglandin E_1 and Prostaglandin E_2 also increased cAMP production in similar dose response relationship. However, maximum effects of Prostaglandins obtained at 10^{-6}M were less than 50% of that achieved by 10^{-8}M hPTH1-34. On the other hand, Eel calcitonin had no effect on the cAMP production even at a high concentration of 10^{-6}M.

Using this assay system, we characterized ACSF in extracts of esophageal and lung carcinoma from patients with typical findings of humoral hypercalcemia of malignancy. The tumors

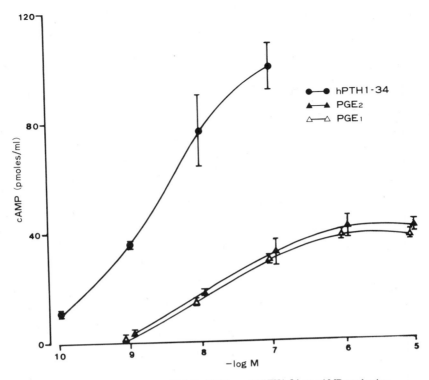

Fig. 1 Comparison of Effect of PG E_1, PG E_2, and hPTH1-34 on cAMP production of bone fragments.

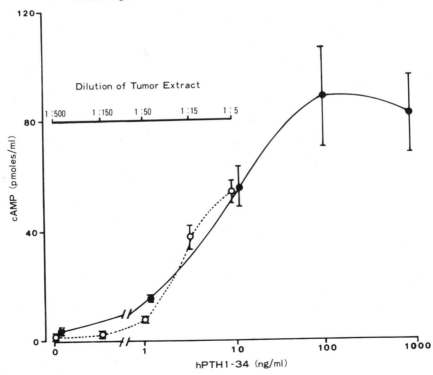

Fig. 2 Effect of hPTH1-34 or tumor extract on cAMP production of bone fragments.

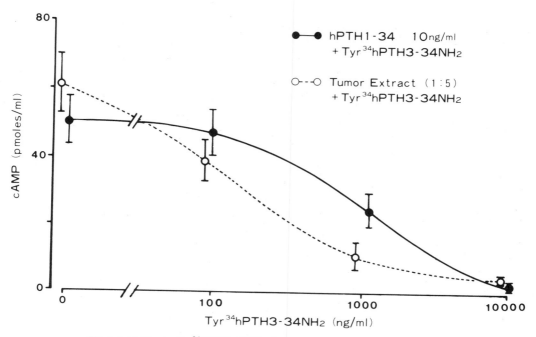

Fig. 3 Inhibition by Try[34]hPTH3-34NH₂ of cAMP production of bone fragments stimulated by tumor extract or hPTH1-34.

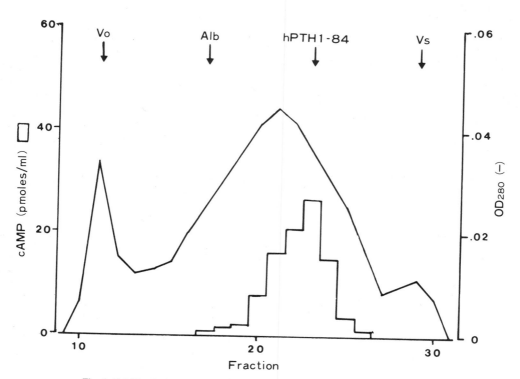

Fig. 4 Gel filtration of extract on sephadex G-200.
Fractions were assayed for adenylate cyclase stimulating activity using chick bone fragments. Vo: void volume, Vs: salt volume, Alb: albumin.

obtained at autopsy were extracted with 8M Urea – 0.2N HCL and centrifuged at 10,000 X G. The supernatant was dialysed against 0.05M NH_4HCO_3 and lyophlized. The extracts were finally reconstituted with medium, and added to the above system. Fig. 2 shows the dose-related production of cAMP by bone fragments incubated with the extract of an esophageal carcinoma, which were parallel to that caused by hPTH1-34. The increase of cAMP production induced by the extract was inhibited by a PTH antagonist Tyr^{34}hPTH3-34, indicating that a factor in the extract stimulates adenylate cyclase through binding to the PTH-receptor (Fig. 3).

Another extract from a lung carcinoma, which had a PTH-like ACSF activity was subjected to gel filtration on Sephadex G-200 (Fig. 4). The ACSF assayed in our system was eluted to a position close to that of hPTH1-84 used in calibration of the column. Thus it was infered that the molecular weight of the ACSF in the tumor was approximately 10,000 daltons.

DISCUSSION

The chick tibiae, at the embryonic stage they were used in our experiments, are known to be rich in osteoblasts and chondrocytes, but not in osteoclasts (3). It has also been shown that both osteoblasts and chondrocytes respond to PTH with increase of cAMP. Therefore, we suspect that the cells participating in the cAMP production in our system are both osteoblasts and chondrocytes.

In respect to the sensitivity to hPTH, our system is equal or superior to the cultures of renal cortical cells or osteoblastic cells so far reported (4), (5). In addition, it dose not require sterile procedures and the results can be obtained even next day of incubation. Taken these into account, the system described here appears to be useful for detecting ACSFs in tumors.

REFERENCE

1. A. F. Stewart, R. Horst, A. E. Broadus et al., N Engl J Med. 303: 1377–1383 (1980)
2. J. M. Mosely, M. Kubota, T. J. Martin et al., Parathyroid Hormone-Related Protein Purified from a Human Lung Cancer Cell Line, Proc. Natl. Acad. Sci. USA, 84: 5043–5052 (1987)
3. R. T. Turner, J. E. Puzas, D. J. Baylink et al., *In vitro* synthesis of 1-alpha, 25 dihydroxycholecalciferol and 24, 25-dihydrocholecalciferol by isolated calvarial cells, Proc. Natl. Acad. Sci. USA. 77: 5720–5724 (1980)
4. R. Zonefrati, M. L. Brandi, R. Toccafondi et al., Prathyroid Hormone Bioassay Using Human Kidney Cortical Cells in Primary Culture, Acta Endocrinologica. 100: 398–405 (1982)
5. R. J. Majeska, S. B. Rodan, G. A. Rodan, Parathyroid Hormone-Responsive Clonal Cell Lines from Rat Osteosarcoma, Endocrinology. 107: 1494–1503 (1980)

BONE MINERAL DENSITY IN CHRONIC RENAL FAILURE

M. Fukunaga and R. Morita

Department of Nuclear Medicine, Kawasaki Medical School
Kurashiki, Japan

INTRODUCTION

Recently non-invasive techniques such as photodensitometry using X-ray
films, single or dual photon absorptiometry (SPA or DPA) and quantitative
computed tomography for correctly assessing bone mass have been developed.
Therefore, bone mineral density (BMD) in not only appendicular bone, predominantly cortical bone, but also axial bone, predominantly trabecular
bone, could be measured.
It is well-known that there occurred a variety of skeletal lesions
(osteitis fibrosa, osteomalacia, osteosclerosis or osteoporosis) in
chronic renal failure (CRF)(1). Although bone histological, blood biochemical and hormonal examinations in CRF have been widely performed,
less attention is focused in BMD. It is also suggested that, under the
diseased situations, metabolic bone disease, the change of bone mineral
might appear more prominent and earlier in trabecular bone than in cortical bone. In this study, in order to evaluate changes of bone mineral
in CRF, BMD in appendicular bone by SPA and axial bone by DPA have been
measured.

Outline of newly developed DPA instrument

In this study, newly developed DPA instrument, DUALOMEX HC-1, was used.
This unit is devised with its detector component consisting of a scintillation camera system, instead of the scintiscanner employed in conventional instruments (2)-(5). The detector has one NaI (Tl) scintillation
crystal backed with a matrix of 22 photomultiplier tubes. With an effective field of view of 12.5X15.6 cm, it enables simultaneous measurement
of more than 3 vertebrae. The uniformity in 80% of the field size is
less than $\pm$ 10%. The intrinsic spatial resolution is 9.0 mm(FWHM) at a
44 keV and 5.0 mm (FWHM) at a 100 key keV photon energy. The distance
between the source and detector is 100 cm. The scintillation camera is
positioned with the subject sitting on the chair set by the side of the
detector. The entire procedure of measurement takes 6 min. for body
thickness of 20 cm. The precision assessed from inter-assay reproduci-
bility was 1.6%(C.V.) for phantom and 3.5%(C.V.) for human studies (N=6,
respectively). Data collection and processing were done by personal
computer. The radioactive source used ^{153}Gd, its dose (50 mCi) being
lower than that in conventional instruments. The irradiation is as
limited as less than 2 mR.

Methods and Materials

BMD at 3rd lumbar vertebra (L_3), predominantly composing trabecular bone, was measured by DUALOMEX HC-1, and BMD at 1/3 distal radius, predominantly composing cortical bone, was measured by SPA (Norland). The procedure of bone mineral analysis of L_3 is below; upon termination of data acquisition, an image of the lumbar vertebrae in antero-posterior view is displayed, and the upper and lower ends of L_3 are then identified by moving image cursors. In the area of L_3, mean bone mineral content (BMC), mean bone width (BW) and mean BMD (BMC/BW) were obtained.

Since BMD values were greatly influenced by age and sex, and index of % BMD was used in this study. % BMD was defined as the percentage of BMD in individual to mean BMD value corresponding to age and sex-matched controls.

Fifty-nine patients with CRF (10 patients prior to hemodialysis (HD) and 49 on HD) were used in this study. Patients on HD were divided to 4 groups depending on durations of HD (10 patients; less than 1 year history of HD, 10; 1-5 yrs., 15:5-10 yrs., and 14; more than 10 yrs). In these patients, % BMDs were compared.

In 24 patients with long history, 6-13 yrs., of HD, relation between secondary hyperparathyroidism (SHP) state and % BMD values were studied. SHP was diagnosed from findings as follows; 1) subperiosteal resorption on X-ray films of hands, 2) on bone scintigraphy, increased accumulation of 99mTc labelled phosphorus compound in skull and mandible, 3) carboxyl terminal parathyroid hormone (PTH) concentration showing higher than 10 ng/ml. Based on these criteria, 9 patients (9.2 ± 2.4 yrs. of duration of HD) were found to be free of SHP. Furthermore, SHP was divided into 2 groups; 7 mild - 10 to 20 ng/ml of PTH, and 8 severe - higher than 20 ng/ml of PTH (9.7 ± 3.2 yrs. and 9.8 ± 2.3 yrs. of duration of HD, respectively).

Results

Relation between durations of HD and % BMD values in CRF was shown in Table 1. % BMD values at L_3 were distributed more widely than those at distal radius (20.5-30.4% (C.V.) for L_3 vs. 8.1-81.4% (C.V.) for distal radius). As to vertebral % BMD, a group with 1 to 5 yrs.,-history of HD showed significantly high % BMD value (112.7%, $p < 0.01$), while other groups showed normal to slightly low % BMD values (91.0-99.7%). In regard to distal radius, except for a non-HD group (%BMD of 99.7%), % BMD values decreased with increasing durations of HD, especially in cases with more than 10 yrs.-history of HD (%BMD of 79.8%).

Relation between SHP state and % BMD values was shown in Fig. 1. In cases without SHP, % BMD values at L_3 (92.4 ± 18.1%) were slightly low. In mold SHP, higher % BMD values were observed, while in severe SHP, % BMD values (82.8 ± 38.4%) tended to decrease. In contrast to L_3, % BMD values at distal radius in both mild and severe SHP, markedly decreased, especially in severe cases (90.0 ± 10.0% for cases without SHP, 77.7 ± 9.3% for mild SHP and 69.5 ± 16.1% for severe SHP).

Discussion

With this preliminary study, it was shown that in most of cases with CRF BMD values at both trabecular and cortical bone were low, leading to decreased BMD on whole skeleton. However, under conditions which were in a relatively short lapse of time after initiation of HD or in mild SHP, discrepancy between axial bone and appendicular bone was observed; high BMD in trabecular bone and low BMD in cortical bone. Furthermore, in-

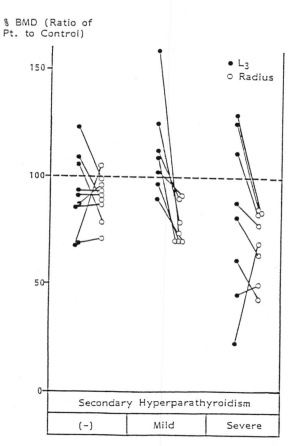

% BMD (Ratio of
Pt. to Control)

Fig. 1.   % BMD values at L_3 and distal radius in SHP.

Table 1. Relation between durations of HD and % BMD at L_3 and distal radius. A group with 1 to 5 yrs.-history of HD showed significantly high % BMD values (p<0.01).

	N	% BMD	
		L_3	Radius
Hemodialysis			
(−)	10	95.6±30.4	99.7±10.1
− 1 yrs.	10	92.6±23.3	95.2±17.0
− 5	10	112.7±20.5	96.7± 8.1
− 10	15	99.7±26.9	82.3±14.3
10 −	14	91.0±29.2	79.8±18.4

teresting enough, no significant increased of BMD was seen in cortical bone.

Although the causes of bone lesions in CRF were multi-factorial, PTH might play an important role. It is reported that PTH has not only catabolic effects, but also anabolic effects. The former effect leads to bone resorption, and the latter effect contributes to bone formation. This anabolic effect is also reported in PTH-treated animal experiment increase in total calcium, hydroxyproline and dry weight in trabecular bone, associated without no significant increase in cortical bone (6). This animal study was coincident with our results of high trabecular BMD and low cortical BMD seen in not severe type of SHP but mild type of SHP with CRF.

Therefore, I might suggest that trabecular bone balance between bone formation and resorption was positive in mild SHP, and negative in severe SHP. However, the reason for high vertebral BMD in cases with 1-5 yrs.-history of HD was definitely unknown, though the existence of mild SHP was suggested.

Thus, it still remain to be clarified completely. Therefore, further investigations including those close related to bone histological findings or parameter relfecting activity of osteoblast (osteocalcin) will be required.

References

1. Sherrad, D., Ott, S., Malony, N., et al (1983) Clinical Disorders of Bone and Mineral Metabolism, Frame, B., Potts, J.T. Jr., eds., Excerpta Medica, Amsterdam, p. 254-258.
2. Tomomitsu, T., Fukunaga, M., Otsuka, N., et al (1986) Jap. J. Nucl. Med. 23, 499-503.
3. Tomomitsu, T., Fukunaga, M., Otsuka, N., et al (1987) Jap. J. Nucl. Med. 24, 171-175.
4. Fukunaga, M., Otsuka, N., Ono, S., et al (1987) Jap. J. Nucl. Med. 24, 469-473.
5. Fukunaga, M., Otsuka, N., Ono, S., et al (1987) Jap. J. Nucl. Med. 24, 1399-1404.
6. Gunness-Hey, M., Hock, J.M. (1984) Metab. Bone Dis. & Relat. Res. 5, 177-182.

COMBINATION-THERAPY WITH 1-38 hPTH AND CALCITONIN INCREASES VERTEBRAL

DENSITY IN OSTEOPOROTIC PATIENTS

RD Hesch, U Busch, M Prokop, G Delling and EF Rittinghaus

Abteilung fur Klinische Endokrinologie (R.D.H., U.B., E.F.R)
und Abteilung fur Radiologie (M.P.), Medizinische Hochschule
Hannover, Hannover; Institut fur Pathologie (G.D.)
Universitatskrankenhaus Eppendorf, Hamburg

INTRODUCTION

We have investigated a combined PTH-Calcitonin therapy to enhance reduced bone mass in osteoporotic patients. Previous therapy protocols
using calcium, vitamin D, estrogen, sodium fluoride, or combinations of
these drugs, have not been successful in enhancing bone mass more than
10% in one year especially in low turn-over states. Studies using anabolic doses of the PTH fragment 1-34 hPTH have produced modest gains
documented by histmorphometry. A recent report of Slovik et al. (1)
clearly showed PTH to be effective in enhancing vertebral bone density,
measured by quantitated computed tomography (QCT). Rasmussen et al. (2)
proposed to additionally reduce bone resorption by combing the phosphate
stimulated endogenous PTH secretion with calcitonin injections. This concept was effective in enhancing trabecular bone mass on histomorphometric
analysis. Others described the addition of calcitonin to PTH treatment
not being effective (3, 1). The objective of our study was to develop a
novel approach to combination therapy (see patient and study design). N-
terminal PTH and nasally applied calcitonin were used to induce a positive
bone balance in osteoporotic patients. Changes in bone density were
monitored by quantitative CT-methods (QCT).

PATIENTS AND STUDY DESIGN

Patients: We studies 8 patients (6 male, 2 female) with osteoporosis, documented by bone biopsy of the iliac crest, x-ray and bone density measurements. The females were postmenopausal, but the etiology of
the disease in the male subjects was unclear. In one case alcohol abuse
may be a causal factor (patient 1). Informed consent was obtained from
each patient after ethical committee approval to the study.

Study design: The whole treatment period lasted nearly 14 months including 4 therapeutic cycles of 104 days. 1 cycle consisted of 70 day treatment with PTH (1-38 hPTH s.c. 720-750 U daily) followed by 2 weeks of
calcitonin (100 IU nasal spray twice daily) and a 3 week medication free
pause. During PTH treatment calcitonin was added for periods of 14 days
starting on day 15 and 43 respectively.

New Actions of Parathyroid Hormone
Edited by S. G. Massry and T. Fujita
Plenum Press, New York

MATERIALS AND METHODS

Peptides: The 1-38 hPTH peptide was from Bachem, Torrance, California, one ampoule containing 720-750 U compared with the standard NIBSC 82/508 by bioassay monitoring the cAMP production of renal cortical membranes (4). Salmon calcitonin nasal spray was from Sandoz AG, Freiburg, FRG, one bottle providing 100 U/stroke, 40% reaching the circulation.

Bone density: Bone density was determined for cortical bone at the lower forearm by single photon absorbtiometry (SPA) and for trabecular bone of the spine by quantitated computed tomography (QCT) with the single (SEQCT) and dual energy (DEQCT) technique (the latter method was additionally used in pat. 4-8) using the UCSF calibration phantom.

Vertebral height: To exclude further wedging of vertebral bodies we calculated the indeed of vertebral deforming events described by Kleerekoper et al. (5).

RESULTS

Bone density: We observed increases of vertebral density (QCT) in the range of 10-36 mg/ccm mineral equivalent (12-89% of initial values) (see Fig. 1). Increases of density could be shown with the first QCT-control after 7 months of therapy. The individual vertebrae of a single patient responded differently. There was no loss of cortical bone (SPA measurements).

Vertebral height: The index of vertebral deforming events (5) did not indicate further wedging, and excludes this as a reason of increased bone density.

Bone turn-over: The serum alkaline phosphatase increased not before the addition of calcitonin on day 15. Statistically significances was reached with day 55 (p 0,025) and day 258 (p 0,005). Serum osteocalcin levels paralleled the AP pattern tightly.

DISCUSSION

Since low doses of PTH clearly show anabolic actions on bone we combined PTH injections with calcitonin nasal spray to enhance bone mass in osteoporotic patients. This concept was proposed by Rasmussen in 1976 who used oral phosphate instead of bone active N-terminal PTH. Our study shows the combination of 1-38 hPTH and calcitonin nasal spray to be very effective in enhancing trabecular bone mass. Results are comparable to those described by Slovik et al (1) adding 1,25(OH)$_2$ vitamin D to 1-34 hPTH injections for 12 months. Because a shift of calcium from cortical to trabecular bone might occur we exclude this by SPA measurements. Furthermore, progressive wedging can mimic therapy induced increases of bone density. We excluded this by measurements of vertebral height. From this we conclude that the dramatic improvement in bone density in our patients is only due to anabolic actions of PTH and calcitonin. Interestingly, the vertebral bodies of each individual patient responded quite different, suggesting they represent different stages in the development of osteoporosis. The increase of AP with the addition of calcitonin may show that both hormones act together at the osteoblast level but it is not clear from these results if it is direct or indirect. In future, futher studies must be undertaken to optimize the rhythm and dose of hormone application. Maintaining the newly won bone mass is essential. If this is physiological bone it should be estrogen depended. In our female patients studies to demonstrate this are under way. In males androgen application should be considered, since there is growing evidence

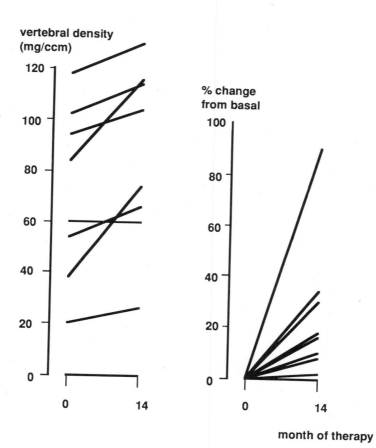

Figure 1.   The Increases of Vertebral Density are Shown by SE QCT.
Absolute (left) and Relative (right) Changes.

evidence testosterone is effective in conserving bone in males. The interrelationship between androgen-deficiency and bone loss is not as clear as the estrogen dependency of female bone. Other drugs like diphosphonates may also be of value.

REFERENCES

1. Slovik DM, Rosenthal DI, Doppelt SH, Potts JT., Jr, Daly MA, Campbell JA, Neer RM. (1986). Restoration of spinal bone in osteoporotic men by treatment with human parathyroid hormone (1-34) and 1,25-dihydroxy-vitamin D. J. Bon. Min. Res. 1(4):377-381.

2. Rasmussen H, Bordier P. (1974). The physiological and cellular basis of metabolic bone disease. William and Wilkins, Baltimore: 305-314.

3. Parsons JA, Meunier P, Podbesek R, Reeve J, Stevenson RW. (1961). Pathological and therapeutic implications of the cellular and humoral responses to parathyrin. Biocem. Soc. Trans. 9:383-386.

4. Niepel B, Radeke H, Atkinson MJ, Hesch RD. (1983). A homologous biological probe for parathyroid hormone in human serum. J. Immuno-assay 4:21-49.

5. Kleerekoper M, Parfitt AM, Ellis BI. (1984). Measurement of vertebral fracture rates in osteoporosis. Proceedings of the Copenhagen Intern Symposium on Osteoporosis: 103-109.

mRNA, 19, 20
Rous sarcoma virus, 427

Salmon, 131
Salt, dietary, and hypertension, 146-149
Saponin, 70
Sarcoma, human, cell lines, 204, 207, 208, 435-440, 447, 448
Scatchard plot analysis, 111
Sclerosis, amyotrophic, lateral (ALS), 173
SDS-PAGE chromatography, 105, 107
Seawater elements in the human body, 349
Seizure, epileptiform, 383
Serotonin, 69, 341
Shock, septic, and hypocalcemia, 193
Signal
  hypothesis, 19
  peptidase, 20, 24, 25
  peptide, 20, 23
    assay, 21
    effect, biological, 22
    synthetic, 21, 24, 25
  pathway, 419-422
  recognition particle, 19
    ribonucleoprotein *11*S, 19
Snail, freshwater -, 131
Sodium, 145, 221, 250, 280, 311, 317-319, 352, 371
Sodium azide, 403
Sodium fluoride, 459
Sodium nitroprusside, 34, 35, 128
Sodium-potassium ATPase, 302, 303 305, 308, 311-313, 317
Soy protein, 358, 359
Southern blot analysis, 96
Spermidine, 435
Spermine, 435
Staphylococcus epidermidis, 194
  and PTH, 194
Stenosis, aortic, 161
Succinate, 320
Sucrose density gradient
  analysis, 110, 111
Synaptosome, 301-328, 371
  model for CNS function, 318
  preparation, 302

Tachycardia, ventricular, 159, 16
  and hemodialysis, 161
T-cell, 35
Testosterone, 272-275, 462
Tetany, 383
Tetrakiaphosphate, 448
Tetrodotoxin, 189
Theophylline, 290, 293, 294

Thioester derivative, 29
Thiol, 29
Thiophosphate, *see* WR-*2721*
Thymocyte of rat, 54
Thyroidectomy, 383
Thyroparathyroidectomy, 167, 247-250
Thyroxine, 221
Tissue
  adipose, 199, 203, 209
  gastrointestinal, 130
  neural, 130-131
    and PTH, 130-131
  tracheal, 130
  uterine, 130
  vas deferens, 130
Toad bladder, 254-257
Translation, 20-24
Translocation, 20-24
Trifluoperazine, 259-261
Triglyceride of serum, 213-217
Triglyceride lipase, hepatic, 204
Triolein, 200, 204, 209
Trout, 131
Trypsin, 110
Tuberculosis, 194
Tumor, human
  hypercalcemia, 95-99
  peptide, common, 64
Tyrosine hydroxylase, 312
Tyrosine kinase
  autophosphorylation, 14

UMR*106* cell line, *see* Cell line
Urea nitrogen of blood (in rat), 204
Uremia, 137-139, 157, 208, 219-245, 265, 271, 273, 278, 311, 317-328, 395, 403-406
  and PTH, 137, 139, 157, 301
Urethane, 120
Uric acid, 352
Urine
  acidification, 247
  osmolality, 253

Vasodilation by PTH, 113, 119-125
Vasopressin, 69, 253-256, 265, 396, 399
Vasorelaxation, 107, 115, 116
  by PTH, 128
Verapamil, 237-241, 256, 396, 397, 403-406
Vitamin C, 426
Vitamin D, 105, 251-254, 272, 352, 459
  deficiency, 83, 370, 371, 382, 384, 385
  interaction, 371-374
  intoxication, 144
  metabolite, 373-374, 385, 412-414, *see* separate metabolites
  and PTH, 371-374, 412-414